Quality Improvement in Neonatal and Perinatal Medicine

Guest Editors

ALAN R. SPITZER, MD
DAN L. ELLSBURY, MD

CLINICS IN PERINATOLOGY

www.perinatology.theclinics.com

March 2010 • Volume 37 • Number 1

SAUNDERS an imprint of ELSEVIER, Inc.

W.B. SAUNDERS COMPANY
A Division of Elsevier Inc.

Elsevier, Inc. • 1600 John F. Kennedy Blvd. • Suite 1800 • Philadelphia, PA 19103-2899

http://www.theclinics.com

CLINICS IN PERINATOLOGY Volume 37, Number 1
March 2010 ISSN 0095-5108, ISBN-13: 978-1-4377-1856-0

Editor: Carla Holloway
Developmental Editor: Theresa Collier

Clinics in Perinatology (ISSN 0095-5108) is published quarterly by Elsevier Inc., 360 Park Avenue South, New York, NY 10010-1710. Months of issue are March, June, September, and December. Business and Editorial Offices: 1600 John F. Kennedy Blvd., Ste. 1800, Philadelphia, PA 19103-2899. Customer Service Office: 3251 Riverport Lane, Maryland Heights, MO 63043. Periodicals postage paid at New York, NY and additional mailing offices. Subscription prices are $239.00 per year (US individuals), $347.00 per year (US institutions), $281.00 per year (Canadian individuals), $441.00 per year (Canadian institutions), $345.00 per year (foreign individuals), $441.00 per year (foreign institutions) $116.00 per year (US students), and $168.00 per year (Canadian and foreign students). Foreign air speed delivery is included in all Clinics subscription prices. All prices are subject to change without notice. **POSTMASTER:** Send address changes to *Clinics in Perinatology*, Elsevier Health Sciences Division, Subscription Customer Service, 3251 Riverport Lane, Maryland Heights, MO 63043. **Customer Service: Telephone: 1-800-654-2452** (U.S. and Canada); **1-314-447-8871** (outside U.S. and Canada). **Fax: 1-314-447-8029. E-mail: journalscustomerservice-usa@elsevier.com** (for print support); **journalsonlinesupport-usa@elsevier.com** (for online support).

Reprints. For copies of 100 or more, of articles in this publication, please contact the Commercial Reprints Department, Elsevier Inc., 360 Park Avenue South, New York, NY 10010-1710. Tel. (212) 633-3812; Fax: (212) 482-1935; email: reprints@elsevier.com.

Clinics in Perinatology is also pubilshed in Spanish by McGraw-Hill Interamericana Editores S.A., P.O. Box 5-237, 06500 Mexico D.F., Mexico.

Clinics in Perinatology is covered in *MEDLINE/PubMed (Index Medicus) Current Contents, Excepta Medica, BIOSIS and ISI/BIOMED.*

Printed and bound in the United Kingdom
Transferred to Digital Print 2011

Contributors

GUEST EDITORS

ALAN R. SPITZER, MD
Senior Vice President and Director, The Center for Research, Education, and Quality, Pediatrix Medical Group, Sunrise, Florida

DAN L. ELLSBURY, MD
Director, Continuous Quality Improvement, The Center for Research, Education, and Quality, Pediatrix Medical Group, Sunrise, Florida; Mercy Medical Center, Des Moines, Iowa

AUTHORS

NICHOLAS E. BRUNS, BA
Rush Medical College, Rush University Medical Center, Chicago, Illinois

REESE H. CLARK, MD
Director of Neonatal Research, The Center for Research, Education, and Quality Improvement, Pediatrix Medical Group, Sunrise, Florida

WILLIAM H. EDWARDS, MD
Vermont Oxford Network, Burlington, Vermont; Professor of Pediatrics, Dartmouth Medical School, Hanover, New Hampshire

DAN L. ELLSBURY, MD
Director, Continuous Quality Improvement, The Center for Research, Education, and Quality, Pediatrix Medical Group, Sunrise, Florida

JANET L. ENGSTROM, RN, PhD, CNM, WHNP-BC
Department of Women, Children and Family Nursing, Rush University Medical Center, Chicago, Illinois

NEIL N. FINER, MD
Professor of Pediatrics, Director, Division of Neonatology, University of California San Diego Medical Center, San Diego, California

JAY P. GOLDSMITH, MD
Clinical Professor, Department of Pediatrics, Tulane University Medical School, New Orleans, Louisiana

JEFFREY B. GOULD, MD, MPH
Robert L. Hess Professor of Pediatrics, Principal Investigator, California Perinatal Quality Care Collaborative, Director, Perinatal Epidemiology and Health Outcomes Research Unit, Division of Neonatal and Developmental Medicine, Stanford University Medical Center, Palo Alto, California

JAMES GRAY, MD, MS
Division of Newborn Medicine, Harvard Medical School; Division of Clinical Informatics, Department of Neonatology, Beth Israel Deaconess Medical Center, Boston, Massachusetts

DARREN HANDLER, BS
Data Warehouse Manager and New Product Development, The Center for Research, Education, and Quality Improvement, Pediatrix Medical Group, Sunrise, Florida

JAMES HANDYSIDE, BSc
Principal Consultant, Improvision Healthcare, Ontario, Canada; Quality Improvement Leader - NICQ Projects, Vermont Oxford Network, Burlington, Vermont

JEFFREY D. HORBAR, MD
Professor of Pediatrics, University of Vermont College of Medicine; Vermont Oxford Network, Burlington, Vermont

BRIANA J. JEGIER, PhD
Department of Women, Children and Family Nursing, Rush University Medical Center, Chicago, Illinois

SUSAN LANDERS, MD, FAAP, FABM
Neonatalogist, Medical Director, NICU Nutrition and Lactation Services, Seton Family of Hospitals, Pediatrix Medical Group, Seton Medical Center, Austin, Texas

TINA LEONE, MD
Assistant Professor of Pediatrics, Division of Neonatology, University of California San Diego, San Diego, California

ROBERT C. LLOYD, PhD
Executive Director Performance Improvement, Institute for Healthcare Improvement

PAULA P. MEIER, RN, DNSc, FAAN
Department of Women, Children and Family Nursing; Section of Neonatology, Department of Pediatrics, Rush University Medical Center, Chicago, Illinois

ALOKA L. PATEL, MD
Section of Neonatology, Department of Pediatrics, Rush University Medical Center, Chicago, Illinois

ROBERT H. PFISTER, MD
Assistant Professor, Department of Pediatrics, The University of Vermont; Fletcher Allen Health Care, Burlington, Vermont

RICHARD J. POWERS, MD
Director, Pediatrix Neonatology Medical Group of San Jose; Medical Director, Good Samaritan Hospital, Newborn Intensive Care Unit, San Jose, California

DALE P. REISNER, MD
Associate Director, CQI for Maternal Fetal Medicine, Pediatrix Medical Group/MEDNAX; Division of Perinatal Medicine, Swedish Medical Center/Seattle, Seattle, Washington

WADE D. RICH, RRT, CCRC
Research Coordinator, Division of Neonatology, University of California San Diego, San Diego, California

ROGER F. SOLL, MD
Professor of Pediatrics, Division of Neonatal-Perinatal Medicine; Director, Neonatal Intensive Care Unit, Fletcher Allen Health Care; Coordinating Editor, Cochrane Neonatal Review Group, University of Vermont College of Medicine, Burlington, Vermont

ALAN R. SPITZER, MD
Senior Vice President and Director, The Center for Research, Education, and Quality, Pediatrix Medical Group, Sunrise, Florida

GAUTHAM SURESH, MD
Associate Professor of Pediatrics, Children's Hospital at Dartmouth, Dartmouth-Hitchcock Medical Center, One Medical Center Drive, Lebanon, New Hampshire

ROBERT URSPRUNG, MD, MMSc
Associate Director, Continuous Quality Improvement, The Center for Research, Education, and Quality, Pediatrix Medical Group, Sunrise, Florida

DAVID W. WIRTSCHAFTER, MD
David Wirtschafter, MD, Inc, Valley View, California

WADE D. RICH, RRT, CCRC
Research Coordinator, Division of Neonatology, University of California San Diego, San Diego, California

ROGER F. SOLL, MD
Professor of Pediatrics, Division of Neonatal-Perinatal Medicine; Director, Neonatal Intensive Care Unit, Fletcher Allen Health Care; Coordinating Editor, Cochrane Neonatal Review Group, University of Vermont College of Medicine, Burlington, Vermont

ALAN R. SPITZER, MD
Senior Vice President and Director, The Center for Research, Education, and Quality, Pediatrix Medical Group, Sunrise, Florida

GAUTHAM SURESH, MD
Associate Professor of Pediatrics, Children's Hospital at Dartmouth, Dartmouth-Hitchcock Medical Center, One Medical Center Drive, Lebanon, New Hampshire

ROBERT URSPRUNG, MD, MMSc
Associate Director, Continuous Quality Improvement, The Center for Research, Education, and Quality, Pediatrix Medical Group, Sunrise, Florida

DAVID W. WIRTSCHAFTER, MD
David Wirtschafter, MD, Inc., Valley View, California

Contents

The Pediatrix BabySteps® Data Warehouse and the Pediatrix QualitySteps Improvement Project System—Tools for "Meaningful Use" in Continuous Quality Improvement 49

Alan R. Spitzer, Dan L. Ellsbury, Darren Handler, and Reese H. Clark

The Pediatrix BabySteps Clinical Data Warehouse (CDW) is a rich and novel tool allowing unbiased extraction of information from an entire neonatal population care by physicians and advanced practice nurses in Pediatrix Medical Group. Because it represents the practice of newborn medicine ranging from small community intensive care units to some of the largest neonatal intensive care units in the United States, it is highly representative of scope of practice in this country. Its value in defining outcome measures, quality improvement projects, and research continues to grow annually. Now coupled with the BabySteps QualitySteps program for defined clinical quality improvement projects, it represents a robust methodology for meaningful use of an electronic health care record, as designated during this era of health care reform. Continued growth of the CDW should result in continued important observations and improvements in neonatal care.

The Role of Regional Collaboratives: The California Perinatal Quality Care Collaborative Model 71

Jeffrey B. Gould

Improving the outcome of the infants cared for in one's neonatal intensive care unit is the main objective of improvement projects that are pursued independently or as a member of a national collaborative. Regional quality improvement collaborations represent the intersection of hospital-based and community-based medicine offering the possibility of coordinated improvement efforts conducted at both the hospital and community level. This article discusses the aspirations, workings, and achievements of the California Perinatal Quality Care Collaborative, a regional collaboration formed to improve perinatal care. While it is never easy to align the often differing fundamental positions held by the various member factions and stakeholder groups, the common goal of a universally agreed-upon mission statement can act as a magnet drawing the various components together. Rapid development of a first quality improvement initiative is an effective strategy to engage the participants in a way that allows them to demonstrate, share, and build upon their individual expertise, and provides them a strong sense of professional accomplishment.

A Primer on Quality Improvement Methodology in Neonatology 87

Dan L. Ellsbury and Robert Ursprung

This article provides a systematic and pragmatic approach to quality improvement in the neonatal intensive care unit setting. The "model for improvement" serves as the foundation for the approach, and is based on three core questions, followed by cycles of testing: What are we trying to accomplish? How will we know that a change represents an improvement? What changes can we make that will result in continuous improvement? This article reviews these questions in detail and provides specific examples to highlight the practical use of this methodology.

Navigating in the Turbulent Sea of Data: The Quality Measurement Journey **101**

Robert C. Lloyd

This article provides a roadmap for your quality measurement journey. It begins with a discussion of 3 approaches to measurement (improvement, accountability and research) and challenges readers to be clear about why they are measuring. Key milestones along the quality measurement journey are then presented and a framework for selecting measures, developing clear operational definitions, building data collection plans, and understanding the variation that exists in data is outlined. The article ends with a discussion of why data need to be linked to improvement strategies.

Human Factors and Quality Improvement **123**

James Handyside and Gautham Suresh

Human factors analysis (HFE) presents a formidable contribution to quality improvement (QI) in the neonatal intensive care unit (NICU). The science behind the fundamental principles concerning the design of work systems that match the needs of the people who work in them is sound and is applied widely in other safety critical situations. Early application of HFE in NICUs has shown the usefulness of these methods for frontline teams working to improve quality, reliability, and safety. The inclusion of human factors considerations in the design of structure and process has the potential to improve outcomes for patients and families and to improve the comfort and usability of work systems for providers who work in them. New technologies and continual change must be informed and designed through the application of HFE methods and principles to realize the full potential of QI.

Random Safety Auditing, Root Cause Analysis, Failure Mode and Effects Analysis **141**

Robert Ursprung and James Gray

Improving quality and safety in health care is a major concern for health care providers, the general public, and policy makers. Errors and quality issues are leading causes of morbidity and mortality across the health care industry. There is evidence that patients in the neonatal intensive care unit (NICU) are at high risk for serious medical errors. To facilitate compliance with safe practices, many institutions have established quality-assurance monitoring procedures. Three techniques that have been found useful in the health care setting are failure mode and effects analysis, root cause analysis, and random safety auditing. When used together, these techniques are effective tools for system analysis and redesign focused on providing safe delivery of care in the complex NICU system.

Pay for Performance in Neonatal-Perinatal Medicine—Will the Quality of Health Care Improve in the Neonatal Intensive Care Unit? A Business Model for Improving Outcomes in the Neonatal Intensive Care Unit **167**

Alan R. Spitzer

Because neonatal medicine is such an expensive contributor to health care in the United States—with a small population of infants accounting

for very high health care costs—there has been a fair amount of attention given to this group of patients. An idea that has received increasing attention in this discussion is pay for performance. This article discusses the concept of pay for performance, examines what potential benefits and risks exist in this model, and investigates how it might achieve the desired goals if implemented in a thoughtful way.

Part II: Specific Applications of Quality Improvement Methodology in Neonatal and perinatal Medicine

Collaboration Between Obstetricians and Neonatologists: Perinatal Safety Programs and Improved Clinical Outcomes **179**

Dale P. Reisner and Susan Landers

Although collaboration between obstetricians and neonatologists may seem an obvious way to provide the best quality care to infants and their mothers, this has not always occurred. This article highlights the experiences of several recently published efforts demonstrating how coordinated care resulted in improved clinical outcomes.

Delivery Room Intervention: Improving the Outcome **189**

Wade D. Rich, Tina Leone, and Neil N. Finer

The authors have conducted video review of neonatal resuscitations since 1999. Over this 10-year period 3 phases of our experience have been recognized. Our early reviews helped us recognize what we were doing in the delivery room, an area that had been ignored in improved intervention. It was noted that on many occasions multiple people were trying to accomplish the same task, that bag and mask ventilation was almost exclusively the purview of the respiratory therapists and was not performed well by others, and that infants with low birth weight were often hypothermic on admission. After determining what was being done and how well it was being done, we moved on to how to do it better. This period included making environmental changes by warming the room, the use of occlusive wrap, determining the effectiveness of bag and mask ventilation with colorimetric CO_2 detectors, and the introduction of crew resource management to develop consistent and effective communication. The third and current phase of our experience is to determine how these interventions affect delivery room and potentially later outcomes. Well-designed clinical trials are still needed to further establish the most optimal resuscitation interventions.

Comprehensive Oxygen Management for the Prevention of Retinopathy of Prematurity: The Pediatrix Experience **203**

Dan L. Ellsbury and Robert Ursprung

Comprehensive oxygen management, focused on avoiding hyperoxia and repeated episodes of hypoxia-hyperoxia in very low birth weight infants, has been successfully used for the reduction of retinopathy of prematurity. Building on this experience, the Comprehensive Oxygen Management for

the Prevention of Retinopathy of Prematurity quality improvement initiative was developed to facilitate the spread and refinement of these techniques. The initiative focused on staff education and evaluation and redesign of the processes and practices involving oxygen use. Monitoring of the effectiveness of the system changes was supported through audits of clinical practice changes, use of oxygen saturation trending data, and the incidence of retinopathy of prematurity.

Improving the Use of Human Milk During and After the NICU Stay **217**

Paula P. Meier, Janet L. Engstrom, Aloka L. Patel, Briana J. Jegier, and Nicholas E. Bruns

The feeding of human milk (milk from the infant's own mother; excluding donor milk) during the newborn intensive care unit (NICU) stay reduces the risk of costly and handicapping morbidities in premature infants. The mechanisms by which human milk provides this protection are varied and synergistic, and appear to change over the course of the NICU stay. The fact that these mechanisms include specific human milk components that are not present in the milk of other mammals means that human milk from the infant's mother cannot be replaced by commercial infant or donor human milk, and the feeding of human milk should be a NICU priority. Recent evidence suggests that the impact of human milk on improving infant health outcomes and reducing the risk of prematurity-specific morbidities is linked to specific critical exposure periods in the post-birth period during which the exclusive use of human milk and the avoidance of commercial formula may be most important. Similarly, there are other periods when high doses, but not necessarily exclusive use of human milk, may be important. This article reviews the concept of "dose and exposure period" for human milk feeding in the NICU to precisely measure and benchmark the amount and timing of human milk use in the NICU. The critical exposure periods when exclusive or high doses of human milk appear to have the greatest impact on specific morbidities are reviewed. Finally, the current best practices for the use of human milk during and after the NICU stay for premature infants are summarized.

Decreasing Central Line Associated Bloodstream Infection in Neonatal Intensive Care **247**

Richard J. Powers and David W. Wirtschafter

Central Line Associated Bloodstream Infections (CLABSIs) have come to be recognized as preventable adverse events that result from lapses in technique at multiple levels of care. CLABSIs are associated with increased mortality and adverse outcomes that may have lifelong consequences. This review provides a summary of evidence-based strategies to reduce CLABSI in the newborn intensive care unit that have been described in the literature over the past decades. Implementation of these strategies in "bundles" is also discussed, citing examples of successful quality improvement collaboratives. The methods of implementation require an understanding of the scientific data and technical developments, as well as knowledge of how to influence change within the unique and complicated milieu of the newborn intensive care unit.

Quality Improvement in Respiratory Care: Decreasing Bronchopulmonary Dysplasia **273**

Robert H. Pfister and Jay P. Goldsmith

Chronic lung disease (CLD) is one of the most common long-term complications in very preterm infants. Bronchopulmonary dysplasia (BPD) is the most common cause of CLD in infancy. Modern neonatal respiratory care has witnessed the emergence of a new BPD that exhibits decreased fibrosis and emphysema, but also decreased alveolar septation, and microvascular development. CLD encompasses the classic and the new BPD, and recognizes that lung injury can occur in term infants who need aggressive ventilatory support and who develop lung injury as a result, and that CLD is a multisystem disease. Controversy exists on whether quality improvement (QI) methods that implement multiple interventions will be effective in limiting pathology with multiple causes. Caution in generalization of QI findings is encouraged. QI methods toward improvement in CLD or any other outcome should be considered as a tool for implementing evidence and studying the effects of change in complex adaptive systems.

Index **295**

GOAL STATEMENT

The goal of *Clinics in Perinatology* is to keep practicing neonatologists and maternal-fetal medicine specialists up to date with current clinical practice in perinatology by providing timely articles reviewing the state of the art in patient care.

ACCREDITATION

The *Clinics in Perinatology* is planned and implemented in accordance with the Essential Areas and Policies of the Accreditation Council for Continuing Medical Education (ACCME) through the joint sponsorship of the University of Virginia School of Medicine and Elsevier.

The University of Virginia School of Medicine is accredited by the ACCME to provide continuing medical education for physicians. The University of Virginia School of Medicine designates this educational activity for a maximum of 15 *AMA PRA Category 1 Credits*™ for each issue, 60 credits per year. Physicians should only claim credit commensurate with the extent of their participation in the activity.

The American Medical Association has determined that physicians not licensed in the US who participate in this CME activity are eligible for a maximum of 15 *AMA PRA Category 1 Credits*™ for each issue, 60 credits per year.

Credit can be earned by reading the text material, taking the CME examination online at http://www.theclinics.com/home/cme, and completing the evaluation. After taking the test, you will be required to review any and all incorrect answers. Following completion of the test and evaluation, your credit will be awarded and you may print your certificate.

FACULTY DISCLOSURE/CONFLICT OF INTEREST

The University of Virginia School of Medicine, as an ACCME accredited provider, endorses and strives to comply with the Accreditation Council for Continuing Medical Education (ACCME) Standards of Commercial Support, Commonwealth of Virginia statutes, University of Virginia policies and procedures, and associated federal and private regulations and guidelines on the need for disclosure and monitoring of proprietary and financial interests that may affect the scientific integrity and balance of content delivered in continuing medical education activities under our auspices.

The University of Virginia School of Medicine requires that all CME activities accredited through this institution be developed independently and be scientifically rigorous, balanced and objective in the presentation/discussion of its content, theories and practices.

All authors/editors participating in an accredited CME activity are expected to disclose to the readers relevant financial relationships with commercial entities occurring within the past 12 months (such as grants or research support, employee, consultant, stock holder, member of speakers bureau, etc.). The University of Virginia School of Medicine will employ appropriate mechanisms to resolve potential conflicts of interest to maintain the standards of fair and balanced education to the reader. Questions about specific strategies can be directed to the Office of Continuing Medical Education, University of Virginia School of Medicine, Charlottesville, Virginia.

The faculty and staff of the University of Virginia Office of Continuing Medical Education have no financial affiliations to disclose.

The authors/editors listed below have identified no professional or financial affiliations for themselves or their spouse/partner:

Robert Boyle, MD (Test Author); Nicholas E. Bruns, BA; William H. Edwards, MD; Neil N. Finer, MD; Jay P. Goldsmith, MD; James Gray, MD; Darren Handler, BS; James Handyside, BSc; Carla Holloway (Acquisitions Editor); Susan Landers, MD; Tina Leone, MD; Aloka L. Patel, MD; Robert H. Pfister, MD; Wade D. Rich, RRT, CCRC; and Gautham Suresh, MD.

The authors/editors listed below identified the following professional or financial affiliations for themselves or their spouse/partner:

Reese H. Clark, MD is employed by Pediatrix Medical Group.
Dan L. Ellsbury, MD (Guest Editor) is employed by Pediatrix Medical Group.
Janet L. Engstrom, RN, PhD, CNM, WHNP-BC is an industry funded research/investigaor for Medela, Inc.
Jeffrey B. Gould, MD, MPH serves on the Advisory Committee for Paradigm Health.
Jeffrey D. Horbar, MD is employed by Vermont Oxford Network.
Briana J. Jegier, PhD is an industry funded research/investigaor for Medela, Inc.
Robert C. Lloyd, PhD is employed by the Institute for Healthcare Improvement; is on the Advisory Committee/Board Institute for Healthcare Improvement and Advocate Health; and is a consultant for Principal of R. C. Lloyd & Associates.
Paula P. Meier, RN, DNSc, FAAN is an industry funded research/investigator and consultant for Medela, Inc.
Richard J. Powers, MD serves on the Speakers Bureau for MedImmune and Ovation Pharmaceuticals.
Dale P. Reisner, MD is employed by and owns stock in Mednax/Obstetrix.
Roger F. Soll, MD is president of the Vermont Oxford Network, and is the coordinating editor for the Cochrane Review Group.
Alan R. Spitzer, MD (Guest Editor) is employed by and owns stock in Mednax.
Robert Ursprung, MD, MMSc is employed by Mednax, and is on the Advisory Committee/Board for Vermont Oxford Network.
David W. Wirtschafter, MD is President of David D Wirtschafter, MD, Inc., and is a consultant for California Children's Services, Department of Healthcare Services, State of California.

Disclosure of Discussion of Non-FDA Approved Uses for Pharmaceutical Products and/or Medical Devices.

The University of Virginia School of Medicine, as an ACCME provider, requires that all faculty presenters identify and disclose any off-label uses for pharmaceutical and medical device products. The University of Virginia School of Medicine recommends that each physician fully review all the available data on new products or procedures prior to clinical use.

TO ENROLL

To enroll in the Clinics in Perinatology Continuing Medical Education program, call customer service at 1-800-654-2452 or visit us online at www.theclinics.com/home/cme. The CME program is available to subscribers for an additional fee of $195.00

FORTHCOMING ISSUES

June 2010

Early Onset Neonatal Sepsis
Richard Polin, MD and
Karen Fairchild, MD,
Guest Editors

September 2010

Health Care Associated Infections in the Neonatal Intensive Care Unit
Richard Polin, MD and
Karen Fairchild, MD,
Guest Editors

December 2010

Perinatal HIV/AIDS
Athena P. Kourtis, MD, PhD, MPH and
Marc Bulterys, MD, PhD,
Guest Editors

RECENT ISSUES

December 2009

Neurology of the Newborn Infant
Adré J. du Plessis, MBChB, MPH,
Guest Editor

September 2009

Fetal Neurology
Adré J. du Plessis, MBChB, MPH,
Guest Editor

June 2009

Fetal Surgery
Hanmin Lee, MD,
Guest Editor

RELATED INTEREST

Pediatric Clinics of North America, August 2009 (Volume 56, Issue 4)
Pediatric Quality
Leonard G. Feld, MD, PhD, MMM, FAAP and Shabnam Jain, MD, FAAP,
Guest Editors
www.pediatric.theclinics.com

Preface

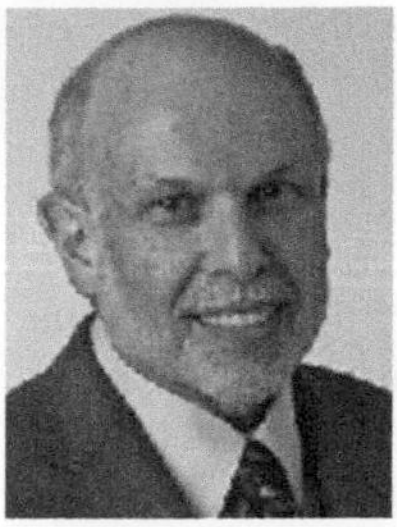 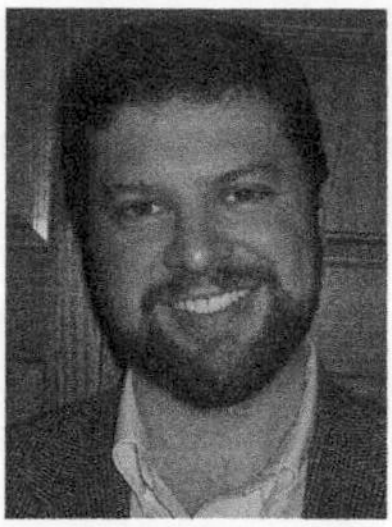

Alan R. Spitzer, MD Dan L. Ellsbury, MD
Guest Editors

As we enter the second decade of the new millennium, the breathtaking changes occurring in medicine represent some of the most significant advances in the delivery of health care since World War II. Not only does the science of medicine continue to progress at an astonishing pace, but the manner in which patients receive the benefits of this science is also changing dramatically. Transparency is the key word in this process. No longer is a paternalistic physician attitude acceptable; "Trust me, I'm the doctor" has now transformed into "show me the data." Patients and families expect to be informed not only of the options in care, but the likely outcomes of those options so that they can become active participants in the decision-making process. To evaluate outcomes, therefore, the clinician now requires information that was previously often only anecdotally collected, namely accurate outcomes of specific conditions for large groups of patients and comparative results of different treatments of those conditions in significant patient populations. The development of methods for collecting and storing this information is quickly becoming a basic part of the physician's daily life, and underlies much of quality improvement (QI). Furthermore, with health care reform integrating the electronic health record (EHR) and the concept of meaningful use of the EHR into medical practice, data evaluation and transparency of outcomes move to the forefront of patient care. The PDSA (Plan, Do, Study, Act) Cycle of collecting information, developing a methodology of intervention for a specific problem, intervening as planned, evaluating the results, then acting on the data gathered, thereby becomes an inevitable practice approach for much of medicine.

Maternal-fetal medicine and the neonatal intensive case unit (NICU) are no strangers to these processes. Since the introduction of neonatal medicine as a subspecialty and the appearance of the first NICUs during the 1960s and 1970s, outcome evaluation has been an elemental part of practice and has resulted in plummeting mortality for even the tiniest neonates during the subsequent 4 decades. But improved survival does not suffice for most neonatologists, and all of us remain deeply committed to our infants surviving with the fewest possible adverse outcomes as well. The agenda of QI, therefore, has been an essential tradition in the NICU, and one that will ideally continue to move neonatal outcomes in a positive direction. The fact that the American Board of Pediatrics has made QI part of its program for

Clin Perinatol 37 (2010) xv–xvi
doi:10.1016/j.clp.2010.01.017

Maintenance of Certification (MOC) highlights the core value of QI in medical care, and the March of Dimes has also designated QI as an important program in its effort to reduce premature births. Our own organization, Pediatrix Medical Group, has made meaningful QI participation mandatory for all of our physician groups. In addition, Pediatrix enthusiastically supports an extensive Clinical Data Warehouse and 3 Quality Improvement Summit Meetings annually for our physicians to attend. This issue of *Clinics in Perinatology* was designed to provide the reader with all the tools and concepts necessary to understand QI methodology and to initiate QI projects within their own practices and their NICUs. The outstanding contributors to this volume are some of the world's leading experts in QI and all have done a superb job in succinctly summarizing their areas of expertise. We are pleased to have had the opportunity to edit this edition of *Clinics in Perinatology* and hope that the reader finds many fertile ideas within these pages that will further enhance the outcomes for all neonates.

Alan R. Spitzer, MD
Pediatrix Medical Group
1301 Concord Terrace
Sunrise, FL 33323, USA

Dan L. Ellsbury, MD
CQI, Pediatrix Medical Group
1301 Concord Terrace
Sunrise, FL 33323, USA

Mercy Medical Center
Des Moines, IA, USA

E-mail addresses:
Alan_Spitzer@pediatrix.com (A.R. Spitzer)
Dan_Ellsbury@pediatrix.com (D.L. Ellsbury)

Crossing the Quality Chasm in Neonatal-Perinatal Medicine

Dan L. Ellsbury, MD

KEYWORDS

- Quality chasm • Quality improvement
- Complex adaptive systems • Neonatal medicine

WHAT IS THE QUALITY CHASM?

In its landmark report, *Crossing the Quality Chasm*, the Institute of Medicine summarized the current state of quality in The American health care system[1]: *"Between the health care we have and the care we could have lies not just a gap, but a chasm."*

What is the genesis of the quality chasm? At no time in history has the growth in medical science and technology been so rapid. Since the publication of the first randomized clinical trials more than 50 years ago,[2] there has been an explosion of research activity in medicine. Over the past 30 years, these trials have increased from 100 per year to more than 10,000 annually.[3,4] New medications, medical devices, and other technologies have demonstrated a similar escalation in number and complexity, resulting in an increasingly vast array of therapies that clinicians must assimilate and translate into state-of-the-art care.

Faced with such rapid changes, the health care delivery system has fallen far short in its ability to translate this knowledge into daily clinical practice. On average, 17 years is required for new knowledge generated by randomized controlled trials to be incorporated into general practice.[5] A quality chasm is evident in all health care populations, including adult, pediatric, and newborn patients. Underuse, overuse, and misuse of therapies is commonplace and some patients are harmed as a result.[6–11]

THE QUALITY CHASM IN NEONATOLOGY

There is ample evidence of a quality chasm in neonatal intensive care. Large variations in use of established therapies exist and medical errors are frequent. Unexplained center-to-center variability in outcomes is present in multiple neonatal networks throughout the world.[6,9,10,12–14] This article discusses a few examples of treatments that are underused, overused, or misused in current neonatal intensive care.

The Center for Research, Education, and Quality, Pediatrix Medical Group, 1301 Concord Terrace, Sunrise, FL 33323, USA
E-mail address: Dan_Ellsbury@pediatrix.com

Clin Perinatol 37 (2010) 1–10
doi:10.1016/j.clp.2010.01.001

Breast Milk

A large volume of data supports breast milk as the optimal nutritional source for premature infants. Its use is associated with improved neurodevelopmental outcome and reduced rates of necrotizing enterocolitis and nosocomial infections. Despite this knowledge, fewer than half of very low-birth-weight infants receive breast milk at the time of discharge from neonatal ICUs (NICUs). Significant intercenter variability in breast milk use has been demonstrated.[15,16]

Antenatal Corticosteroids

Treatment with antenatal corticosteroids is associated with an overall reduction in neonatal death, respiratory distress syndrome, intraventricular hemorrhage, necrotizing enterocolitis, respiratory support, intensive care admissions, and systemic infections in the first 48 hours of life. Antenatal corticosteroid use has improved since the National Institutes of Health consensus statement,[17] but suboptimal administration rates persist.[18–23]

Surfactant

Infants with established respiratory distress syndrome who receive animal-derived surfactant treatment have a decreased risk of pneumothorax, pulmonary interstitial emphysema, mortality, and bronchopulmonary dysplasia. Despite this evidence, its use remains suboptimal and variable.[24–27]

Central Line Bundles

Central line bundles are a small group of key procedures and processes that, when done together, decrease the rate of catheter-associated blood stream infections. The bundle is simply a concept that has been successfully used to maximize compliance with sterile technique during central catheter insertion and care. The bundles have been successfully used in adult and pediatric ICUs and similar success is now seen in the neonatal ICU setting.[28–33]

Oxygen

Supplemental oxygen is a heavily used medication in NICUs. High blood oxygen levels contribute to oxidative injuries in premature infants, including the development of retinopathy of prematurity and bronchopulmonary dysplasia. Despite this knowledge, it is common practice to functionally remove the ability of oxygen saturation monitoring systems to detect hyperoxia by setting the alarm limits to greater than 95% or even by functionally disabling the alarms. Oxygen management strategies to avoid hyperoxia have been successfully implemented but variation in oxygen use persists.[34–43]

Thermal Support

Silverman and colleagues[44] linked cold stress with mortality more than 50 years ago. Cold stress can lead to harmful side effects, including hypoglycemia, respiratory distress, hypoxia, metabolic acidosis, coagulation defects, and delayed transition from fetal to newborn circulation. Simple interventions to improve the thermal environment at birth are available. Despite the known association between cold stress and poor outcomes, and the ready availability of simple thermal support interventions hypothermia on admission to NICUs remains common in premature infants.[44–49]

Antibiotic Duration

Antibiotics are heavily used in NICU care for the treatment of sepsis, pneumonia, and other infections. Prolonged exposure to antibiotics is associated with the development of resistant organisms, fungal infections, and necrotizing enterocolitis. Despite these concerns, many infants continue to receive antibiotics after initial cultures are found to be negative and the infants appear clinically well.[50–53]

Metoclopramide

Metoclopramide is heavily used in premature infants for the treatment of gastroesophageal reflux, apnea-associated reflux, and bowel dysmotility despite a significant lack of evidence of efficacy or safety. The known central nervous system adverse effects in the adult and pediatric populations are particularly concerning with the use of this medication. Despite this information, the drug remains heavily used in NICUs.[54–65]

H_2-Blockers

H_2-blocking drugs are commonly used in premature infants for the treatment of gastroesophageal reflux associated apnea. However, evidence does not support a major role for gastroesophageal reflux in the etiology of apnea of prematurity. Treatment of reflux with H2-blockers will not prevent apnea, and may expose the infant to adverse medication effects. Of great concern, H_2-blocker use has been associated with development of necrotizing enterocolitis, possibly due to alteration of gut micribiota from the modification of gastric pH.[60,61,63,65,66]

Cefotaxime

Cefotaxime is one of the most commonly used antibiotics in NICUs. Cefotaxime use with ampicillin, as compared with ampicillin and gentamicin, however, was associated with higher mortality when used as empiric treatment for sepsis in the first 3 days of life.[67] Cefotaxime and other third-generation cephalosporin use is a significant risk factor for the development of invasive candidiasis in extremely low-birth-weight infants. Cefotaxime use is associated with the development and spread of extended-spectrum β-lactamases, which confer resistance to all penicillins and cephalosporins.[65,68–72]

The Quality Chasm Exists in Neonatology

As demonstrated by these examples, a quality chasm exists in neonatology, and, unfortunately, this list is by no means complete. All of the therapies on this list are important targets for NICU quality improvement efforts and several have already been the subjects of successful quality initiatives.

SYSTEMS THINKING

Health care has safety and quality problems because it relies on outmoded systems of work. Poor designs set the workforce up to fail, regardless of how hard they try. If we want safer, higher-quality care, we will need to have redesigned systems of care.
Institute of Medicine[1]

Central Law of Improvement: "Every system is perfectly designed to achieve the results it achieves."
Donald Berwick[73]

Systems thinking is a key element of quality improvement. Without a clear grasp of basic systems theory, attempts at improvement are impeded. It is critically important to understand that the system drives the outcome (central law of improvement). If outcomes are poor in a NICU, it is because that NICU's system is perfectly designed to generate that poor outcome. Changing the outcome first requires changing the system.

Deming defined a system as a network of interdependent components that work together to try to accomplish a specific aim.[74,75] Systems may be simple or complex and may be further described as mechanical or naturally adaptable systems.[76–82]

Simple Systems

Simple systems possess minimal components with simple relationships. For example, a home apnea monitor detects apnea in an infant and triggers an audible alarm. The electrodes are designed to detect the apnea event; the alarm is designed to alert the caregiver. These two components function together as a simple system to detect and report an event.

Complex Systems

Complex systems possess multiple, interrelated components that work together for a specific purpose. A central monitoring station in a NICU is a complex system that displays multiple measurements on several patients, displays audio and visual alarm events, and records, stores, and displays data trends. The components function together to enable NICU staff to detect a variety of physiologic abnormalities in several patients simultaneously, enabling them to intervene before harm occurs.

Mechanical Systems

Mechanical systems are highly predictable systems. The stimulus and response are well understood, and the outcome can be anticipated, even in a variety of circumstances and environments. The previous monitor examples are also examples of mechanical systems—simple mechanical systems and complex mechanical systems.

Adaptive Systems

The components of adaptive systems are capable of responding in multiple unpredictable ways, and these responses may then interact in multiple unpredictable ways. The introduction of living beings (from humans to microorganisms) introduces an element of chaos into any system. In the monitoring scenario, if the purpose of central monitoring is to minimize the duration of time with oxygen saturation levels above 95%, then the human elements—the baby's physiologic responses and the nurses' responses to the alarm data—create an adaptive system.

COMPLEX ADAPTIVE SYSTEMS

All of these system types exist in health care but generally function together as components of a complex adaptive system. Why bother to categorize systems? If a system model is not understood, system redesign may be ineffective or even counterproductive. If the human parts of a system are expected to behave like components of a mechanical system, system redesign is flawed and the outcome poor.

For example, consider this medical error: breast milk is given intravenously to an infant. A mechanical systems viewpoint of this error is to consider the nurse the "defective" part of the system and the correction to "remove the faulty part." From a complex adaptive systems perspective, the analysis and correction of the problem is different: the syringes used for breast milk and for intravenous lipids are identical, the milk and lipids are similar in appearance, and the double-check system was not used due to unavailability of a second nurse. System redesign includes modification of the syringe types, such that the enteral syringe is visibly different from the intravenous syringe in design and unable to physically connect to intravenous tubing. Nurse staffing design during high activity periods are assessed and modifications designed to enable double checks to occur as planned during high activity time periods.

TYPES OF CHANGE: TINKERING AND SYSTEM CHANGE

Two general categories of change are tinkering and system change. Tinkering (also known as first-order change) generally refers to simple changes imposed on individuals, such as trying harder or being more careful. These effort-based changes, although sometimes useful, are unlikely to yield sustained improvement.[73]

System change (also known as second-order change) refers to redesign of a system to always produce the desired outcome. Additional individual effort is not the primary design of the change. Over time, system changes are more likely to yield sustained improvement than tinkering. For examples of system change and tinkering in NICUs, see **Table 1**. Any change introduced into a complex adaptive system can have unintended and unpredictable results. It is imperative that changes be tested and refined via plan-do-study-act cycles (see the article by Ellsbury and Ursprung elsewhere in this issue) to avoid unintended consequences.

USING SIMPLICITY TO CROSS THE CHASM OF COMPLEXITY

Despite the labyrinthine processes and pathways of complex adaptive systems, it is heartening to realize that simplicity is a key factor in modification of these systems. Plsek[76] describes three simple rules for human complex adaptive system modification: (1) general direction pointing, (2) prohibitions, and (3) resource or permission providing. This approach is counterintuitive from a mechanistic perspective—more

Table 1
A comparison of tinkering and system change

Problem	Tinkering	System Change
Physicians orders are illegible, causing medication errors	Chastise physicians, tell them to try harder	Computerize order entry or use typed standardized order sets to minimize the need for handwriting
Breast milk use is low in premature infants	Suggest that the hospital hire more lactation consultants	Evaluate NICU staff opinions, correct opinions that formula and breast milk are equivalent; create process to provide breast pumps shortly after delivery
Oximeter alarms are not set as ordered	Sanction nurses who are noncomplaint	Establish a root cause for noncompliance (education, alarm defaults), provide education, modify preset alarm defaults
Surfactant is not always available when needed in the delivery room	Ask nursing staff to remember to order the drug from pharmacy when a delivery may occur	Establish a ward stock of surfactant that is immediately available for any delivery

complexity should require more rules. But for complex adaptive systems, it is the case that "less is more." Systematic breakdown and control of all component parts is not possible; the adaptive components and interrelationships are not predictable. Simple rules must be established for a system, rules that create the conditions for purposeful self-organizing behavior under which widespread and diverse natural experimentation occurs focused on generating the desired outcome.[76–82]

An example of this approach is the Pediatrix Comprehensive Oxygen Management for the Prevention of Retinopathy of Prematurity initiative. A few simple rules were used to govern this project: educate the NICU staff, redesign the system to avoid hyperoxia, and monitor compliance with the changes. Each NICU was encouraged to adapt the program to the specific environment of that NICU. The details of implementation varied between the NICUs, which often found different paths to the same outcome. The result was that in a large national network of NICUs, severe retinopathy of prematurity showed a marked and sustained decrease (see the article by Ellsbury and Ursprung elsewhere in this issue).

SUMMARY

A quality chasm exists in neonatal intensive care. Despite years of clinical research in neonatology, many therapies continue to be underused, overused, or misused. A key concept in crossing the quality chasm is the central law of improvement (every system is perfectly designed to achieve the results it achieves). An appreciation of the NICU as a complex adaptive system is integral to successful system redesign. The unpredictability of human factors and the dynamic complexity of the NICU system are not amenable to rigid reductionist control and redesign. Change is best accomplished in this complex adaptive system by use of simple rules, such as (1) general direction pointing, (2) prohibitions, and (3) resource or permission providing. These rules create the conditions for purposeful self-organizing behavior under which widespread natural experimentation occurs focused on generating the desired outcome.

A great opportunity exists in neonatology. Years of knowledge, obtained from the hard and insightful work of many researchers, sit uselessly on the shelf, ready and waiting to be applied in daily neonatal intensive care.

Knowing is not enough; we must apply. Willing is not enough; we must do.
–Goethe[83]

REFERENCES

1. Institute of Medicine. Crossing the quality chasm: a new health system for the 21st century. Washington, DC: National Academy Press; 2001.
2. Daniels M, Hill AB. Chemotherapy of pulmonary tuberculosis in young adults; an analysis of the combined results of three Medical Research Council trials. Br Med J 1952;1(4769):1162–8.
3. Chassin MR, Galvin RW. The urgent need to improve health care quality. Institute of Medicine National Roundtable on Health Care Quality. JAMA 1998;280(11): 1000–5.
4. Chassin MR. Is health care ready for Six Sigma quality? Milbank Q 1998;76(4): 565–91, 510.
5. Balas EA, Boren SA. Managing clinical knowledge for health care improvement. In: Bemmel J, McCray AT, editors. Yearbook of medical informatics. Bethesda (MD): National Library of Medicine; 2000. p. 65–70.

6. Chedoe I, Molendijk HA, Dittrich ST, et al. Incidence and nature of medication errors in neonatal intensive care with strategies to improve safety: a review of the current literature. Drug Saf 2007;30(6):503–13.
7. Takata GS, Mason W, Taketomo C, et al. Development, testing, and findings of a pediatric-focused trigger tool to identify medication-related harm in US children's hospitals. Pediatrics 2008;121(4):e927–35.
8. Brennan TA, Leape LL, Laird NM, et al. Incidence of adverse events and negligence in hospitalized patients. Results of the Harvard Medical Practice Study I. N Engl J Med 1991;324(6):370–6.
9. Suresh G, Horbar JD, Plsek P, et al. Voluntary anonymous reporting of medical errors for neonatal intensive care. Pediatrics 2004;113(6):1609–18.
10. Snijders C, van Lingen RA, Molendijk A, et al. Incidents and errors in neonatal intensive care: a review of the literature. Arch Dis Child Fetal Neonatal Ed 2007;92(5):F391–8.
11. Kohn LT, Corrigan JM, Donaldson MS, editors. To err is human: building a safer health system. Washington, DC: National Academy Press; 2000. p. 26–48.
12. Gill AW, Australian and New Zealand Neonatal Network. Analysis of neonatal nosocomial infection rates across the Australian and New Zealand Neonatal Network. J Hosp Infect 2009;72(2):155–62.
13. Kusuda S, Fujimura M, Sakuma I, et al. Neonatal Research Network, Japan. Morbidity and mortality of infants with very low birth weight in Japan: center variation. Pediatrics 2006;118(4):e1130–8.
14. Aziz K, McMillan DD, Andrews W, et al. Canadian Neonatal Network. Variations in rates of nosocomial infection among Canadian neonatal intensive care units may be practice-related. BMC Pediatr 2005;5:22.
15. Powers NG, Bloom B, Peabody J, et al. Site of care influences breastmilk feedings at NICU discharge. J Perinatol 2003;23(1):10–3.
16. Gartner LM, Morton J, Lawrence RA, et al. American Academy of Pediatrics Section on Breastfeeding. Breastfeeding and the use of human milk. Pediatrics 2005;115(2):496–506.
17. NIH consensus development panel on the effect of corticosteroids for fetal maturation on perinatal outcomes. Effect of corticosteroids for fetal maturation on perinatal outcomes. JAMA 1995;273:413–8.
18. Roberts D, Dalziel S. Antenatal corticosteroids for accelerating fetal lung maturation for women at risk of preterm birth. Cochrane Database Syst Rev 2006;(3):CD004454.
19. Howell EA, Stone J, Kleinman LC, et al. Approaching NIH guideline recommended care for maternal-infant health: clinical failures to use recommended antenatal corticosteroids. Matern Child Health J 2009. [Epub ahead of print]. DOI:10.1007/s10995-009-0480-3.
20. Bronstein JM, Goldenberg RL. Practice variation in the use of corticosteroids: a comparison of eight datasets. Am J Obstet Gynecol 1995;173:296–8.
21. Bronstein JM, Cliver SP, Goldenberg RL. Practice variation in the use of interventions in high risk obstetrics. Health Serv Res 1998;32:825–39.
22. Wright LL, Horbar JD, Gunkel H, et al. Evidence from multicenter networks on the current use and effectiveness of antenatal corticosteroids in low birth weight infants. Am J Obstet Gynecol 1995;173:263–9.
23. Wirtschafter DD, Danielsen BH, Main EK, et al. California Perinatal Quality Care Collaborative. Promoting antenatal steroid use for fetal maturation: results from the California Perinatal Quality Care Collaborative. J Pediatr 2006;148(5):606–12.

24. Halliday HL. Surfactants: past, present and future. J Perinatol 2008;28(Suppl 1): S47–56.
25. Seger N, Soll R. Animal derived surfactant extract for treatment of respiratory distress syndrome. Cochrane Database Syst Rev 2009;(2):CD007836. DOI: 10.1002/14651858. CD007836.
26. Engle WA. American Academy of Pediatrics Committee on Fetus and Newborn. Surfactant-replacement therapy for respiratory distress in the preterm and term neonate. Pediatrics 2008;121(2):419–32.
27. Horbar JD, Carpenter JH, Buzas J, et al. Vermont Oxford Network. Timing of initial surfactant treatment for infants 23 to 29 weeks' gestation: is routine practice evidence based? Pediatrics 2004;113(6):1593–602.
28. Koll BS, Straub TA, Jalon HS, et al. The CLABs collaborative: a regionwide effort to improve the quality of care in hospitals. Jt Comm J Qual Patient Saf 2008; 34(12):713–23.
29. Jeffries HE, Mason W, Brewer M, et al. Prevention of central venous catheter-associated bloodstream infections in pediatric intensive care units: a performance improvement collaborative. Infect Control Hosp Epidemiol 2009;30(7):645–51.
30. Costello JM, Morrow DF, Graham DA, et al. Systematic intervention to reduce central line-associated bloodstream infection rates in a pediatric cardiac intensive care unit. Pediatrics 2008;121(5):915–23.
31. McKee C, Berkowitz I, Cosgrove SE, et al. Reduction of catheter-associated bloodstream infections in pediatric patients: experimentation and reality. Pediatr Crit Care Med 2008;9(1):40–6.
32. Wirtschafter DD, Pettit J, Kurtin P, et al. A statewide quality improvement collaborative to reduce neonatal central line-associated blood stream infections. J Perinatol 2009. [Epub ahead of print]. DOI:10.1038/jp.2009.172.
33. Pronovost P. Interventions to decrease catheter-related bloodstream infections in the ICU: the Keystone Intensive Care Unit Project. Am J Infect Control 2008; 36(10):S171.e1–5.
34. Chow LC, Wright KW, Sola A. CSMC Oxygen Administration Study Group. Can changes in clinical practice decrease the incidence of severe retinopathy of prematurity in very low birth weight infants? Pediatrics 2003;111(2):339–45.
35. Ellsbury DL. Quality improvement program for the reduction of retinopathy of prematurity [abstract]. E-PAS 2006;59:3602.469.
36. Sears JE, Pietz J, Sonnie C, et al. A change in oxygen supplementation can decrease the incidence of retinopathy of prematurity. Ophthalmology 2009; 116(3):513–8.
37. Deulofeut R, Critz A, Adams-Chapman I, et al. Avoiding hyperoxia in infants < or = 1250 g is associated with improved short-and long-term outcomes. J Perinatol 2006;26(11):700–5.
38. Vanderveen DK, Mansfield TA, Eichenwald EC. Lower oxygen saturation alarm limits decrease the severity of retinopathy of prematurity. J AAPOS 2006;10(5): 445–8.
39. Wright KW, Sami D, Thompson L, et al. A physiologic reduced oxygen protocol decreases the incidence of threshold retinopathy of prematurity. Trans Am Ophthalmol Soc 2006;104:78–84.
40. Hagadorn JI, Furey AM, Nghiem TH, et al. AVIOx Study Group. Achieved versus intended pulse oximeter saturation in infants born less than 28 weeks' gestation: the AVIOx study. Pediatrics 2006;118(4):1574–82.
41. Clucas L, Doyle LW, Dawson J, et al. Compliance with alarm limits for pulse oximetry in very preterm infants. Pediatrics 2007;119(6):1056–60.

42. O'Donovan DJ, Fernandes CJ. Free radicals and diseases in premature infants. Antioxid Redox Signal 2004;6(1):169–76.
43. Sola A, Rogido MR, Deulofeut R. Oxygen as a neonatal health hazard: call for détente in clinical practice. Acta Paediatr 2007;96(6):801–12.
44. Silvermam WA, Fertig JW, Berger AP. The influence of the thermal environment upon the survival of newly born premature infants. Pediatrics 1958;22(5): 876–86.
45. McCall EM, Alderdice FA, Halliday HL, et al. Interventions to prevent hypothermia at birth in preterm and/or low birthweight infants. Cochrane Database Syst Rev 2008;(1):CD004210.
46. Laptook AR, Watkinson M. Temperature management in the delivery room. Semin Fetal Neonatal Med 2008;13(6):383–91.
47. Laptook AR, Salhab W, Bhaskar B, Neonatal Research Network. Admission temperature of low birth weight infants: predictors and associated morbidities. Pediatrics 2007;119(3):e643–9.
48. Knobel RB, Vohra S, Lehmann CU. Heat loss prevention in the delivery room for preterm infants: a national survey of newborn intensive care units. J Perinatol 2005;25(8):514–8.
49. Cramer K, Wiebe N, Hartling L, et al. Heat loss prevention: asystematic review of occlusive skin wrap for premature neonates. J Perinatol 2005;25(12):763–9.
50. Spitzer AR, Kirkby S, Kornhauser M. Practice variation in suspected neonatal sepsis: a costly problem in neonatal intensive care. J Perinatol 2005;25(4):265–9.
51. Cotten CM, Taylor S, Stoll B, et al. NICHD Neonatal Research Network. Prolonged duration of initial empirical antibiotic treatment is associated with increased rates of necrotizing enterocolitis and death for extremely low birth weight infants. Pediatrics 2009;123(1):58–66.
52. Cordero L, Ayers LW. Duration of empiric antibiotics for suspected early-onset sepsis in extremely low birth weight infants. Infect Control Hosp Epidemiol 2003;24(9):662–6.
53. Bizzarro MJ, Gallagher PG. Antibiotic-resistant organisms in the neonatal intensive care unit. Semin Perinatol 2007;31(1):26–32.
54. Hibbs AM, Lorch SA. Metoclopramide for the treatment of gastroesophageal reflux disease in infants: a systematic review. Pediatrics 2006;118(2):746–52.
55. Wheatley E, Kennedy KA. Cross-over trial of treatment for bradycardia attributed to gastroesophageal reflux in preterm infants. J Pediatr 2009;155(4):516–21.
56. Clark RH, Spitzer AR. Patience is a virtue in the management of gastroesophageal reflux. J Pediatr 2009;155(4):464–5.
57. Paturi B, Ryan RM, Michienzi KA, et al. Galactorrhea with metoclopramide use in the neonatal unit. J Perinatol 2009;29(5):391–2.
58. Malcolm WF, Gantz M, Martin RJ, et al. National Institute of Child Health and Human Development Neonatal Research Network. Use of medications for gastroesophageal reflux at discharge among extremely low birth weight infants. Pediatrics 2008;121(1):22–7.
59. Mejia NI, Jankovic J. Metoclopramide-induced tardive dyskinesia in an infant. Mov Disord 2005;20(1):86–9.
60. Finer NN, Higgins R, Kattwinkel J, et al. Summary proceedings from the apnea-of-prematurity group. Pediatrics 2006;117(3 Pt 2):S47–51.
61. Di Fiore JM, Arko M, Whitehouse M, et al. Apnea is not prolonged by acid gastroesophageal reflux in preterm infants. Pediatrics 2005;116(5):1059–63.
62. Poets CF. Gastroesophageal reflux: a critical review of its role in preterm infants. Pediatrics 2004;113(2):e128–32.

63. Peter CS, Sprodowski N, Bohnhorst B, et al. Gastroesophageal reflux and apnea of prematurity: no temporal relationship. Pediatrics 2002;109(1):8–11.
64. Kenney C, Hunter C, Davidson A, et al. Metoclopramide, an increasingly recognized cause of tardive dyskinesia. J Clin Pharmacol 2008;48(3):379–84.
65. Clark RH, Bloom BT, Spitzer AR, et al. Reported medication use in the neonatal intensive care unit: data from a large national data set. Pediatrics 2006;117(6):1979–87.
66. Guillet R, Stoll BJ, Cotten CM, et al. National Institute of Child Health and Human Development Neonatal Research Network. Association of H2-blocker therapy and higher incidence of necrotizing enterocolitis in very low birth weight infants. Pediatrics 2006;117(2):e137–42.
67. Clark RH, Bloom BT, Spitzer AR, et al. Empiric use of ampicillin and cefotaxime, compared with ampicillin and gentamicin, for neonates at risk for sepsis is associated with an increased risk of neonatal death. Pediatrics 2006;117(1):67–74.
68. Cotten CM, McDonald S, Stoll B, et al. The association of third-generation cephalosporin use and invasive candidiasis in extremely low birth-weight infants. Pediatrics 2006;118(2):717–22.
69. Benjamin DK Jr, DeLong ER, Steinbach WJ, et al. Empirical therapy for neonatal candidemia in very low birth weight infants. Pediatrics 2003;112(3 Pt 1):543–7.
70. Benjamin DK Jr, Stoll BJ, Fanaroff AA, et al. Neonatal candidiasis among extremely low birth weight infants: risk factors, mortality rates, and neurodevelopmental outcomes at 18 to 22 months. Pediatrics 2006;117(1):84–92.
71. Zaoutis TE, Goyal M, Chu JH, et al. Risk factors for and outcomes of bloodstream infection caused by extended-spectrum beta-lactamase-producing Escherichia coli and Klebsiella species in children. Pediatrics 2005;115(4):942–9.
72. Linkin DR, Fishman NO, Patel JB, et al. Risk factors for extended-spectrum beta-lactamase-producing Enterobacteriaceae in a neonatal intensive care unit. Infect Control Hosp Epidemiol 2004;25(9):781–3.
73. Berwick DM. A primer on leading the improvement of systems. BMJ 1996;312(7031):619–22.
74. Deming WE. Out of the crisis. Cambridge (MA): Massachusetts Institute of Technology; 1986.
75. Deming WE. The new economics for industry, government, education. 2nd edition. Cambridge (MA): Massachusetts Institute of Technology; 2000.
76. Plsek P. Redesigning healthcare with insights from the science of complex adaptive systems. Institute of Medicine. Crossing the quality chasm: a new health system for the 21st century. Washington, DC: National Academy Press; 2001. 309–22.
77. Plsek PE, Greenhalgh T. Complexity science: the challenge of complexity in health care. BMJ 2001;323(7313):625–8.
78. Plsek PE, Wilson T. Complexity, leadership, and management in healthcare organisations. BMJ 2001;323(7315):746–9.
79. Wilson T, Holt T, Greenhalgh T. Complexity science: complexity and clinical care. BMJ 2001;323(7314):685–8.
80. Fraser SW, Greenhalgh T. Coping with complexity: educating for capability. BMJ 2001;323(7316):799–803.
81. Stacey RD. Complexity and creativity in organizations. San Francisco (CA): Berrett-Koehler; 1996.
82. Nelson EC, Batalden PB, Godfrey MM. Quality by design: a clinical microsystems approach. San Francisco (CA): Jossey-Bass; 2007.
83. Goethe JW, Saunders TB. The maxims and reflections of Goethe. New York (NY): MacMillan; 1906. p. 144.

Evaluating the Medical Evidence for Quality Improvement

Roger F. Soll, MD[a,b,c,d,*]

KEYWORDS

- Evidence-based medicine • Randomized controlled trials
- Neonatology

Advances in neonatal care have led to significant improvement in survival and quality of life of newborn infants.[1] That said, Neonatal-Perinatal Medicine has also participated in the introduction of untested drugs and interventions that have led to disastrous complications. The past several decades in Neonatal-Perinatal Medicine have seen their share of therapeutic misadventures: the epidemic of retinopathy attributable to the indiscriminate use of supplemental oxygen; gray baby syndrome attributable to chloramphenicol; and an increase in the incidence of kernicterus attributable to the introduction of sulfonamide drugs.[2] To avoid these disasters, clinicians must practice medicine based on the strong support of the available evidence. This review builds on the principles of evidence-based medicine (EBM) discussed in a previous review of the subject[3] and discusses how to practice EBM and how EBM can be used in quality improvement. Examples from Neonatal-Perinatal Medicine are given for which these principles were, or were not, adhered to.

On evaluation of the use of commonly used interventions, a tremendous variation in practice is discerned. A review of the Vermont Oxford Network database of infants weighing 401 to 1500 g demonstrates large variation in a variety of common

The author is Professor of Pediatrics at the University of Vermont College of Medicine, President of the Vermont Oxford Network, and Coordinating Editor of the Cochrane Neonatal Review Group. He has received no direct support regarding any of the interventions discussed in the article.

[a] Division of Neonatal-Perinatal Medicine, University of Vermont College of Medicine, Smith 552A, 111 Colchester Avenue, Burlington, VT 05401, USA

[b] Neonatal Intensive Care Unit, Fletcher Allen Health Care, University of Vermont College of Medicine, Smith 552A, 111 Colchester Avenue, Burlington, VT 05401, USA

[c] Vermont Oxford Network, University of Vermont College of Medicine, Smith 552A, 111 Colchester Avenue, Burlington, VT 05401, USA

[d] Cochrane Neonatal Review Group, University of Vermont College of Medicine, Smith 552A, 111 Colchester Avenue, Burlington, VT 05401, USA

* Division of Neonatal-Perinatal Medicine, University of Vermont College of Medicine, Smith 552A, 111 Colchester Avenue, Burlington, VT 05401.

E-mail address: Roger.Soll@vtmednet.org

Clin Perinatol 37 (2010) 11–28
doi:10.1016/j.clp.2010.01.002
0095-5108/10/$ – see front matter

practices.[4] Practices such as the use of nasal continuous positive airway pressure (CPAP) and high-frequency ventilation vary greatly between centers. In very low birth weight infants, the median use of nasal CPAP is 67%, but the interquartile range is broad (52%–79%).[5] Similar variation in practice is observed with more recent technological innovations such as high-frequency ventilation (HFV). The median use rate of HFV is 22%, but the interquartile range is 9% to 28%. If these and other practices are based on the best evidence, why is our practice so varied? And if these practices truly matter, why are some of us putting our infants at risk?

To avoid these problems, we need to learn to evaluate the medical evidence and base our practice on the best available evidence. EBM is the integration of clinical expertise, patient values, and the best evidence into the decision-making process for patient care.[6] EBM requires personal commitment, institutional commitment, and societal commitment. These factors are reflected in personal practice choices as well as the development of guidelines that may influence practice on a local or national level. EBM cannot be expected to provide answers to all our questions, but EBM will allow us to improve the quality of care by identifying and promoting practices that work, while eliminating those that are ineffective or harmful.[7] In his primer on EBM, Sackett and colleagues[8] proposed 6 simple steps that are essential to practicing EBM. These steps are detailed in this article.

FORMULATING THE QUESTION

Although it seems obvious, formulating the question is critical to the practice of EBM. Questions must be searchable (ie, having a reasonable expectation that some research has attempted to answer the question) and clinically relevant. The question must be explicit regarding the patient or problem being considered, the intervention being considered, the comparison intervention, and the clinical outcome of interest.[9] The question could deal with any aspect of care, including etiology, diagnosis, prevention, treatment, or prognosis. For the purpose of this review, the focus is on evaluating the efficacy of new therapies.

The clinical question should be structured in the PICO format (Patient or Problem, Intervention, Comparison, Outcomes). For the "Patient or Problem," the specific characteristics of the patient (or in the case of guidelines or recommendations, the population or group of patients) in whom the intervention takes place must be defined. Issues such as the patient's age, disease severity, or coexisting conditions need to be considered. For this discussion, the "Intervention" will involve treatment choices. Both the "Intervention" and the "Comparison" need to be specifically defined. Are you considering treatment or nontreatment, or the comparison between 2 different drugs or surgical interventions? The "Outcome" chosen should be of consequence either to the patient or society, not merely a surrogate for clinical or physiologic improvement.

For example, imagine you had a 2-week-old, 27-week gestational age infant who remained on assisted ventilation with worsening respiratory status. You wonder whether corticosteroid administration might improve your ability to extubate this infant and enhance his chances for survival. The key components for your clinical question would include:

Patient or Problem:	2-week-old ex– 27-week gestational age infant on assisted ventilation
Intervention:	Corticosteroids
Comparison:	No corticosteroids
Outcomes:	Ability to wean from ventilation and survival

The 4-part clinical question could be formulated as follows: "In a 2-week-old, 27-week gestation baby on assisted ventilation with worsening respiratory status, does the administration of corticosteroids compared with not giving corticosteroids decrease the risk of developing chronic lung disease?"

FINDING THE EVIDENCE

Once you have formulated the clinical question, the next step is to search for relevant evidence that may help answer the question. This process has changed dramatically since the advent of computer databases and the Internet. Long gone are the days of sitting in the library poring through volumes of Index Medicus. Today, there are multiple resources for access to the general medical literature and some resources that are unique to Neonatal-Perinatal Medicine. Searching the medical literature is now widely available through the Internet, including several bibliographic databases such as the Cochrane Library database, MEDLINE, EMBASE, and CINAHL. MEDLINE is the premier biomedical database produced by the National Library of Medicine. MEDLINE includes journals published from 1966 to the present, indexes over 5200 international biomedical journals, and contains more than 18 million references. A variety of MEDLINE search engines are available, including Ovid and PubMed. PubMed is freely available on the Internet through the National Library of Medicine (http://www.ncbi.nlm.nih.gov/pubmed/). Practitioners must learn effective search strategies in MEDLINE, including the use of the National Library of Medicine subject index (MeSH headings), and a variety of limits, including publication types (eg, clinical trial, letter, review) and text words to create the most efficient literature searches. Haynes and colleagues[10] offer simple strategies to locate the best studies of treatment, diagnosis, prognosis, or etiology with the greatest precision. Depending on your needs, you may want your search to be more sensitive (including the greatest number of relevant articles but also including some less relevant articles) or more specific (including mostly relevant articles but omitting a few relevant articles). Search engines such as PubMed have incorporated these "filters" into specialized search engines (refer to the "Clinical queries using research methodology filters" in PubMed).

Other databases include EMBASE and CINAHL. EMBASE (published by Elsevier Science) covers the biomedical literature from 7000 journals, and is particularly strong in pharmaceutical and toxicologic studies. CINAHL is the Cumulative Index to Nursing and Allied Health Literature, and represents the most comprehensive resource for Nursing and Allied Health Sciences publications. For a comprehensive literature search, such as the search needed to create a systematic overview, knowledge and use of these search engines is essential. However, for the busy clinician, certain shortcuts may be useful. Although not comprehensive, quick questions can be answered by simple searches through Google Scholar or other readily available search engines.

There are a variety of other resources that may be important in the practice of EBM, particularly in Neonatal-Perinatal Medicine. The Cochrane Library of Databases (which includes the Cochrane Database of Systematic Reviews, the Databases of Abstracts of Reviews and Effectiveness, and the Cochrane Control Trials Registry) is maintained by the Cochrane Collaboration, an international initiative that designs, prepares, maintains, and disseminates systematic reviews of health care interventions. The Cochrane Review Group creates systematic overviews for the Cochrane Library.[11] These reviews are available through the Cochrane Library or through the National Institute of Child Health and Human Development (NICHD) Web site (http://www.nichd.nih.gov/COCHRANE/).

CONDUCTING THE SEARCH

Each database has its own specific way to search the literature. A familiarity with the most basic portals and databases (eg, using PubMed to search MEDLINE) is critical for success. To successfully pair down the search, an understanding of the use of the Boolean operators "AND" and "OR" is essential. If you are combining 2 terms "AND" allows only articles containing both terms to be retrieved while "OR" allows articles containing either term to be retrieved. In addition, certain specific limits (such as publication type, publication dates, or study population) may be very useful in refining your search.

Given the PICO question asked earlier, a simple search of MEDLINE using PubMed might include the following: chronic lung disease AND corticosteroids OR steroids OR glucocorticoids OR prednisone OR dexamethasone. Limits might include "clinical trial" or "randomized controlled trial" and an age group, for example, "all infants." More sophisticated searches can be done, but these require greater expertise and, frequently, the help of a research librarian.[12]

APPRAISING THE EVIDENCE

Once you have located potentially relevant articles through your search, you must learn how to evaluate the available evidence. Although all the articles may contain some useful information, all are not equally valid. The quality (also known as the strength or validity) of the evidence ranges from extensively researched issues using methodologically sound study designs (such as systematic reviews or large, well-designed randomized controlled trials [RCTs]) to the opinion of respected authorities (based on clinical evidence, descriptive studies, or reports of expert committees). Many groups have attempted to help practitioners and guideline developers evaluate the strength of the evidence. One useful approach on which to base the "validity" or "strength" of the available evidence is the hierarchy of evidence created by the US Preventive Services Task Force (http://www.ahrq.gov) (**Box 1**).[13]

You may not always find the highest level of evidence to answer your question. In the absence of the best evidence, you then need to consider moving down the pyramid to other types of studies. The Task Force has placed the "opinions of respected authorities" at the base of the pyramid, implying that this represents the lowest level of evidence. While that may be true, it must be remembered that many

Box 1
Judging the strength of the evidence

I: Properly powered and conducted RCT; well-conducted systematic review or meta-analysis of homogeneous RCTs

II-1: Well-designed controlled trial without randomization

II-2: Well-designed cohort or case-control analytical study

II-3: Multiple time series with or without the intervention; dramatic results from uncontrolled experiments

III: Opinions of respected authorities, based on clinical experience; descriptive studies or case reports; reports of expert committees

From US Preventive Services Task Force hierarchy of evidence (http://www.ahrq.gov).

of the most important breakthroughs in medical care began with the observation and opinions of experts. The often quoted story of Sir Alexander Fleming's observation that a substance produced by the fungus *Penicillium notatum* had bactericidal properties led to the eventual discovery of the antibiotic penicillin.[14] However, even as great an idea as a new antibiotic needs to be vigorously tested, as demonstrated by the disastrous introduction of sulfonamides in newborns leading to an increase in the incidence of kernicterus.

Other study designs contribute to our understanding of new interventions. Case series and case reports consist of reports on the treatment of an individual patient or groups of patients. In the hierarchy of the US Preventive Task Force pyramid, these studies would be classified as II-3. No statistical comparisons can be done because these are only reports of cases that do not use a control group for comparison. That is not to say that important scientific insight has not been gained from such studies. If a specific new intervention is associated with a bizarre and previously unseen complication (eg, the effects of thalidomide when given to pregnant women), such reports provide essential and actionable information.[15]

Well-designed cohort or case-control analytical study are combined in the Task Force pyramid (classified as II-2). Case-control studies are studies in which patients who have a specific condition are compared with people who do not have the condition. The evaluation is fairly straightforward; individuals who have the outcome of concern are compared with individuals who have not experienced that outcome to reveal the frequency that each group has been exposed to the intervention in question. Cohort studies compare 2 "cohorts" of patients from the same time period, one of whom has a received a particular treatment and the other who has not. The classic example of a cohort study in perinatal medicine is the report of decreased mortality in women cared for by the midwifery service at the Second Obstetric Clinic of the Vienna General Hospital, associated with hand-washing practices.[16] Although potentially useful, cohort studies are prone to bias. Unlike RCTs, the groups may not be similar and may differ in ways other than exposure to the intervention under study.

The most valid evidence comes from RCTs. The methodology of RCTs seeks to minimize bias at all points of the study and thereby gives the most accurate and reproducible estimates of effect. Random allocation of study subjects is essential to minimize bias at the time of study entry (selection bias) and provides the basis for all traditional statistical comparisons used in the analysis of trial results. Bias can also occur after patient allocation. Bias can occur regarding the exposure to the intervention (performance bias), completeness of follow-up (exclusion bias), and measurement of outcomes (detection or assessment bias).[17] RCTs are limited in their ability to evaluate the long-term consequences of therapy and have no use in evaluating issues, such as complex processes of care or environmental issues, as seen with exposure to chemical or industrial hazards.[18] Even with these limitations, it is critical that clinicians familiarize themselves with the methodological issues involved in the proper conduct of RCTs to appreciate the validity of the evidence.

Methodological quality of RCTs does impact on the interpretation of results. Both groups in the trial must be treated the same except for administration of the experimental treatment. If "cointerventions" (interventions other than the study treatment) exist, they should be applied in a similar fashion to both groups. In trials in which treatment allocation has been inadequately concealed, treatment effects are commonly overestimated.[19] In trials without a placebo, there may be greater reported effects.[20] All subjects entered into a trial should be accounted for at the end of the trial (intention to treat analysis). Failure of a subject to receive the assigned intervention may be due to the difficulty of delivering the intervention (eg, immediate intubation and surfactant treatment in the delivery room) or patient noncompliance (eg, refusal to take a foul tasting medicine or stopping taking a medicine because the patient perceives no benefit). These situations will skew the results of the study by leaving subjects in the study that had a more positive response to treatment. Similarly, loss to follow-up may skew results. Subjects who do not make themselves available for follow-up could theoretically be quite different from those that do (either having experienced a poor response or adverse event, or perhaps because they are completely cured and see no reason to seek further medical advice). All of these issues must be formally addressed to understand the validity of the trial (**Box 2**).[8]

Box 2
Assessing the validity and importance of a clinical trial

Are the results of this therapy study valid?

1. Was the assignment of patients to treatment randomized?

   The assignment of patients to either group (treatment or control) must be done by in a random fashion; this might include a coin toss (heads to treatment/tails to control) or use of randomization tables, often computer generated.

2. Were all the patients who entered the trial properly accounted for at its conclusion? Was follow-up complete?

   All patients who started the trial should be accounted for at the end of the trial. If patients are not accounted for, the validity of the study may be jeopardized. A good study will have better than 80% follow-up for their patients. Patients may drop out of a study for various reasons, including because of adverse events related to the treatment. If these patients are not included in the results, they can make the treatment look better than it really is (and vice versa).

3. Were patients analyzed in the groups to which they were (originally) randomized?

   Patients should be analyzed within their assigned groups. This is called "intention to treat" analysis. Patients who are noncompliant with treatment or follow-up should not be eliminated from the study analysis. Excluding noncompliant patients leaves behind those that may be more likely to have a positive outcome, creating bias.

4. Were patients, clinicians, and study personnel "blind" to treatment allocation?

   "Blinding" or "masking" means that the study subject and study personnel do not know which treatments were received. Blinding eliminates bias and any preconceived notions as to how the treatments should be working. When it is difficult or unethical to blind patients to a treatment, such as a surgical treatment, then a "blinded" researcher is needed to interpret the results.

5. Were the groups similar at the start of the trial?

   Based on random assignment, the treatment and the control group should be similar for most prognostic characteristics except for whether they received the experimental treatment. If there are known factors that highly influence outcome, equal distribution of these factors can be addressed by stratification at the time of randomization.

6. Aside from the experimental intervention, were the groups treated equally?

   Both groups must be treated the same except for administration of the experimental treatment. All "cointerventions" must be applied in a similar fashion to both study groups.

Systematic reviews are an extremely useful tool to evaluate the entirety of the high-order evidence available to address a specific question. To perform a systematic review, an extensive literature search must be conducted to identify all eligible methodologically sound studies. The studies are reviewed, assessed, and the results summarized according to the predetermined criteria. The reviews published in the Cochrane Library are a prime example of this process.

Systematic reviews are potentially even more powerful than individual RCTs. Systematic reviews limit the bias inherent to traditional overviews by conducting a comprehensive search of all potentially relevant articles and using explicit, reproducible criteria in the selection of articles for review.[21] Qualitative systematic reviews summarize the data but do not perform further statistical analyses. Quantitative systematic reviews, or meta-analyses, are systematic reviews that use statistical methods to combine the results of multiple RCTs. The statistical methods for pooling results are similar to the statistical methods used in analyzing the data from multicenter trials. Pooling the results of previous similar RCTs increases the statistical power lacking in the individual smaller trials, and enables the clinician to have greater security in accepting or rejecting treatment differences demonstrated by the trials.[22,23]

Meta-analysis has its critics. Any attempt at pooling results from various studies will not only incorporate the biases of the primary studies but will also add additional bias attributable to study selection and the inevitable heterogeneity of the selected studies. LeLorier and colleagues[24] compared the findings of 12 large RCTs with the results of meta-analyses conducted earlier on the same topics. There was only fair agreement between the meta-analyses and the large clinical trials. However, differences in the point estimate between the RCTs and the meta-analyses were statistically significant in only 12% of the comparisons. The discrepancies noted by LeLorier may be attributable to a variety of biases that may be incorporated in the meta-analysis. There are several plausible explanations of how a meta-analysis might obtain a positive result that is not confirmed by subsequent large, well-designed RCTs. Publication bias, the tendency for investigators to preferentially submit studies with positive results, and the tendency of editors to choose positive studies for publication skews the medical literature toward favorable reports of treatment. Unless the authors of the meta-analysis have done a scrupulous search of all available resources, these studies will not be located and the meta-analysis stands a good chance of reporting a falsely positive finding. This problem is further compounded by the greater chance that this false positive finding will itself be published. Meta-analysis can offer false negative conclusions because of inappropriate study selection. If the studies selected are not groupable (heterogeneous), the positive effects observed with one specific treatment or in one specific population may be lost. To minimize bias, the authors of the meta-analysis and the readers of the review must demand the same methodological quality from these analyses that they would from an individual RCT. It is essential that all meta-analyses include a prospectively designed protocol, a comprehensive and extensive search strategy, strict criteria for inclusion of studies, standard definitions of outcomes, and standard statistical techniques.

Once the evidence has been found, the importance of the evidence must be assessed. Clinical trials may use a variety of statistical techniques in reporting their results. Just because a reported difference is "statistically significant," does not make the finding automatically clinically relevant. To assess whether the results of a trial are, in fact, clinically relevant, one needs to calculate some simple statistics from the study findings (**Table 1**).[5] The relative and absolute risk reductions are useful statistics in understanding the clinical impact of the therapy. The relative risk reduction (RRR) is the control event rate (CER) minus the experimental event rate (EER) over the

Table 1 Key terminology for estimating the size of the treatment effect			
	Outcome		
	Positive	Negative	Risk of Outcome
Treated (Y)	a	b	Y = a/(a + b)
Control (X)	c	d	X = c/(c + d)

Relative Risk (RR) is the risk of the outcome in the treated group (Y) compared with the risk in the control group. RR = Y/X.

Relative Risk Reduction (RRR) is the percent reduction in risk in the treated group (Y) compared with the control group (X). RRR = 1 − Y/X × 100% or 1 − RR × 100%.

Absolute Risk Reduction (ARR) is the difference in risk between the control group (X) and the treatment group (Y). ARR = X − Y.

Number Needed to Treat (NNT) is the number of patients that must be treated over a given period of time to prevent one adverse outcome. NNT = 1/(X − Y) or 1/ARR.

control event rate. The absolute risk reduction (ARR) is the CER minus the EER. The RRR indicates the relative but not absolute reduction in event rate. The ARR (also known as the event rate difference) indicates the absolute reduction in the event rate. If the overall incidence of the event is low, the ARR will be very low as well, even if there is a relatively large difference between the study groups. Understanding both the RRR and the ARR is essential to making any clinical judgment. The relative risk (RR) compares the risk or chance of an occurrence given the presence of a risk factor, to the chance of the occurrence given the absence of the risk factor. An RR of approximately 1 means that the particular outcome is no more likely to be associated with the exposure to the intervention than with the lack of exposure. Risk difference is a more straightforward statistic. The ARR or risk difference is the difference between the probability of the event with and without the exposure. A positive risk difference suggests that there may be a positive association between the risk factor and the disease. If the risk difference is close to zero, there is likely to be no association. Also of use is the number needed to treat (NNT). The NNT is calculated by dividing 1 by the ARR. For example, if the ARR is 20%, the NNT would be 5. In other words, 5 infants would need to be treated to prevent one theoretical event.

Many studies publish *P* values to evaluate statistical significance. In reality, all that the *P* value tells the reader is whether the event was likely to be random or not. Confidence intervals are more useful in quantitating the uncertainty of the estimated value of an effect measurement. A 95% confidence interval (CI) reflects 95% certainty that the true value of the measure lies within the bounds of the interval.

APPLICABILITY

Once the appropriate research articles are in hand and the data have been summarized in ways that are clinically relevant, it is necessary to decide how to integrate this evidence into clinical practice or, in the case of institutions, into practice guidelines. In the individual patient, one must assess whether the results of the randomized trial apply to the treatment of that particular individual. A variety of characteristics (age, sex, comorbidity, and disease severity) may be substantially different from the characteristics of the patients enrolled in the trial. These differences may make it unclear that the extrapolation of the results of the evidence to the individual patient is appropriate. A typical example would be the use of a treatment in a patient with a condition similar, but not identical, to the condition of patients treated in the trial. This situation frequently needs to be addressed with respect to issues of timing or disease severity. In these situations, Sackett and colleagues[8] ask us to use common sense. They pose the question in reverse, asking "Is my patient so different from those in the trial that the results cannot help me make my treatment decision?" In reality, there are few situations in which you would expect that an intervention would produce qualitatively different results in patients who do not strictly fit eligibility criteria. Only in these situations should you consider rejecting the results.

Another common mistake in applying the evidence occurs with inappropriate subgroup analyses. If there was some prior reason for expecting differential responses to the intervention among different subgroups of patients, this analysis should be prospectively planned as part of the study. If not, these analyses are nothing more than "fishing" expeditions. It is very likely that differences will emerge, but it is impossible to distinguish between real effects and chance events.[15] Unless there is some persuasive biologic reason to believe that the treatment would be totally ineffective or detrimental to the patient (compared with patients enrolled in the study), one should assume a similar direction of effect in the patient's illness.

GRADE Recommendations

Evidence must be used not only in the care of individual patients but also in the creation of clinical policies or guidelines. In creating policies or guidelines, one must consider the evidence regarding the impact of the disease, barriers to implementing the clinical policy, safety, acceptability, and cost effectiveness.[25] Even in situations where the evidence is extensive, formulating a clinical policy can be a difficult task. Decisions regarding clinical policies and guidelines involve a series of compromises that take both the individual and societal values into account.

The process of developing guidelines lacks any standardization or consistency. Guyatt and colleagues[26–29] recommend use of the GRADE system (Grades of Recommendation, Assessment, Development, and Evaluation), a method for categorizing and communicating information regarding the quality of evidence. The GRADE system has been adopted by organizations worldwide. To achieve transparency and simplicity, the GRADE system classifies the quality of evidence into 1 of 4 levels: high, moderate, low, or very low.[26] High-quality evidence means that the current evidence is methodologically sound and provides a very precise estimate of effect, such that further research is very unlikely to change the estimate of effect; moderate quality denotes that further research is likely to have an important impact on interpretation of the estimate of effects and may change the estimate; low quality notes that future research is very likely to have an important impact on our interpretation of the estimate of effect and is likely to change the estimate; and very low quality denotes that the estimate of effect is very uncertain. There are limitations to such a simplified approach. Quality of evidence is a continuum; any discrete characterization involves some degree of arbitrariness. However, Guyatt and colleagues argue that given the difficulties in disseminating evidence-based recommendations, the advantages of simplicity, transparency, and clarity outweigh these limitations.

Making GRADE recommendations requires a sophisticated sense of the methodological issues that affect the validity of RCTs. Evidence derived from RCTs is the highest quality evidence, but as noted in the previous discussion, confidence in the evidence may be decreased for several reasons, including methodological limitations of the study, inconsistencies of results across studies, lack of precision (from inappropriately small sample size), and reporting or publication bias.[26] The GRADE system offers 2 grades of recommendations: either "strong" or "weak." Strong recommendations can be made in situations where the risk/benefit ratio is clear (where the benefits clearly outweigh the risks or vice versa). On the other hand, when the balance of risks and benefits are less certain, either because of low-quality evidence or because the evidence suggests that the risks and benefits are closely balanced, only weak recommendations can be made. Using the GRADE system potentially provides a system for rating quality of evidence and strength of recommendations that is explicit, comprehensive, transparent, and pragmatic.

EVALUATING PERFORMANCE: THE ROLE OF QUALITY IMPROVEMENT

In Sackett's primer on EBM, the final step to the practice of EBM is to evaluate our own performance.[5] Of all the steps in evidence-based medicine, this seems to receive the least attention. However, this is as important a step as there is in the practice of EBM.

EBM helps us to find and understand the evidence of "efficacy" of a given intervention; the results that were found in an idealized experimental situation. If these results are valid, we need to give careful attention to how we will integrate these interventions in our practice and monitor our practice to assure that these new practices are "effective."

The original concept of evaluating performance implied that this performance was based on an individual patient or provider. However, in Neonatology, it makes more sense to see this in the context of the complex system of the Neonatal Intensive Care Unit (NICU). The Vermont Oxford Network has applied a team approach to health care improvement, with the goal of improving the effectiveness and efficiency of neonatal care.[30] The various Neonatal Intensive Care Quality (NIC/Q) projects have used a collaborative model of quality improvement and benchmarking that was originally developed by industry and has now been applied successfully to health care.[31] The major components of the NIC/Q project include:

1. Multidisciplinary collaboration within and among hospitals
2. Feedback of information from the network database regarding clinical practice and patient outcome
3. Training and quality improvement methods
4. Site visits to project NICUs
5. Benchmarking visits to superior performers within the network
6. Identification and implementation of "potentially better practices"
7. Evaluation of the results.

The original project involved ten NICUs and was funded by the Center for the Future of Children of the David and Lucille Packard Foundation, and was performed in collaboration with the Rand Corporation.[32] In the original NIC/Q project, teams from the 10 hospitals worked together in cross-institutional improvement groups. These groups participated in an intensive series of large group meetings, site visits, and conference calls. Two major clinical quality indicators were chosen: nosocomial infection and chronic lung disease. Six NICUs focused on reducing nosocomial infection and 4 units focused on reducing chronic lung disease. The "potentially best practices" that were proposed were based on an evidence review and careful analysis of other practices at "best performing" centers. In the original NIC/Q project, reductions were seen in both chronic lung disease and nosocomial infection. In the second NIC/Q collaborative, a more formalized system for teaching quality improvement skills was put in place.[33] Four key habits for clinical improvement became the focus of this project: the habit for change, the habit for clinical practices and processes, the habit for collaborative learning, and the habit for evidence-based practice. The openness and urgency for change (the habit for change), the belief that productive work is accomplished through a variety of well thought out processes (the habit for clinical practice and process), and the willingness to assist in collaborative learning (the habit for collaborative learning) all address behavioral issues. Of importance is that the habit for evidence-based practice is an integral part of these improvement projects. Teaching EBM, including all of the previously discussed issues regarding finding evidence and validating evidence, was incorporated in this stage. The success of these improvement projects is studied in the Plan Do Study Act cycles (PDSA cycle) used to test and implement the changes. Each individual cycle's specific plans are developed (Plan), conducted (Do), results are evaluated (Study), and actions are taken based on what has been learned (Act). Evidence provides the cornerstone for all of these plans. As simple as these steps seem, organizations need training and assistance to integrate them into their routine behavior, and these changes can lead to measurable improvement in clinical outcomes.

Examples of EBM in Neonatal-Perinatal Medicine

When EBM tells us what to do to: antenatal steroids

The ability for EBM to influence perinatal practice is clearly illustrated in a variety of situations. An often quoted example of this impact is the history of the adoption of antenatal corticosteroids as standard of care for women with impending preterm delivery. Following preclinical studies by Liggins and Howie,[34] RCTs of antenatal corticosteroids undertaken during the 1970s and 1980s provided consistent evidence of benefit for preterm infants. Despite availability of this evidence, most women with impending preterm delivery during that era did not receive antenatal steroids and further controlled trials continued to be approved, funded, and undertaken. A systematic review published by Crowley and colleagues[35] in the 1990s confirmed that antenatal steroids substantially reduced the risk of respiratory distress syndrome, neonatal mortality, and neonatal morbidity, without increasing the rate of adverse maternal outcome. This original meta-analysis included a total of 18 RCTs (enrolling more than 3700 infants) studying the effect of antenatal corticosteroids on promoting lung maturity. This review has since been updated by Roberts and Dalziel[36] in 2006 and now includes 21 studies. In a cumulative meta-analysis, Sinclair asked the question, "At what point in the history of trials of antenatal corticosteroids for fetal lung maturation was the aggregated evidenced sufficient to show that this treatment reduces the incidence of respiratory distress syndrome (RDS) and neonatal death?"[37] In this analysis, trials were ordered by their date of publication and meta-analyses were performed sequentially. As previously noted, the initial trial of Liggins and colleagues[34] demonstrated a significant reduction in the risk of RDS and the risk of neonatal death. As each new trial was added to the cumulative meta-analysis, the risk reduction remained statistically significant. The point estimate of the risk reduction changed little with the addition of each new trial; however, the 95% CI narrowed, giving increased precision to the estimate to effect. One is hard pressed to justify the need for so many clinical trials. Despite overwhelming evidence from RCTs, use of antenatal steroids in very low birth weight infants remained low throughout the 1980s. The lack of acceptance of the data on antenatal steroids was, in part, attributable to inappropriate subgroup analyses. Clinicians were concerned that antenatal corticosteroids were ineffective in twin gestation, male infants, prolonged rupture of membranes, and a variety of other clinical situations. The meta-analysis conducted by Crowley and colleagues[35] evaluated the effect of antenatal steroids in several of these subgroups, and established that antenatal steroids were effective in a broad range of clinical situations and were not affected by issues such as multiple gestation and gender.

The evidence from the systematic review provided the cornerstone of the National Institutes of Health's consensus statement regarding the use of antenatal corticosteroids. The consensus statement recommends the use of antenatal corticosteroids for women at risk in a broad range of gestational ages with few exceptions.[38] Wright and colleagues[39] demonstrated improved understanding of the impact of corticosteroids by obstetricians in the NICHD Network before and after the National Institutes of Health Consensus Development Conference and by increased use of steroids within the NICHD Network. In 1999, more than 79% of at-risk infants were treated with either a partial or full course of antenatal corticosteroids compared with 16% in 1987.[40]

When EBM tells us what not to do: postnatal corticosteroids

Corticosteroid therapy may decrease lung injury after birth through a variety of mechanisms, including stabilization of lysosomal membranes, decrease in inflammatory response, and decrease in pulmonary edema.[41] corticosteroids potentially could improve lung function, decrease the need for supplemental oxygen, decrease the need for ventilator support, decrease lung injury and chronic lung disease, and ultimately decrease mortality.

Multiple trials have been conducted to assess the use of postnatal corticosteroids for the prevention of chronic lung disease. The best estimates of the risks and benefits of postnatal corticosteroid therapy are provided by the systematic overviews of Halliday and Erhenkranz published in the Cochrane Library.[42] Twenty-eight RCTs enrolling a total of 3740 participants are included in this analysis. Although the trials of postnatal corticosteroid represent a heterogeneous group of studies, differing in time of treatment, steroid preparation, steroid dosage, and length of treatment, the meta-analysis provides a useful springboard to understand the strengths of weaknesses of the therapy. Interpretation of the results are further complicated by the fact that many of the trials allowed for later "rescue" treatment of control infants who had evolving chronic lung disease. This approach complicates any interpretation of the data; late or selective treatment in the control group will allow for an underestimate of both the potential benefits and the potential risks. That said, the meta-analysis of these trials clearly shows that there are strong benefits to the early use (age <8 days) of postnatal corticosteroids in preterm infants at risk of developing chronic lung disease. Fewer infants require supplemental oxygen at 28 days or at 36 weeks postmenstrual age. Although mortality alone seems unaffected by early treatment, more infants survive with chronic lung disease at 36 weeks postmenstrual age (22 studies, 3320 infants; typical RR 0.89, 95% CI 0.84, 0.95). The typical estimate of effect suggests that, for every 4 infants treated with steroids early in the course of evolving chronic lung disease, one additional infant without chronic lung disease will survive.

Although postnatal corticosteroids lead to clinical improvement, there is great concern regarding both the short-term and long-term complications of therapy. Many complications of corticosteroid therapy have been reported, including hypertension, hyperglycemia, infection, hypertrophic cardiomyopathy, gastrointestinal bleeding, gastrointestinal perforation, and decrease in somatic growth. Of most concern are the long-term problems regarding growth and neurodevelopment. Although fewer studies contribute to the meta-analysis, it is clear that there is an increased risk of cerebral palsy (12 studies, 1452 infants; typical RR 1.45, 95% CI 1.06, 1.98) and poor neurodevelopmental outcome.

The findings concerning poor neurodevelopmental outcome have led to strong statements from the American Academy of Pediatrics and the Canadian Pediatric Society.[43] These statements recommend severe restriction in the use of postnatal corticosteroids in the prevention and treatment of chronic lung disease, noting that "outside the context of a randomized, controlled trial, the use of corticosteroids should be limited to exceptional clinical circumstances (eg, an infant on maximal ventilator support and oxygen support)." These evidence-based recommendations have led to significant change in clinical practice. The exposure of at-risk babies has decreased dramatically. In the Vermont Oxford Network, up to 28% of very low birth weight infants were exposed to postnatal corticosteroids before the Academy statement (in 1997) and only 8% were exposed after (though there is variation in practice with the interquartile difference from 2% to 11%).[1,44]

When EBM provides abundant evidence but the course of action is still unclear: prophylactic indomethacin

Applying EBM to practice becomes more complicated when the value of the outcome is less clear (virtually any time the outcome is something other than mortality) and there are actual or theoretical concerns of competing risk. Such is the case regarding the use of prophylactic indomethacin in the prevention of intraventricular hemorrhage. In current practice, 26% of all very low birth weight infants experience intraventricular hemorrhage, 9% of which are of the more severe grades.[5] Prophylactic indomethacin has been evaluated in the prevention of patent ductus arteriosus and in the prevention of intraventricular hemorrhage. Indomethacin, a cyclooxygenase inhibitor of prostaglandin synthesis, has been demonstrated to modulate cerebral blood flow, decrease serum prostaglandin levels, and promote germinal matrix maturation.[45]

Multiple clinical trials have suggested that indomethacin lowers the risk of intraventricular hemorrhage in very low birth weight infants. Fowlie and Davis[46] conducted a systematic review of 19 RCTs of prophylactic indomethacin involving 2872 infants. The meta-analysis suggests a decrease in the risk of patent ductus arteriosus (typical RR 0.44, 95% CI 0.38, 0.50) and severe intraventricular hemorrhage (typical RR 0.66, 95% CI 0.53, 0.82) associated with prophylactic indomethacin administration. In clinical terms, one needs to treat 5 infants with prophylactic indomethacin to prevent one patent ductus arteriosus, 12 infants to prevent one intraventricular hemorrhage, and 26 infants to prevent one severe intraventricular hemorrhage. However, use of prophylactic indomethacin is not widespread because of concern regarding possible side effects of treatment, including cerebral ischemia and necrotizing enterocolitis. In addition, the long-term effects of indomethacin are not well known.

Schmidt and colleagues[47] conducted a large, pragmatic trial of indomethacin, which showed similar effects to those of previous smaller trials regarding the short-term outcomes. However, little difference was noted in neurodevelopmental follow-up. This result leaves families and clinicians with difficult decisions to make. This situation is potentially ideal for applying decision analysis. Decision analysis is useful in situations whereby competing risks allow for a probabilistic quantitative framework to aid in decision making.[48] Decision analysis requires one to structure the problem, assign probabilities to chance events, assign utility or value to all outcomes, evaluate the utility of each strategy, and perform a sensitivity analysis. At each step along the way, there are a variety of assumptions. In this case, 3 possible decisions can be evaluated: prophylactic indomethacin for all at-risk infants, cranial ultrasound screening for baseline intraventricular hemorrhage and indomethacin to at-risk infants without severe hemorrhage, or indomethacin administration only to infants with symptomatic patent ductus arteriosus. The decision tree incorporates estimates derived from the clinical literature regarding the baseline risks of intraventricular hemorrhage, patent ductus arteriosus, and the theoretical risks associated with indomethacin therapy. The results of the decision analysis help inform the clinician regarding the decision to use prophylactic indomethacin. Obviously, if there are no ischemic complications, the decision analysis will support the results of the meta-analysis and prophylactic indomethacin will be favored. However, concerns about possible side effects or the risk of side effects in the face of limited developmental improvement will lead different families and clinicians to make different decisions.

When we ignore EBM: high-frequency ventilation

In an attempt to prevent chronic lung disease, techniques of ventilation that theoretically decrease lung injury have been introduced. HFV is perhaps one of the most promising of these newer technologies. High-frequency ventilators apply continuous distending pressure and deliver small tidal volumes (less than the anatomic dead space) superimposed on an extremely rapid rate.[49] Experimental work in animal models suggests that ventilation strategies using high-frequency oscillatory ventilation may prevent lung injury in preterm infants. However, individual clinical trials demonstrate little clinical benefit and there are possibilities of adverse effects, including increased risk of intraventricular hemorrhage and poor neurologic development.

Cools and colleagues[50] reviewed the RCTs comparing elective use of high-frequency oscillatory ventilation (HFOV) to conventional ventilation (CV) in preterm infants mechanically ventilated for pulmonary dysfunction. Studies that enrolled preterm or low birth weight infants with pulmonary dysfunction mainly due to RDS who were thought to require intermittent positive pressure ventilation (IPPV) were considered eligible for inclusion in the review. Studies were only included if randomization to either elective HFOV or CV occurred early in the course of RDS soon after mechanical ventilation was begun.

In their search of the literature, the investigators found 17 RCTs (enrolling 3652 infants) that met the criteria. The size of the studies varied considerably, ranging from 43 infants to 273 infants. Although all studies included preterm infants, the upper limit for birth weight and gestational age differed between the studies. The age and randomization varied from less than 1 hour to 9 hours of age. In addition, a heterogeneous group of ventilators was used to deliver HFOV.

In an overall analysis, surprisingly few changes in clinical outcome were noted. No individual trial reported a decrease in pulmonary air leak. In fact, the meta-analysis of 12 trials suggests a slight increase in the risk of pulmonary air leak (12 studies, 2766 infants; typical RR 1.19 95% CI 1.05, 1.34). None of the individual trials demonstrated any difference in mortality, and the overall analysis demonstrated no difference in the risk of death at 28 to 30 days (9 studies; typical RR 1.09, 95% CI 0.88, 1.35) or at approximately term equivalent age (15 studies; typical RR 0.98, 95% CI 0.83, 1.14). The effect of elective HFOV on the combined outcome death or chronic lung disease at 36 to 37 weeks postmenstrual age or discharge was marginal (9 studies; typical RR 0.92, 95% CI 0.85, 1.00). No differences in mortality were noted in a variety of subgroup analyses, including evaluation of ventilation strategy (high lung volume strategy).

Some of the possible risks of HFOV were not apparent in the meta-analysis. No effect was seen in the risk of intraventricular hemorrhage or white matter damage. Few trials have addressed long-term neurodevelopmental status. Although only 2 trials reported on neurodevelopmental outcome at 1 to 3 years, an increased risk of neurodevelopmental problems was reported (typical RR 1.26, 95% CI 1.01, 1.58).

Based on the results of the systematic overview, Cools and colleagues concluded that there was no clear evidence that elective HFOV, as compared with CV, offered important advantages when used as an initial ventilation strategy to preterm babies with acute pulmonary dysfunction. Yet HFV has come into widespread use. As noted earlier, 22% of all very low birth weight infants in the Vermont Oxford Network are placed on HFV at some point in their hospital stay.[5] It is difficult to understand the diffusion of expensive technology in the face of so little positive evidence.

Can EBM tell us when to begin new therapies: cooling therapy for hypoxic ischemic encephalopathy

Mild hypothermia for infants with moderate to severe hypoxic ischemic encephalopathy has shown great promise in individual RCTs. Jacobs and colleagues[51] have conducted a meta-analysis of these trials that demonstrates a strong effect on mortality and severe neurodevelopmental problems. Eight RCTs were included in this review, comprising 638 term infants with moderate to severe encephalopathy and evidence of intrapartum asphyxia. Therapeutic hypothermia resulted in a statistically significant and clinically important reduction in mortality (typical RR 0.74, 95% CI 0.58, 0.94), neurodevelopmental disability (typical RR 0.68, 95% CI 0.51, 0.92), and the combined outcome of mortality or major neurodevelopmental disability to 18 months of age (typical RR 0.76, 95% CI 0.65, 0.89). The point estimate of these important clinical outcomes suggest that for every 7 infants with moderate to severe hypoxic ischemic encephalopathy treated with cooling therapy, one additional infant will survive without neurodevelopmental disability.

Debate remains, however, regarding whether there is enough evidence for widespread introduction of this therapy. Concerns include the relatively small sample size of the completed studies and the uncertainty regarding longer term follow-up. It will be interesting to track the dissemination and "effectiveness" of therapeutic hypothermia as the neonatology community attempts to integrate this new therapy into practice.

SUMMARY

Neonatal-Perinatal Medicine has developed sufficient resources to help support the practice of EBM. Commitment to practicing evidence-based medicine, including mastering the 5 steps recommended by Sackett and colleagues, is essential to developing expertise in EBM. An institutional commitment and collaborative learning between institutions is critical to successfully practice EBM in the complex world of Neonatal-Perinatal Medicine.

ACKNOWLEDGMENTS

I would like to thank Susan Hayward for her assistance in preparing the manuscript.

REFERENCES

1. Horbar JD, Badger GJ, Carpenter JH, et al. Members of the Vermont Oxford Network. Trends in mortality and morbidity for very low birth weight infants, 1991–1999. Pediatrics 2002;110(1 Pt 1):143–51.
2. Silverman WA. Human experimentation in perinatology. Clin Perinatol 1987;14: 403–16.
3. Soll RF, Andruscavage L. Section 1: evidence-based quality improvement, principles, and perspectives: the principles and practice of evidence-based neonatology. Pediatrics 1999;103(1 Suppl E):215–24.

4. Horbar JD, Badger GJ, Lewit EM, et al. Hospital and patient characteristics associated with variation in 28-day mortality rates for very low birth weight infants. Vermont Oxford Network. Pediatrics 1997;99(2):149–56.
5. VON Annual Data 2008. Available at: http://www.vtoxford.org.
6. Sackett DL, Rosenberg WM, Gray JA, et al. Evidence-based medicine what it is and what it isn't [editorial]. Br Med J 1996;312:71–2.
7. Akobeng AK. Principles of evidence based medicine. Arch Dis Child 2005;90: 837–40.
8. Sackett DL, Richardson WS, Rosenberg W, et al. Evidence-based medicine. How to practice and teach EBM. 2nd edition. London, England: Churchill Livingston; 2000.
9. Richardson WS, Wilson MC, Nishikawa J, et al. The well-built clinical question: a key to evidence-based decisions. ACP J Club 1995;123:Al2–13.
10. Haynes RB, Wilczynski NL, McKibben KA, et al. Developing optimal search strategies for detecting clinically sound studies in MEDLINE. J Am Med Inform Assoc 1994;1:447–58.
11. Sinclair JC, Bracken MB, Horbar JD, et al. Introduction to neonatal systematic reviews. Pediatrics 1997;100:892–5.
12. Higgins JPT, Green S. Cochrane handbook for systematic reviews of interventions version 5.0.2 [updated September 2009]. The Cochrane Collaboration. 2009. Available at: http://www.cochrane-handbook.org. Accessed November 15, 2009.
13. Preventive Services Resource Links. U.S. Preventive services task force. Agency for healthcare research and quality. Rockville (MD), 2009. Available at: http://www.ahrq.gov/clinic/uspstf/resource.htm. Accessed November 15, 2009.
14. Fleming A. On the antibacterial action of cultures of a penicillium, with special reference to their use in the isolation of *B. influenzae.* Br J Exp Pathol 1929; 10(31):226–36.
15. Chalmers I, Enkin M, Keirse MJNC. Effective care in pregnancy and childbirth. Oxford, UK: Oxford University Press; 1989.
16. Nuland Sherwin B. The doctors' plague: germs, childbed fever, and the strange story of Ignác Semmelweis. Great discoveries series. New York: W.W. Norton; 2003.
17. Ohlsson A. Randomized controlled trials and systematic reviews: a foundation for evidence-based perinatal medicine. Acta Paediatr 1996;85:647–55.
18. Feinstein AR. An additional basic science for clinical medicine: II. The limitations of randomized trials. Ann Intern Med 1983;99:544–50.
19. Chalmers TC, Celano P, Sacks HS, et al. Bias in treatment assignment in controlled clinical trials. N Engl J Med 1983;309(22):1358–61.
20. Beecher HK. The powerful placebo. JAMA 1955;159:1602–6.
21. Cook DJ, Mulrow CD, Haynes RB. Systematic reviews: synthesis of best evidence for clinical decisions. Ann Intern Med 1997;126(5):376–80.
22. Cunningham AS. Meta-analysis and methodology review: what's in a name? J Pediatr 1988;113:328–9.
23. Sinclair JC, Bracken MB. Effective care of the newborn infant. Oxford, UK: Oxford University Press; 1992.
24. LeLorier J, Gregoire G, Benhaddad A, et al. Discrepancies between meta-analyses and subsequent large randomized, controlled trials. N Engl J Med 1997; 337:536–42.
25. Muir Gray JA. Evidence-based healthcare. London, England: Churchill Livingstone; 1997.

26. Guyatt GH, Oxman AD, Vist GE, et al. GRADE Working Group. GRADE: an emerging consensus on rating quality of evidence and strength of recommendations. BMJ 2008;336:924–6.
27. Guyatt GH, Oxman AD, Kunz R, et al. GRADE Working Group. What is "quality of evidence" and why is it important to clinicians? BMJ 2008;336:995–8.
28. Guyatt GH, Oxman AD, Kunz R, et al. GRADE Working Group. Going from evidence to recommendations. BMJ 2008;336:1049–51.
29. Guyatt GH, Oxman AD, Kunz R, et al. GRADE Working Group. Incorporating considerations of resources use into grading recommendations. BMJ 2008;336: 1170–3.
30. Horbar JD. The Vermont Oxford Network: evidence-based quality improvement for neonatology. Pediatrics 1999;103(1 Suppl E):350–9.
31. Plsek PE. Quality improvement methods in clinical medicine. An overview of quality improvement methods in healthcare. Pediatrics 1999;103(1 Suppl E): 203–14.
32. Horbar JD, Rogowski J, Plsek PE, et al. Collaborative quality improvement for neonatal intensive care. NIC/Q project investigators of the Vermont Oxford Network. Pediatrics 2001;107(1):14–22.
33. Horbar JD, Plsek PE, Leahy K, NIC/Q 2000. NIC/Q 2000: establishing habits for improvement in neonatal intensive care units. Pediatrics 2003;111(4 Pt 2): e397–410.
34. Liggins GC, Howie RN. A controlled trial of antepartum glucocorticoid treatment for prevention of the respiratory distress syndrome in premature infants. Pediatrics 1972;50(4):515–25.
35. Crowley P, Chalmers I, Keirse MJ. The effects of corticosteroid administration before preterm delivery: an overview of the evidence from controlled trials. Br J Obstet Gynaecol 1990;97(1):11–25.
36. Roberts D, Dalziel SR. Antenatal corticosteroids for accelerating fetal lung maturation for women at risk of preterm birth. Cochrane Database Syst Rev 2006;(3):CD004454. DOI:10.1002/14651858.CD004454.pub2.
37. Sinclair JC. Meta-analysis of randomized controlled trials of antenatal corticosteroids for the prevention of respiratory distress syndrome: discussion. Am J Obstet Gynecol 1995;173:335–44.
38. NIH Consensus development panel on the effect of corticosteroids for fetal maturation on perinatal outcomes. JAMA 1995;273:413–8.
39. Wright LL, Merenstein GB, Goldenberg RL, et al. Impact of the NIH consensus development conference on corticosteroids for fetal maturation: change in obstetric attitudes [abstract]. Pediatr Res 1996;39:254.
40. Fanaroff AA, Hack M, Walsh MC. The NICHD neonatal research network: changes in practice and outcomes during the first 15 years. Semin Perinatol 2003;27:281–7.
41. Bancalari E. Corticosteroids and neonatal chronic lung disease. Eur J Pediatr 1998;157(Suppl 1):S31–7.
42. Halliday HL, Ehrenkranz RA, Doyle LW. Early (< 8 days) postnatal corticosteroids for preventing chronic lung disease in preterm infants. Cochrane Database Syst Rev 2009;(1):CD001146. DOI:10.1002/14651858.CD001146.pub2.
43. Committee on Fetus and Newborn. Postnatal corticosteroids to treat or prevent chronic lung disease in preterm infants. Pediatrics 2002;109(2):330–8.
44. Walsh MC, Yao Q, Horbar JD, et al. Changes in the use of postnatal steroids for bronchopulmonary dysplasia in 3 large neonatal networks. Pediatrics 2006;118: e1328–35.

45. Edwards AD, Wyatt JS, Richardson C, et al. Effects of indomethacin on cerebral haemodynamics in very preterm infants. Lancet 1990;335:1491–5.
46. Fowlie PW, Davis PG. Prophylactic intravenous indomethacin for preventing mortality and morbidity in preterm infants. Cochrane Database Syst Rev 2002;(3):CD000174. DOI:10.1002/14651858.CD000174.
47. Schmidt B, Davis P, Moddemann D, et al. Long-term effects of indomethacin prophylaxis in extremely-low-birth-weight infants. N Engl J Med 2001;344(26): 1966–72.
48. Pauker SG, Kassirer JP. Decision analysis. N Engl J Med 1987;316:250–8.
49. Butler WJ, Bohn DJ, Bryan AC, et al. Ventilation by high-frequency oscillation in humans. Anesth Analg 1980;59:577–84.
50. Cools F, Henderson-Smart DJ, Offringa M, et al. Elective high frequency oscillatory ventilation versus conventional ventilation for acute pulmonary dysfunction in preterm infants. Cochrane Database Syst Rev 2009;(3):CD000104. DOI:10.1002/14651858.CD000104.pub3.
51. Jacobs SE, Hunt R, Tarnow-Mordi WO, et al. Cooling for newborns with hypoxic ischaemic encephalopathy. Cochrane Database Syst Rev 2007;(4):CD003311. DOI:10.1002/14651858.CD003311.pub2.

The Vermont Oxford Network: A Community of Practice

Jeffrey D. Horbar, MD[a,b,*], Roger F. Soll, MD[a,b], William H. Edwards, MD[b,c]

KEYWORDS

• Vermont Oxford Network • Newborn • Safety • Quality

The Vermont Oxford Network is a not-for-profit organization established in the late 1980s with the goals of improving the quality and safety of medical care for newborn infants and their families through a coordinated program of research, education, and quality improvement.[1] In this paper the authors discuss the activities and programs sponsored by the Network to achieve those goals.

In support of its mission, the Vermont Oxford Network maintains databases including information on interventions and outcomes for infants cared for at member institutions. The primary goal of the databases is to assist member hospitals in understanding their performance for purposes of quality improvement. All members participate in the very-low-birth-weight (VLBW) database and have the option to participate in the expanded database for all neonatal intensive care unit (NICU) infants and the Registry for infants with neonatal encephalopathy. The Manuals of Operation for the databases and samples of all data forms and data item definitions are available on the Network's Internet site (http://www.vtoxford.org).

Network membership and enrollment in Network databases has increased steadily (**Fig. 1**). In 2008, the Vermont Oxford Network included more than 800 institutions around the world (**Table 1**).

VLBW DATABASE

Infants are eligible for the VLBW database if they have a birth weight from 401 to 1500 g, or a gestational age between 22 and 29 weeks, and are born at the member hospital or are transferred to it within 28 days of birth. Infants born at a participating hospital who die in the delivery room or before NICU admission are included.

Drs Horbar, Soll and Edwards are the Directors of the Vermont Oxford Network.
[a] Department of Pediatrics, University of Vermont College of Medicine, Burlington, VT, USA
[b] Department of Pediatrics, Vermont Oxford Network, Burlington, VT, USA
[c] Department of Pediatrics, Dartmouth Medical School, Hanover, NH, USA
* Corresponding author. Department of Pediatrics, University of Vermont College of Medicine, Burlington, VT.
E-mail address: horbar@VTOXFORD.org

Clin Perinatol 37 (2010) 29–47
doi:10.1016/j.clp.2010.01.003 perinatology.theclinics.com
0095-5108/10/$ – see front matter

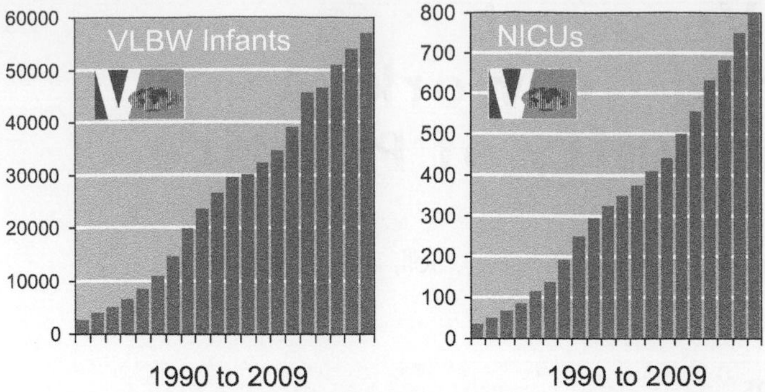

Fig. 1. The number of VLBW infants enrolled (*left*) and the number of NICUs participating (*right*) each year in the Vermont Oxford Network database from 1990 to 2009.

The characteristics of infants weighing 501 to 1500 g born in 2008 reported by the 750 institutions participating in the Network for that year are shown in **Table 2**, stratified in 250-g birth weight categories. **Table 3** shows hospital level percentiles for several key performance measures reported by the Network. As an example, for the outcome, nosocomial bacterial infection, 10% of hospitals have rates for infants weighing 501 to 1500 g of 3.7% or less, whereas 10% of hospitals have rates of 31.7% or more. This represents nearly a 10-fold range of nosocomial infection rates between hospitals with the lowest and highest rates. Marked variation among hospitals is apparent for many, if not most, interventions and outcomes reported in the Vermont Oxford Network Database.

EXPANDED DATABASE FOR ALL NICU INFANTS

In 2008, 241 hospitals participated in the Vermont Oxford Network Expanded Database and reported on nearly 106,000 infants born in the hospital who were treated in the NICU or died before admission, or who were transferred to the NICU from another hospital within 28 days of birth. The respiratory interventions and outcomes by birth weight category for these infants are shown in **Table 4**. Again, marked variation among hospitals is apparent for many of the items.

It is important to recognize that the data examples discussed so far for the VLBW and Expanded Databases are unadjusted for patient factors that may influence outcomes. In subsequent sections, the approaches to risk adjustment taken by the Vermont Oxford Network in research and for member reporting are discussed.

DATA SUBMISSION

All Vermont Oxford Network members have free access to eNICQ, a locally installed application that supports the collection, editing, and submission of Vermont Oxford Network data. Only de-identified data are exported to the Vermont Oxford Network. Currently more than 650 members are using eNICQ to manage Network data collection and submission. eNICQ is compatible with other NICU information systems and in the future will be integrated with electronic health records of specific systems.

RISK ADJUSTMENT

Variation has been found in almost every area of medical practice that has been studied.[2,3] The NICU is no exception. There are several potential sources for the

Table 1
Geographic distribution of member centers 2008

	N	%
United States Region		
New England	20	3
Middle Atlantic	68	9
East North Central	87	12
West North Central	44	6
South Atlantic	84	11
East South Central	36	5
West South Central	61	8
Mountain	26	3
Pacific	149	20
Puerto Rico	1	0
Total United States	576	77
International		
Austria	10	1
Belgium	1	0
Brazil	2	0
Canada	5	1
Chile	3	0
China	1	0
Finland	5	1
Germany	3	0
Ireland	7	1
Italy	56	7
Kuwait	1	0
Malaysia	1	0
Namibia	1	0
Portugal	4	1
Saudi Arabia	3	0
Singapore	1	0
Slovenia	1	0
South Africa	33	4
Spain	11	1
Turkey	2	0
United Arab Emirates	2	0
United Kingdom	21	3
Total international	174	23
Total all hospitals	750	100

Reprinted from Vermont Oxford Network 2008 VLBW database summary; with permission.

observed variations in intervention and outcome. These include differences in the severity of illness (case mix), chance, and differences in the quality or effectiveness of care. If the differences due to case mix and chance can be adequately account for the residual unexplained variation may be a valuable indicator of differences in the quality or effectiveness of care.

Table 2
Infant characteristics by birth weight and overall (53,440 infants weighing 501–1500 g born in 2008 in 750 NICUs participating in the Vermont Oxford Network VLBW Database)

	N or Percent (First and Third Network Quartiles)				
Infant Characteristics	**All**	**501–750 g**	**751–1000 g**	**1001–1250 g**	**1251–1500 g**
Total infants (N)	53440	9963	12341	13950	17186
Inborn (%)	85 (83, 97)	84 (83, 100)	83 (80, 100)	85 (80, 100)	87 (82, 100)
Outborn (%)	15 (3, 18)	16 (0, 17)	17 (0, 20)	15 (0, 20)	13 (0, 18)
Male (%)	51 (46, 55)	50 (38, 60)	51 (41, 61)	51 (43, 60)	51 (42, 58)
Race (%)					
Black	25 (3, 35)	30 (0, 43)	26 (0, 36)	23 (0, 34)	21 (0, 32)
Hispanic	17 (1, 26)	17 (0, 29)	17 (0, 26)	17 (0, 28)	16 (0, 25)
White	51 (29, 77)	46 (20, 80)	50 (25, 76)	52 (27, 79)	55 (29, 80)
Asian	5 (0, 5)	4 (0, 3)	5 (0, 6)	5 (0, 5)	5 (0, 6)
Native American	1 (0, 0)	0 (0, 0)	1 (0, 0)	1 (0, 0)	1 (0, 0)
Other	2 (0, 2)	2 (0, 0)	2 (0, 0)	2 (0, 0)	2 (0, 0)
Prenatal care (%)	95 (93, 99)	94 (92, 100)	94 (92, 100)	95 (93, 100)	96 (94, 100)
Antenatal steroids (%)	76 (68, 84)	71 (57, 83)	78 (67, 90)	78 (67, 89)	75 (65, 86)
Chorioamnionitis	11 (4, 14)	18 (0, 25)	14 (0, 19)	10 (0, 14)	7 (0, 10)
Maternal hypertension	26 (20, 32)	22 (7, 29)	25 (14, 33)	28 (18, 38)	28 (19, 36)
Cesarean section (%)	71 (66, 79)	63 (50, 77)	73 (64, 86)	74 (67, 86)	73 (64, 84)
Multiple gestations (%)	28 (21, 34)	25 (7, 33)	25 (12, 33)	29 (16, 38)	32 (21, 40)
Congenital malformation (%)	5 (2, 7)	4 (0, 6)	5 (0, 7)	5 (0, 8)	5 (0, 8)
Small for gestational age (%)	20 (15, 25)	16 (0, 24)	14 (5, 21)	19 (11, 27)	27 (19, 35)
Temperature <36°C (%)	28 (13, 40)	45 (24, 67)	29 (10, 50)	24 (7, 38)	21 (5, 33)

Reprinted from Vermont Oxford Network 2008 VLBW Database Summary with permission.

Table 3
Percentile values for key performance measures (53,440 infants weighing 501–1500 g born in 2008 in 750 NICUs participating in the Vermont Oxford Network VLBW Database)

	Percentile Distribution				
Measure	**10th**	**25th**	**50th**	**75th**	**90th**
Pneumothorax (%)	0.0	1.4	3.6	5.9	8.6
PVL (%)	0.0	0.0	2.4	4.6	7.6
CLD (%)	5.0	12.5	21.4	30.6	40.5
NEC (%)	0.0	2.6	5.3	9.1	13.2
IVH (%)	10.6	16.7	23.0	31.9	39.5
Severe IVH (%)	0.0	4.3	8.1	11.1	15.7
ROP (%)	9.1	17.7	31.3	44.4	57.1
Severe ROP (%)	0.0	0.0	5.4	10.2	14.4
Infections (%)					
Late bacterial	0.0	4.3	8.8	13.6	20.0
Coagulase-negative staph	0.0	3.3	8.1	14.0	20.7
Nosocomial	3.7	9.1	15.4	22.3	31.7
Fungal	0.0	0.0	0.8	2.9	5.1
Mortality excluding early deaths (%)	2.6	5.7	9.1	13.0	17.1
Mortality overall (%)	5.1	8.6	12.5	16.7	22.0
Death or morbidity (%)	28.6	37.1	45.8	53.5	61.9
Mean total length of stay (days)[a]	50.5	58.4	64.9	70.6	77.7
Adjusted mean total length of stay (days)	51.0	54.3	57.8	61.8	65.4

Abbreviations: CLD, chronic lung disease; IVH, intraventricular hemorrhage; NEC, necrotizing enterocolitis; PVL, periventricular leukomalacia; ROP, retinopathy of prematurity.

[a] Severe disability is defined as bilateral blindness, hearing requiring amplification, unable to walk 10 steps with support, cerebral palsy, or a Bayley score (BSID-II, MDI or PDI; BSID-III, cognitive language or motor composite) less than 70 or too severely delayed for Bayley assessment.

Reprinted from Vermont Oxford Network 2008 VLBW database summary; with permission.

To adjust for risk the Vermont Oxford Network uses a multivariable risk adjustment model designed to capture important factors related to patient risk. The model includes terms for gestational age (birth weight had been used in some years), gestational age squared, race (African American, Hispanic, white, other), sex, location of birth (inborn or outborn), multiple birth (yes or no), 1-minute Apgar score, small size for gestational age (lowest 10th percentile), major birth defect (using 4 empirically determined severity categories), and mode of delivery (vaginal or cesarean).

The model is used to calculate an expected number of cases for each specific outcome of interest based on the case mix seen at each hospital. Two measures of interest can then be created for each hospital. One is the ratio of the number of observed to expected cases (O/E), called the standardized mortality or morbidity ratio (SMR). The other is the difference between the number of observed and expected cases, O−E (see later discussion). These measures and their confidence intervals are corrected or shrunken using methods that recognize that some of the observed variation is random noise caused by chance.[4] The shrunken values are more stable estimates because they are adjusted for imprecise estimates and filter random variation. These methods for accounting for case mix and chance have been applied in research and member reporting.

Table 4
Respiratory outcomes and interventions by birth weight (105,757 eligible infants born in 2008 in 241 NICUs participating in the Vermont Oxford Network Expanded Database)

	Percent (First and Third Network Quartiles)					
Respiratory Outcomes and Interventions	**All**	**<1001 g**	**1001–1500 g**	**1501–2000 g**	**2001–2500 g**	**>2500**
Respiratory						
Respiratory distress syndrome	30 (20, 40)	91 (88, 100)	64 (54, 81)	35 (24, 48)	24 (15, 35)	16 (8, 27)
Pneumothorax	4 (2, 5)	8 (0, 10)	3 (0, 4)	2 (0, 3)	2 (0, 3)	5 (3, 7)
Oxygen	58 (51, 71)	98 (99, 100)	84 (80, 94)	59 (50, 75)	51 (41, 65)	51 (44, 67)
Nasal continuous positive airway pressure (CPAP)	31 (20, 41)	69 (50, 80)	64 (47, 79)	39 (26, 52)	28 (16, 38)	19 (9, 29)
Early CPAP	57 (34, 74)	20 (0, 31)	49 (25, 67)	67 (42, 86)	71 (46, 91)	68 (50, 89)
Vent after early CPAP	29 (19, 50)	64 (43, 100)	34 (19, 58)	26 (11, 50)	23 (9, 43)	27 (14, 51)
Conventional ventilator	28 (15, 34)	87 (76, 97)	52 (36, 67)	25 (14, 32)	18 (9, 25)	19 (9, 24)
Hifi ventilator	6 (2, 8)	45 (18, 57)	9 (0, 12)	3 (0, 3)	2 (0, 3)	3 (0, 4)
High flow nasal cannula	27 (12, 40)	56 (27, 75)	48 (23, 72)	26 (7, 43)	21 (6, 33)	21 (6, 31)
Nasal intermittent mechanical ventilation or synchronized intermittent mechanical ventilation	3 (0, 3)	16 (0, 27)	7 (0, 10)	3 (0, 2)	2 (0, 1)	1 (0, 1)
Surfactant at any time	22 (15, 29)	82 (73, 93)	55 (43, 70)	25 (14, 35)	15 (8, 22)	9 (4, 15)
Surfactant after 2 h	36 (25, 49)	9 (0, 13)	20 (7, 30)	38 (21, 60)	56 (36, 80)	77 (67, 93)
Extracorporeal membrane oxygenation	0 (0, 0)	0 (0, 0)	0 (0, 0)	0 (0, 0)	0 (0, 0)	1 (0, 1)
Nitric oxide	3 (0, 4)	10 (0, 10)	3 (0, 3)	1 (0, 1)	1 (0, 2)	3 (0, 3)

Chronic lung disease						
Oxygen at 28 days	37 (23, 42)	80 (69, 92)	30 (17, 39)	13 (0, 18)	16 (0, 20)	25 (0, 29)
Oxygen at 36 weeks	23 (12, 28)	57 (33, 67)	19 (7, 25)	9 (0, 11)	13 (5, 19)	32 (15, 46)
CLD 36 weeks <33	20 (8, 22)	53 (27, 62)	14 (5, 19)	5 (0, 7)	5 (0, 0)	8 (0, 0)
Steroids	2 (0, 3)	18 (2, 28)	3 (0, 5)	1 (0, 0)	1 (0, 0)	1 (0, 0)
Meconium						
Aspiration syndrome	2 (1, 2)	0 (0, 0)	0 (0, 0)	0 (0, 0)	1 (0, 1)	3 (1, 4)
Suctioned	69 (50, 100)	75 (0, 100)	71 (50, 100)	89 (100, 100)	77 (50, 100)	67 (50, 100)
Discharge on oxygen						
Home	3 (1, 4)	31 (0, 38)	7 (0, 8)	2 (0, 2)	1 (0, 1)	1 (0, 1)
Transfer	33 (28, 66)	70 (61, 100)	32 (10, 100)	16 (0, 50)	20 (0, 67)	30 (23, 60)
Discharge on monitor						
Home	9 (3, 12)	46 (15, 66)	23 (5, 31)	12 (2, 18)	7 (0, 8)	3 (1, 4)
Transfer	82 (72, 98)	89 (88, 100)	84 (71, 100)	82 (60, 100)	78 (57, 100)	78 (67, 100)

Reprinted from Vermont Oxford Network 2008 Expanded database summary; with permission.

Other investigators have developed alternative methods to adjust for case mix differences specific to the neonatal population. The SNAP, SNAP-II, SNAPPE-II (Score for Neonatal Acute Physiology) scores developed by Richardson and the CRIB (Clinical Risk Index for Babies) use physiologic variables measured in the first 12 to 24 hours after birth to assess the severity of illness and predict the risk of death for infants who are admitted to the NICU.[5–7] One drawback of these scores is the reliance on variables measured after admission to the NICU. Because these variables may be influenced by the treatments provided after admission to the NICU, the scores are not independent of the effectiveness or quality of care. The SNAPPE-II score has been compared with the Vermont Oxford Network risk adjustment models in a study of more than 10,000 infants. The Vermont Oxford Network risk adjustment performed as well as the SNAPPE-II.[8]

DATABASE RESEARCH

The Vermont Oxford Network databases provide a platform for observational studies and outcomes research. These observational studies have addressed trends over time,[9,10] outcomes in various groups of interest,[11–14] and the diffusion, use, and effect of various interventions.[15–18] The Vermont Oxford Network has conducted research to assess the contribution of differences in the structure and organization of the NICU to variations in patient outcomes. These have included studies of the effect of volume of admissions and the minority serving status of the hospital among others.[19–22] Current studies are assessing the role of nurse staffing and nurse work environment as factors to explain variations among NICUs.

A complete list of articles and abstracts by and about the Vermont Oxford Network can be accessed online at the Vermont Oxford Network Internet site.[23]

MEMBER REPORTING

The Vermont Oxford Network provides members with detailed confidential reports that allow them to track their data over time, compare their performance with a large group of NICUs around the world, and with smaller groups of NICUs with characteristics similar to their own. These reports include unadjusted and adjusted data.

All members receive quarterly and annual reports in print or on CD ROM and have access to real-time reporting on the Vermont Oxford Network Internet Reporting System, Nightingale. These reports are useful for benchmarking performance, for identifying opportunities for improvement, and for tracking changes in performance over time. Because the data are collected using uniform and standardized definitions, subjected to rigorous range logic and consistency checks, and because the reports are risk-adjusted in various ways described, the comparisons are reliable and have proved to be of great value for quality improvement.

The Vermont Oxford Network applies several strategies to adjust and account for case mix and chance in its member reporting. Outcomes and interventions are reported stratified by birth weight and gestational age categories and location of birth. For VLBW infants these variables are highly associated with risks for morbidity and mortality. Some outcomes and length of stay are reported by disposition status (home, transfer, died, and so forth.) because transfer and discharge policies may vary systematically among units and be associated with differences in outcome.

An example of risk-adjusted reporting available to members is shown in **Fig. 2**. This figure shows the difference (O−E) between the observed (O) and expected (E) number of cases of nosocomial infection at all Network centers. The expected number of cases is based on a multivariable risk adjustment model described earlier and the

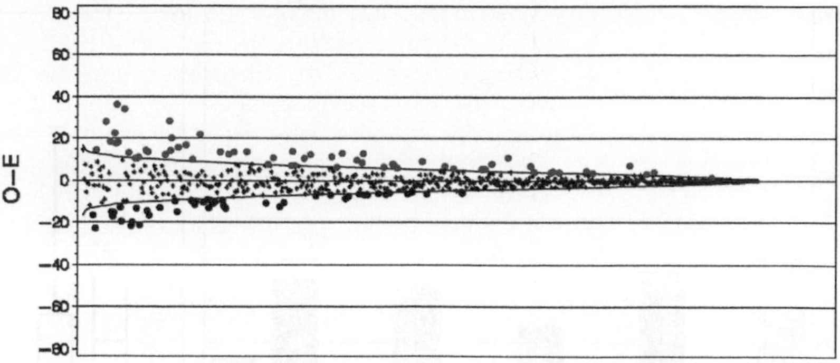

Fig. 2. Shrunken estimates of observed minus expected (O−E) values for bacterial nosocomial infection at all NICUs participating in the Vermont Oxford Network in 2007. Values shown in red indicate hospitals where the O−E is significantly greater than expected; values shown in blue indicate hospitals where the O−E is significantly lower than expected.

O−E values have been shrunken to account for chance. The O−E value for a center can be interpreted as the excess number of cases beyond those expected based on case mix. For centers whose shrunken O−E value lies outside the 95% control limits there is evidence to suggest that the difference between the number of cases expected based on case mix and the number actually observed are significantly different. In Network reports, centers are able to identify their own "dot."

Network reports also allow hospitals to compare their performance with a subgroup of Network hospitals with characteristics similar to their own. By comparing results with other similar hospitals unmeasured differences in case mix may be lessened.

The Vermont Oxford Network provides customized reporting services to established multihospital groups that are geographically and administratively based. These reports allow the members of the group to compare their unit's performance with other units in the group, with the group as a whole, and with the entire Vermont Oxford Network. An example of a figure from a group report for a fictitious group is shown in **Fig. 3**. Several groups have been able to use these reports to support their efforts to establish local improvement groups.

These strategies for minimizing the influence of risk and chance are imperfect; even the best statistical risk models cannot adjust for all of the differences in case mix among centers, nor can they fully account for random events among the small number of observations available at most NICUs. Given these caveats, however, the authors believe that Network reports can be useful to target specific clinical practices and patient outcomes for further in-depth analysis with the goal of identifying potential quality improvement opportunities and tracking performance over time.

NIGHTINGALE

Members have access to their data in real time using the secure and confidential Nightingale Internet Reporting System. A sample screen from Nightingale for a fictitious center 999 is shown in **Fig. 4**. The control menu allows a user to select different populations and years of birth for review. Center-specific data and data for a comparison group are displayed. The comparison group is chosen from a pull-down menu. Choices include the entire Network, NICUs of a specific NICU type, NICUs in the United States only, and for those centers belonging to established groups, a comparison with the aggregated data from all hospitals in that group.

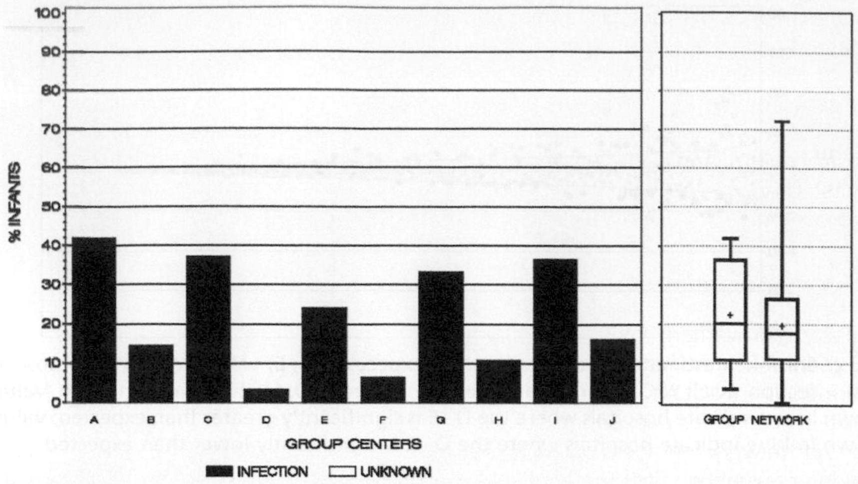

Fig. 3. Example of figure from a group report for a fictitious group comprised of 10 NICUs for the outcome, nosocomial bacterial infection, infants 501 to 1500 g, 2005 (includes late bacterial infections and coagulase-negative staph). Results are shown as bars for each individual NICU (A–J) and as boxplots for the group as a whole (group) and for the entire network.

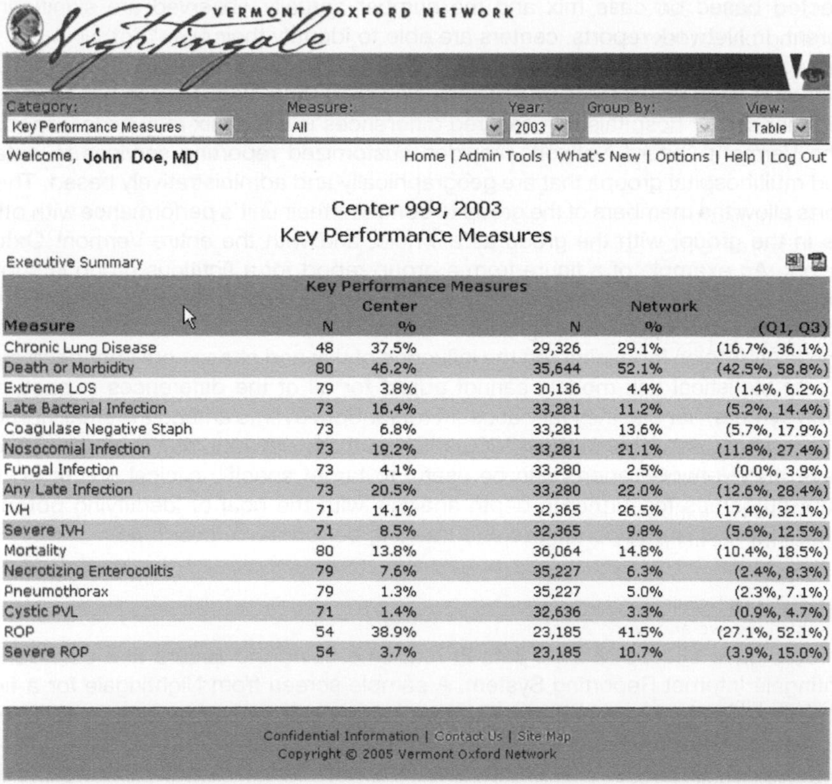

VERMONT OXFORD NETWORK

Nightingale

Category: Key Performance Measures | Measure: All | Year: 2003 | Group By: | View: Table

Welcome, **John Doe, MD**

Home | Admin Tools | What's New | Options | Help | Log Out

Center 999, 2003

Key Performance Measures

Executive Summary

Key Performance Measures					
	Center		Network		
Measure	N	%	N	%	(Q1, Q3)
Chronic Lung Disease	48	37.5%	29,326	29.1%	(16.7%, 36.1%)
Death or Morbidity	80	46.2%	35,644	52.1%	(42.5%, 58.8%)
Extreme LOS	79	3.8%	30,136	4.4%	(1.4%, 6.2%)
Late Bacterial Infection	73	16.4%	33,281	11.2%	(5.2%, 14.4%)
Coagulase Negative Staph	73	6.8%	33,281	13.6%	(5.7%, 17.9%)
Nosocomial Infection	73	19.2%	33,281	21.1%	(11.8%, 27.4%)
Fungal Infection	73	4.1%	33,280	2.5%	(0.0%, 3.9%)
Any Late Infection	73	20.5%	33,280	22.0%	(12.6%, 28.4%)
IVH	71	14.1%	32,365	26.5%	(17.4%, 32.1%)
Severe IVH	71	8.5%	32,365	9.8%	(5.6%, 12.5%)
Mortality	80	13.8%	36,064	14.8%	(10.4%, 18.5%)
Necrotizing Enterocolitis	79	7.6%	35,227	6.3%	(2.4%, 8.3%)
Pneumothorax	79	1.3%	35,227	5.0%	(2.3%, 7.1%)
Cystic PVL	71	1.4%	32,636	3.3%	(0.9%, 4.7%)
ROP	54	38.9%	23,185	41.5%	(27.1%, 52.1%)
Severe ROP	54	3.7%	23,185	10.7%	(3.9%, 15.0%)

Confidential Information | Contact Us | Site Map

Copyright © 2005 Vermont Oxford Network

Fig. 4. Sample screen from the Vermont Oxford Network Internet reporting system, Nightingale, for a fictitious center, 999. Data are shown for the center and for the network. By clicking on measure names users may drill down to more detailed reports. *Courtesy of* the Vermont Oxford Network; with permission.

Data may be displayed in tables or figures that can be saved in a user-specific workspace or exported for inclusion in spreadsheets or slide presentations. Nightingale users may also drill down to lists of cases with specific conditions so that records for cases of interest can be reviewed.

In the near future Nightingale users will also have access to real-time statistical control charts displaying plots of their center data over time with appropriate control limits. These new tools will further enhance the usefulness of Nightingale for quality improvement.

QUALITY IMPROVEMENT

Quality improvement has been a major focus for the Vermont Oxford Network in the last 15 years.[24] The activities have included 6 intensive multidisciplinary Neonatal Intensive Care Quality (NICQ) Collaboratives, and a series of 9 Internet-based iNICQ collaboratives. The activities and work products of these collaboratives are available to Vermont Oxford Network members online and are presented at the Annual Quality Congresses held in conjunction with the annual Vermont Oxford Network Members Meeting. The 2009 Annual Quality Congress was the 10th Congress sponsored by Vermont Oxford Network. These initiatives addressing the education aspect of the Network's mission have included a wide variety of medical, environmental, structural, administrative, and relational issues related to the quality and safety of neonatal intensive care.

The current 2009 NICQ Collaborative brings together multidisciplinary teams including parent representatives from 53 NICUs and leaders of 8 state collaboratives. These teams work with expert faculty for 2 years to fulfill the vision:

> *To be an inclusive Community of Practice that supports the pursuit of shared goals for improvement and the provision of exemplary care for all newborn infants and their families.*

The Manifesto and specific aims of the NICQ 2009 Collaborative are shown in **Box 1**. Providing care that is always family centered, safe, effective, equitable, timely,

Box 1
Manifesto and specific aims adopted by the participants in the Vermont Oxford Network NICQ 2009 Improvement Collaborative

Manifesto: As members of the NICQ Community of Practice we will:

- Provide care that is always family centered, safe, effective, equitable, timely, efficient, and socially and environmentally responsible.
- Apply 4 key habits for improvement in our daily practice: the habit for evidence-based practice, the habit for change, the habit for systems thinking, and the habit for collaborative learning.
- Hold ourselves accountable to patients, families, colleagues, and to the communities in which we live and work by incorporating measurement into our daily practice.
- Treat each other with respect.

Specific aims

- Make measurable improvements in quality and safety
- Engage families as team members for improvement
- Foster a worldwide Community of Practice for newborn care in which knowledge, tools, and resources for improvement are developed, managed, shared, and applied

efficient, and socially and environmentally responsible incorporates the core concepts articulated in the Institute of Medicine's *Crossing the quality chasm: a new health system for the 21st century*.[25] It also adds the important mandate to be socially and environmentally responsible as a commitment to act on the growing concern with stewardship of resources and protecting against harmful and wasteful practices. A forthcoming book, *NICQ 2007: improvement in action*, published by the Vermont Oxford Network shows how multidisciplinary NICU teams address these 7 themes.[26] The 4 key habits of evidence-based practice, change, systems thinking, and collaborative learning were introduced by quality improvement visionary Paul Plsek in the initial NICQ collaborative and have proven durable in multiple projects.[27] The importance of incorporating measurement into daily practice as a means of objectively communicating the results of our care and holding ourselves accountable establishes a commitment to a high level of integrity and accountability. Relationships within care communities and between care providers and patients and their families are only successful when built on a principle of treating each other with respect.

The first formal quality improvement collaborative, the Neonatal Intensive Care Quality (NIC/Q) Benchmarking project, was initiated in 1995 and was based on a successful model of the Northern New England Cardiovascular Disease Study Group (NNECVSG).[28] This first collaborative was conducted with an experimental design that included control centers. The goals of this first project were to demonstrate whether the collaboration resulted in improvement in clinically determined outcomes (nosocomial bacterial infection and chronic lung disease) and/or in costs of care in the centers participating compared with controls. Ten centers working in smaller focus groups underwent a discovery process to review and categorize the evidence for potentially better practices, an acknowledgment that best practices are seldom truly knowable, and verify the applicability by site visits among centers followed by benchmarking site visits to centers with sustained superior outcomes. Changes in practice within the participating centers followed a quality improvement methodology of Planning change, Doing the change, Studying or measuring the results, and Acting on the outcomes (PDSA) by either continuing or modifying the change.[29,30] Studying quality improvement as an intervention is challenging. This initial collaborative demonstrated a significant reduction in the incidence of nosocomial bacterial sepsis in study centers compared with controls, and a perhaps more dramatic finding that costs of care significantly decreased during the collaborative while costs in the control centers increased.[31,32]

NICQ 2000 included an 11-center focus group on family-centered care. In collaboration with the Institute for Family-Centered Care, this group explored the experience of families whose children required neonatal intensive care, and developed potentially better practices and tools for evaluating care from the perspective of families. The focus on families of this collaborative and the ones following led to Vermont Oxford including family participation in quality improvement as integral team members and advocating family-centered care as a core principle, acknowledged by placing families at the center of our improvement efforts (**Fig. 5**).

The NICQ 2007 collaborative added a leadership series to help NICU leaders develop their leadership capabilities through educational sessions with industry experts and shared experiences. The series culminated with a final session where chief executive officers or other top level administrative leaders from each center were invited to create a dialog to develop a better mutual understanding of priorities and challenges between center leaders and NICU teams.

The combined work products of the 6 intensive NICQ and the 9 iNICQ collaboratives are substantial. The commitment of Vermont Oxford Network to share knowledge has

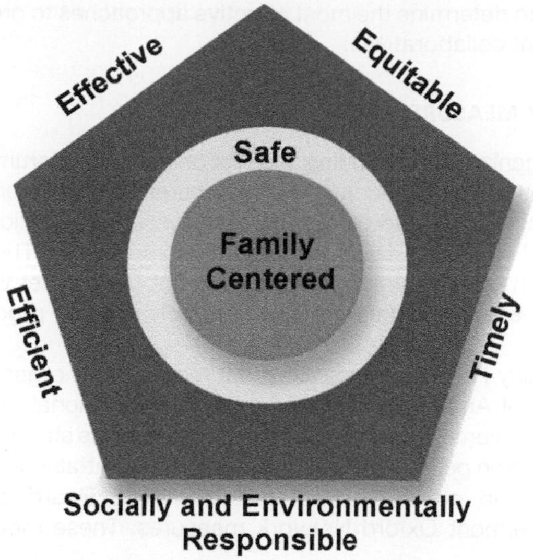

Fig. 5. Seven key themes for quality improvement. (*Adapted from* Battles JB. Quality and safety by design. Qual Saf Health Care 2006;15:i1–13.)

created many challenges in how to effectively make useful information available to the neonatal community. Initially, summaries of the work from the collaboratives were published in a series of online supplements in *Pediatrics*.[33–35] Some quality improvement projects have also been published as peer-reviewed articles. Ideas from the quality improvement work have also led to the design and conduct of clinical trials as described subsequently.

The Vermont Oxford Network is currently developing a web tool, NICQpedia, that will combine access to performance data with simultaneous access to improvement knowledge, tools, and resources. Teams participating in the Network's NICQ 2009 improvement collaborative are using and developing this tool. In a form of peer production,[36] similar to other wiki applications, users including health professionals and families contribute to the creation of a valuable improvement resource by contributing ideas, improvement stories, videos, and other resources and tools focused on improving care for infants and their families. NICQpedia will be available to all Vermont Oxford Network members in 2011.

The effect of quality improvement collaboratives on patient outcomes remains uncertain. A recent systematic review to evaluate the effectiveness of improvement collaboratives concluded that "the evidence underlying quality improvement collaboratives is positive but limited and the effects cannot be predicted with great certainty."[37] This review identified only 12 reports representing 9 studies with a controlled design and only 2 randomized trials. Three of the reports and 1 of the randomized trials were from the Vermont Oxford Network.[31,32,38]

In the past few years a remarkable trend has emerged. Groups of neonatal units are beginning to organize improvement collaboratives at a rapidly increasing rate. Several states, countries, and administrative groups are now organizing improvement collaboratives around various neonatal and perinatal improvement aims. This trend presents a unique opportunity for the field of neonatology. By fostering collaboration and focusing on improvement with colleagues at other institutions, the emerging collaboratives have the potential to speed up our improvement efforts. However, clearly more research is needed to determine the most effective approaches to organizing and conducting improvement collaboratives.

NATIONAL QUALITY MEASURES

Several national organizations including the National Quality Forum (NQF)[39] and the Leapfrog Group[40] have developed standard measures for institutions to use in monitoring and improving quality and safety. Both of these organizations have included Vermont Oxford Network data items as measurement options. The Leapfrog Group allows participants in their survey to use the Vermont Oxford Network data on antenatal steroid treatment for addressing the high-risk delivery process measure for quality.

The National Quality Forum is a not-for-profit membership organization created to improve the quality of American health care by setting national priorities and goals for performance improvement, endorsing national consensus standards for measuring and publicly reporting on performance, and promoting the attainment of national goals through education and outreach programs. The NQF Board of Directors have endorsed several Vermont Oxford Network measures. These measures are shown in **Box 2**.

RANDOMIZED CONTROLLED TRIALS

Trials of health care interventions can be described as either explanatory or pragmatic. Explanatory trials generally measure efficacy: the benefit a treatment produces under ideal conditions, often using carefully defined subjects in a research setting. Pragmatic trials measure effectiveness: the benefit of treatment produced in routine clinical practice. The Vermont Oxford Network is committed to performing pragmatic trials of available therapies to evaluate clinically important outcomes. The first such trial compared 2 surfactants for the treatment of respiratory distress syndrome (RDS).[41] This trial enrolled more than 1300 VLBW infants with RDS diagnosed within 6 hours of birth who were receiving assisted ventilation with more than 40% oxygen. There was no difference in death or bronchopulmonary dysplasia determined at 28 days after birth between treatment groups. Infants treated with the animal-derived surfactant were noted to have a greater improvement in the need for supplemental oxygen in the hours after treatment and had fewer pneumothoraces than the infants treated with the protein-free synthetic surfactant. Before conducting this trial, a trial of nearly identical design was performed by the National Institute of Child Health and Human Development (NICHD) Neonatal Research Network.[42] The results of that study, which enrolled approximately 600 infants, were similar to those of our network trial. The close

Box 2
National Quality Forum endorsed standards from Vermont Oxford Network

NQF 0303: late sepsis or meningitis in neonates

NQF 0304: late sepsis or meningitis in VLBW neonates

NQF 0481: first temperature measured within 1 hour of admission to the NICU

NQF 0482: first NICU temperature <36°C

NQF 0484: infants 22 to 29 weeks treated with surfactant who are treated <2 hours

Source: NQF Endorsed Standards. Available at: http://www.qualityforum.org/Measures_List.aspx

agreement of our results with those of an established, well-funded, academic research network such as the NICHD Neonatal Research Network provide confirmation of the ability of the Vermont Oxford Network to perform valid pragmatic multicenter trials using volunteer investigators at a significantly lower cost.

Subsequent trials have evaluated other important issues in neonatal intensive care. Early postnatal dexamethasone was frequently used in the late 1990s; however, there was little evidence to support this practice. We designed a multicenter, randomized, double-blind controlled trial to evaluate the effect of a 12-day tapering course of dexamethasone compared with saline placebo.[43] Forty-two NICUs enrolled infants weighing between 501 and 1000 g who were on assisted ventilation at 12 hours of age. The study was stopped before completion of sample size goals because of concern regarding serious side effects of the early steroid treatment group. A total of 542 infants were enrolled (early treatment 273, control 269). No differences were noted in chronic lung disease or death at 36 weeks' postmenstrual age. More infants who received early steroid treatment had complications associated with therapy, including increase in hyperglycemia and an increased use of insulin therapy. A trend toward increased gastrointestinal hemorrhage and gastrointestinal perforation was noted. Based on this and other studies, strongly worded guidelines suggesting curtailing the using of postnatal steroids have been drafted.[44]

Another common therapy that has been tested through the Vermont Oxford Network is the effect of prophylactic emollient ointment on nosocomial sepsis and skin integrity in infants with birth weight between 501 and 1000 g.[45] In this study, infants were randomized either to routine use of emollient ointment during the first 14 days or as-needed use of ointment for skin breakdown. The results were surprising. Although no difference was found in the primary outcome of newborn sepsis or death, there was an increase in coagulase-negative staph infections in the infants who received prophylactic ointment therapy.

Perhaps the most innovative trial conducted by Vermont Oxford Network was the cluster trial evaluating a multifaceted collaborative quality improvement intervention designed to promote evidence-based surfactant treatment of preterm infants.[38] The study evaluated changes in the processes of care and clinical outcome. One hundred and fourteen NICUs (which treated 6039 infants of 23–29 weeks' gestation born in 2001) participated. Compared with infants in control hospitals, infants in intervention hospitals improved processes relating to surfactant administration. However, there were no significant differences in clinical outcome.

Currently, trials of delivery room management and trials of mechanisms of heat loss prevention are in progress.

FOLLOW-UP

In keeping with the pragmatic nature of the database and randomized trials, the Vermont Oxford Network has created a pragmatic follow-up program. Many published estimates of death and developmental outcome are from well-funded university programs and may not reflect outcomes of infants from various settings. The goal of the follow-up networks was to describe the neurodevelopmental outcome of extremely low-birth-weight infants from centers in the Vermont Oxford Network and to identify characteristics associated with severe disability. Using predefined measures of living situation, health, and developmental outcome at 18 to 24 months, data were collected for infants born between July 1998 and December 2003 with birth weight between 401 and 1000 g.[46] Thirty-three North American centers in the Vermont Oxford Network participated. Six thousand one hundred and ninety-eight extremely low-birth-weight infants were born and survived until hospital discharge; by the time of follow-up, 1.4% of the infants had died. Of the remaining 6110 infants, 3567 (58.4%) were evaluated. Severe disability occurred in 34% of infants assessed. In the infants at greatest risk (infants <26 weeks' gestation), the overall rate of severe disability was 35.8% (**Table 5**).

Multivariable logistic regression suggested cystic periventricular leukomalacia, congenital malformation, and severe intraventricular hemorrhage were the characteristics most highly associated with severe disability. There was marked variation among the follow-up clinics in attrition rates. Our observation of severe disability risk was less than the risk estimated by the National Institute of Child Health and Development Neonatal Network.[47] It is possible that the difference in risk estimate is because of differences in the populations and families described in these 2 reports. The caregivers of infants in our study were generally 2 parents with 16 or more years of schooling. In contrast, 49% of families of infants in the NICHD Network were single mothers, 28% of whom were not high-school graduates. Such differences in populations in families highlight why, in providing information to parents, physicians should consider the outcome data reported in the current literature and the outcome data based on local experience. Additional work in the follow-up network has included development of simple parental questionnaires that could be administered by nonmedical personnel. These questionnaires have been found to have a high predictive value for severe disability and may prove to be an important screening tool in practice or in trial outcome.

WORLDWIDE COMMUNITY OF PRACTICE

Wenger[48] has defined a community of practice as groups "formed by people who engage in a process of collective learning in a shared domain of human endeavor: a tribe learning to survive, a band of artists seeking new forms of expression, a group of engineers working on similar problems, a clique of pupils defining their identity in the school, a network of surgeons exploring novel techniques, a gathering of first-time managers helping each other cope. In a nutshell: groups of people who share

Table 5
Vermont Oxford Network extremely low birth weight follow-up (2021 infant survivors born 1998 to 2003 after <26 weeks's gestation [1728 assessed] with severe disability)[a]

Gestational Age	Number of Cases with Severe Disability	Number of Infants in Gestational Age Category	Percent with Severe Disability
<23 weeks	11	15	73.3
23 weeks	112	214	52.3
24 weeks	234	531	44.4
25 weeks	261	968	27.0
All (<26 weeks)	618	1728	35.8

[a] Severe disability is defined as bilateral blindness, hearing requiring amplification, unable to walk 10 steps with support, cerebral palsy, or a Bayley score (BSID-II, MDI or PDI; BSID-III, cognitive language or motor composite) less than 70 or too severely delayed for Bayley assessment.

Reprinted from Vermont Oxford Network ELBW follow-up report for infants born in 2006; with permission.

a concern or a passion for something they do and learn how to do it better as they interact regularly."

The authors believe that the neonatology community is an evolving worldwide community of practice in which health professionals and families around the world are engaged in collective learning about our shared domain of human endeavor, providing high-quality and safe care to newborn infants and their families. The Vermont Oxford Network looks forward to providing the tools and resources to help this community of practice continue to grow and flourish.

ACKNOWLEDGMENT

The authors recognize and thank the health professionals and families at member hospitals in Vermont Oxford Network for their dedication to improving the quality and safety of NICU care and for making the work described in this article possible.

REFERENCES

1. The Investigators of the Vermont-Oxford Trials Network Database Project. The Vermont-Oxford Trials Network: very low birthweight outcomes for 1990. Pediatrics 1993;91:540–5.
2. Hartz AJ, Krakauer H, Kuhn EM, et al. Hospital characteristics and mortality rates. N Engl J Med 1989;321:1720–5.
3. The Dartmouth atlas of health care. Available at: http://www.dartmouthatlas.org/. Accessed November 2, 2009.
4. Simpson J, Evans N, Gibberd R, et al. Analysing differences in clinical outcomes between hospitals. Qual Saf Health Care 2003;12:257–62.
5. Richardson DK, Phibbs CS, Gray JE, et al. Birth weight and illness severity: independent predictors of neonatal mortality. Pediatrics 1993;91(5):969–75.
6. Richardson DK, Corcoran JD, Escobar GJ, et al. SNAP-II and SNAPPE-II: simplified newborn illness severity and mortality risk scores. J Pediatr 2001;138(1): 92–100.
7. The International Neonatal Network. The CRIB (clinical risk index for babies) score: a tool for assessing initial neonatal risk and comparing performance of neonatal intensive care units. Lancet 1993;342:193–8 (Erratum 1993;342:626).
8. Zupancic JAF, Richardson DK, Horbar JD, et al. Revalidation of the score for neonatal acute physiology in the Vermont Oxford Network. Pediatrics 2007; 119(1). Available at: http://www.pediatrics.org/cgi/content/full/119/1/e156. Accessed January 26, 2010.
9. Horbar JD, Badger GJ, Carpenter JH, et al. Trends in mortality and morbidity for very low birth weight infants, 1991–1999. Pediatrics 2002;110:143–51.
10. Walsh MC, Yao Q, Horbar JD, et al. Changes in the use of postnatal steroids for bronchopulmonary dysplasia in 3 large neonatal networks. Pediatrics 2006; 118(5):e1328–35.
11. Lucey JF, Rowan CA, Shiono P, et al. Fetal infants: the fate of 4172 infants with birth weights of 401 to 500 grams: the Vermont Oxford Network experience (1996–2000). Pediatrics 2004;113:1559–66.
12. Bernstein IM, Horbar JD, Badger G, et al. Morbidity and mortality in growth restricted very low birth weight newborns. The Vermont Oxford Network. Am J Obstet Gynecol 2000;182:198–206.
13. Suresh GK, Horbar JD, Kenny M, et al, for the Vermont Oxford Network. Major birth defects in very low birth weight infants in the Vermont Oxford Network. J Pediatr 2001;139:366–73.

14. Fitzgibbons SC, Ching Y, Yu D, et al. Mortality of necrotizing enterocolitis expressed by birth weight categories. J Pediatr Surg 2009;44(6):1072–5.
15. Horbar JD, for the Investigators of the Vermont-Oxford Neonatal Network. Antenatal corticosteroid treatment and neonatal outcomes for infants 501 to 1500 grams in the Vermont-Oxford Neonatal Network. Am J Obstet Gynecol 1995; 173:275–81.
16. Horbar JD, for the Vermont Oxford Network. Increasing use of antenatal corticosteroid therapy between 1990 and 1993 in the Vermont Oxford Network. J Perinatol 1997;17:309–13.
17. Finer NN, Horbar JD, Carpenter JH, for the Vermont Oxford Network. Cardiopulmonary resuscitation in the very low birth weight infant: The Vermont Oxford Network experience. Pediatrics 1999;104:428–34.
18. Horbar JD, Carpenter JH, Buzas J, et al, for the members of the Vermont Oxford Network. Timing of initial surfactant treatment for infants 23 to 29 weeks gestation: is routine practice evidence-based? Pediatrics 2004;113:1593–602.
19. Horbar JD, Badger GJ, Lewit EM, et al, for the Vermont Oxford Network. Hospital and patient characteristics associated with variation in 28-day mortality rates for very low birth weight infants. Pediatrics 1997;99:149.
20. Rogowski JA, Horbar JD, Staiger DO, et al. Indirect versus direct hospital quality indicators for very low birth weight infants. JAMA 2004;291:202–9.
21. Rogowski JA, Staiger DO, Horbar JD. Variations in the quality of care for very low birth weight infants: implications for policy. Health Aff 2004;23:88–97.
22. Morales LS, Staiger DO, Horbar JD, et al. Mortality among very low birthweight infants in hospitals serving minority population. Am J Public Health 2005; 95(12):2206–12.
23. Publications related to the Vermont Oxford Network. Available at: http://www.vtoxford.org/about/references.aspx. Accessed November 2, 2009.
24. Horbar JD. The Vermont-Oxford Neonatal Network: integrating research and clinical practice to improve the quality of medical care. Semin Perinatol 1995; 19(2):124–31.
25. Committee on Quality of Health Care in America, Institute of Medicine. Crossing the quality chasm: a new health system for the 21st century. Washington, DC: National Academy Press; 2001. Available at: www.nap.edu/openbook.php?isbn=0309072808. Accessed January 26, 2010.
26. Horbar JD, Leahy K, Handyside J. NICQ 2007: improvement in action. Vermont Oxford Network; 2009. Available at: http://www.vtoxford.org. Accessed January 26, 2010.
27. Plsek PE. Quality improvement methods in clinical medicine. Pediatrics 1999; 103(Suppl):203–12.
28. The Northern New England Cardiovascular Disease Study Group. Available at: http://www.nnecdsg.org. Accessed November 11, 2009.
29. Deming WE. The new economics. 2nd edition. Cambridge (MA): MIT Press; 1994. p. 132.
30. Langley GJ, Nolan KM, Nolan TW, et al. The improvement guide. A practical approach to enhancing organizational performance. San Francisco (CA): Jossey-Bass Publishers; 1996.
31. Horbar JD, Rogowski J, Plsek PE, et al. Collaborative quality improvement for neonatal intensive care. NIC/Q Project Investigators of the Vermont Oxford Network. Pediatrics 2001;107:14–22.
32. Rogowski JA, Horbar JD, Plsek PE, et al. Economic implications of neonatal intensive care unit collaborative quality improvement. Pediatrics 2001;107:23–9.

33. HorbarJD, Gould JB, editors. Evidence-based quality improvement in neonatal intensive care. Pediatrics 1999;103:e202–393. On-line supplement. Available at: http://pediatrics.aappublications.org/content/vol103/issue1/. Accessed November 2, 2009.
34. Horbar JD, Plsek PE, Leahy K, et al. Evidence-based quality improvement in neonatal intensive care: the NICQ 2000 experience. Pediatrics 2003;111: e395–547. On-line supplement. Available at: http://pediatrics.aappublications.org/content/vol111/issue4/. Accessed November 2, 2009.
35. Horbar JD, Plsek PE, Schriefer J, editors. Evidence-based quality improvement in neonatal intensive care: the NICQ 2002 experience. Pediatrics 2006;118: s57–s202. Online supplement. Available at: http://pediatrics.aappublications.org/content/vol118/Supplement_2/. Accessed November 2, 2009.
36. Benkler Y. The wealth of networks: how social production transforms markets and freedom. Available at: http://yupnet.org/benkler/. Accessed November 2, 2009.
37. Schouten LMT, Hulscher MEJL, van Everdingen JJE, et al. Evidence for impact of quality improvement collaborative: systematic review. BMJ 2008; 336:1491–4.
38. Horbar JD, Carpenter JH, Buzas J, et al. Collaborative quality improvement to promote evidence based surfactant for preterm infants: a cluster randomised trial. BMJ 2004;329(7473):1004.
39. NQF National Quality Forum. Available at: http://www.qualityforum.org/. Accessed November 2, 2009.
40. The Leapfrog Group. Available at: http://www.leapfroggroup.org/. Accessed November 2, 2009.
41. Vermont-Oxford Neonatal Network. A multicenter, randomized trial comparing synthetic surfactant with modified bovine surfactant extract in the treatment of neonatal respiratory distress syndrome. Pediatrics 1996;97(1):1–6.
42. Horbar JD, Wright L. Soll RF and the National Institute of Child Health Neonatal Research Network: a multicenter randomized trial comparing two surfactants for the treatment of neonatal respiratory distress syndrome. J Pediatr 1993;123: 757–66.
43. Vermont Oxford Network Steroid Study Group. Early postnatal dexamethasone therapy for the prevention of chronic lung disease. Pediatrics 2001;108(3): 741–8.
44. Committee on Fetus and Newborn. Postnatal corticosteroids to treat or prevent chronic lung disease in preterm infants. Pediatrics 2002;109:330–8.
45. Edwards WH, Conner JM, Soll RF. Vermont Oxford Network Neonatal Skin Care Study Group. The effect of prophylactic ointment therapy on nosocomial sepsis rates and skin integrity in infants with birth weights of 501 to 1000 g. Pediatrics 2004;113(5):1195–203.
46. Mercier CM, Dunn MS, Ferrelli KR, et al. Vermont Oxford Network ELBW Infant Follow-up Study Group. Neurodevelopmental outcome of extremely low birth weight infants from the Vermont Oxford Network: 1998–2003. Neonatology 2009;97:329–38.
47. Vohr BR, Wright LL, Dusick AM, et al. Neurodevelopmental and functional outcomes of extremely low birth weight infants in the National Institute of Child Health and Human Development Neonatal Research Network, 1993–1994. Pediatrics 2000;105:1216–26.
48. Wenger E. Communities of practice: learning, meaning, identity. Cambridge (UK): Cambridge University Press; 1999.

The Pediatrix BabySteps® Data Warehouse and the Pediatrix QualitySteps Improvement Project System—Tools for "Meaningful Use" in Continuous Quality Improvement

Alan R. Spitzer, MD*, Dan L. Ellsbury, MD, Darren Handler, BS, Reese H. Clark, MD

KEYWORDS

- Pediatrix • Neonatal intensive care unit
- Electronic medical records • BabySteps • QualitySteps
- Clinical Data Warehouse

The election of the President Obama in 2008 brought the issue of health care reform to the forefront as part of the administration's agenda. Underlying much of the discussion about improvement in access to health care is the concept that significant change could be implemented with the broader use of electronic medical or health care records (EMR/EHRs). What has been less clear, however, is how EHRs can directly facilitate actual improvement in patient outcomes. To address this issue, the concept of *meaningful use* was also introduced to providers interested in receiving incentive payments from the federal government to establish EHRs, although the phrase was

The Center for Research, Education, and Quality Improvement, Pediatrix Medical Group, 1301 Concord Terrace, Sunrise, FL 33323, USA
* Corresponding author.
E-mail address: alan_spitzer@pediatrix.com

Clin Perinatol 37 (2010) 49–70
doi:10.1016/j.clp.2010.01.016

initially not well defined. The Department of Health and Human Services Web site in June 2009 stated the following:

> *To receive the incentive payments, providers must demonstrate "meaningful use" of a certified EHR. Building upon the work done by the HIT Policy Committee, the Centers for Medicare & Medicaid Services (CMS), along with the Office of the National Coordinator for Health Information Technology (ONC), will be developing a proposed rule that provides greater detail on the incentive program and proposes a definition of meaningful use.*[1]

Subsequently, the Health Information Technology (HIT) Policy Committee developed a phased implementation of meaningful use for the years 2011 to 2015 in the following categories:

- Improve quality, safety, and efficiency, and reduce health care disparities
- Engage patients and families
- Improve care coordination
- Improve population and public health
- Ensure adequate privacy and security protection of personal health information.[2]

In 1996, Pediatrix Medical Group anticipated this issue and began to develop several modalities for care delivery in the neonatal intensive care unit (NICU) that would permit true meaningful use of electronic data collection. A proprietary EHR was initiated to provide a daily medical record note for practicing physicians within the organization. The EHR, initially known as *RDS*, was a modification of an already existing electronic record, and was subsequently replaced by a proprietary system that was developed in-house, called *BabySteps*.

This EHR also served as a tool for data gathering on a rapidly expanding patient population (Pediatrix Medical Group currently cares for approximately 20% of all NICU patients in the United States), while creating a system that would accurately code for the delivery of care according to guidelines developed by the American Academy of Pediatrics Perinatal Section Coding Committee. More importantly, however, serious consideration was given to extracting data from the database that was being developed, ultimately giving rise to the Pediatrix BabySteps Clinical Data Warehouse (CDW). Currently, the CDW is believed to be one of the largest repositories of data on neonates, containing detailed information on more than 600,000 infants and approximately 11,000,000 patient days. Because of the extent and depth of the data collected, it has been queried not only within the organization for novel research observations, but also by the US Food and Drug Administration (FDA), the National Institutes of Health (NIH), and the National Institute of Child Health and Human Development (NICHD), and several academic neonatology programs.[3–6] Many of these queries have resulted in publication in peer-reviewed literature.

Most recently, these tools were complemented by a new electronic module dedicated specifically to clinical quality improvement (CQI) initiatives, known as the QualitySteps System, or Quality Improvement Project System. The QualitySteps System is designed to allow the user to define an area for quality improvement, support a project with dedicated evidence-based literature, measure outcomes to be evaluated, enter and track data with annotated run charts, and then reassess outcome improvement (the Plan, Do, Study, Act cycle for quality improvement). This article describes these tools in detail to provide an understanding of their structure and how they have fulfilled the concept of "meaningful use" for true outcome improvement in the NICU.

BABYSTEPS DEVELOPMENT AND DATA EXTRACTION

In 1996, Pediatrix Medical Group initiated development of a proprietary EHR throughout its practices. Several goals were associated with this project. First, the EHR was intended to create a clear, easily-readable admission, discharge, and daily medical record note that was consistent throughout the expanding number of neonatal practices within the organization (now numbering approximately 200 in 33 states plus Puerto Rico). Beginning in 2004, a series of concepts was defined as being critical for optimal EHR documentation, known as the four "Cs," and are listed in **Box 1**.

Box 1
The four "Cs" of electric health record documentation

Conciseness of notes

- Reduce the daily note to the specific needs of the patient
- Notes should not be so voluminous that they lose readability
- The daily note should, in general, only contain that day's information
- Avoid carryover of excessive amounts of information from previous days
- Excessive verbiage should be excluded, since it tends to breed inconsistency in charting and increases liability

Convey information to other caregivers

- Notes must be easily readable
- Daily changes in the patient's condition or the management plan should be immediately apparent to the reader
- The medical record should accurately chart the progress of care
- Problems should be diagnosed, assessed, treated, resolved, and removed from daily notes as appropriate
- Simple recitation of numbers or laboratory reports does not constitute patient assessment, and further evidence of physician thought processes must be provided in the record
- Spelling and grammatical errors should be eliminated through careful rereading of notes and use of spell-checking

Confirm clinical decisions

- Note should not be simply recount numbers or events, but must assess the patient's clinical condition and provide a cogent and coherent approach to care
- Notes should be read carefully before being placed into the chart
- Confirmation of the clinical plan and the reasons for that plan are essential in assigning proper codes for the care being delivered

Consistent internally

- Notes should be consistent from the physical examination through the management plan. There should not any discrepancies between the physical examination, laboratory values, radiographic studies, the assessment, or the plan for the patient
- Entry of information into fields, rather than as comments, is essential in refining the daily progress note and limiting inconsistency
- A methodology of checking for internal consistency should be a part of everyone's charting
- Inconsistencies are the most common problematic issue within the chart that is difficult to defend in malpractice cases
- Consistency and accuracy in the note supports correct daily coding

Without attentiveness to these issues, there is a tendency within the EHR to add excessive detail that makes evaluation of the daily note difficult, especially for consultants and reviewers, while potentially increasing liability risks. Because parts of notes in many EHRs can be readily cloned and carried over from day to day, it is sometimes erroneously believed that voluminous documentation aids in the care of the patient. Unfortunately, nonrepresentative information is often brought forward unnecessarily, while simply enhancing risks for liability, either through patient error or the potential for malpractice. To offset these risks, Pediatrix has had an extensive corporate-wide documentation training project in place for many years that all physicians are required to review on a regular basis.

The initial EHR was a modification of another program and was called *RDS*. Because of its limitations, it was phased out starting in 2004 and gradually replaced by BabySteps within the Pediatrix practices. Ultimately, the information in both RDS and BabySteps was merged and validated in the CDW, so that the changeover did not result in a loss of information for any of the physicians. **Fig. 1** shows a sample of the front page of the BabySteps admission note.

In planning for automated data extraction, several decisions had to be made that were critical toward obtaining accurate outcome results. These processes are often overlooked during the adoption of the EHR and are most important in the concept of meaningful use. Because the daily medical record note contains a combination of drop down/specific field entry menus and areas for text entry, the question of whether to use both parts of the note for data extraction was debated for some time.

For several reasons, the decision was made to extract data only from the drop down/field entry menu. First, selection of specific diagnoses and other defined parts of the note yields a consistency of information that would otherwise not be possible. Secondly, based on an assessment of how a few specific, common diagnoses were designated in the text areas of the note, great potential variability exists in documentation. As an example, the diagnosis of neonatal intraventricular hemorrhage was found to be mentioned in the text areas in more than 1000 different ways. A partial list of these is shown in **Box 2**, all of which would need to be examined (and any other variations that one might encounter) if the text boxes were to be accurately reviewed. In addition to the increased complexity of the programming that would be needed, this process would slow the data evaluation and extraction to a serious degree, limiting the

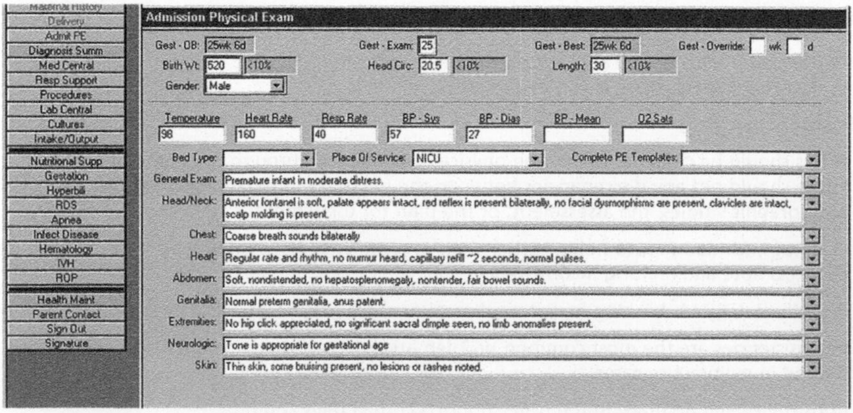

Fig. 1. Part of the BabySteps admission note to the neonatal intensive care unit.

Box 2
Designation variability for intraventricular hemorrhage, partial listing

Intraventricular hemorrhage

IVH

Intracranial hemorrhage

ICH

Gr. 1, 2, 3, or 4

IVH Gr. 1, 2, 3, or 4

ICH Gr. 1, 2, 3, or 4

Grade 1, 2, 3, or 4 IVH

Grade 1, 2, 3, or 4 ICH

Gr. 1, 2, 3, or 4 IVH

Gr. 1, 2, 3, or 4 ICH

Head bleed (with or without grading; all listed also may be graded)

CNS bleed

Periventricular hemorrhage

Ventricular bleed

Vent. Bleed

Periventricular bleed

White matter bleed

WM bleed

Brain bleed

Br. Bleed

Possible bleed

Possible CNS bleed

Possible IVH

Probable IVH

Probable IVH bleed

Probable CNS bleed

Indeterminate bleed

Numerous other combinations and abbreviations of this event were noted.

Abbreviations: Br, brain; CNS, central nervous system; Gr, grade; ICH, intracranial hemorrhage; IVH, intraventricular hemorrhage; Vent, ventricular; WM, white matter

value of the CDW itself. The developers therefore believed that limiting extraction to the drop down menu fields, accompanied by a strong documentation education effort, would be the optimal approach.

GOALS FOR DATA EXTRACTION FROM BABYSTEPS, THE BABYSTEPS DATA WAREHOUSE

The ultimate goals for the data were also discussed in great detail and several key objectives were identified. Most importantly, outcome data needed to be extracted from the electronic record automatically. This approach would have several benefits. Physicians would not be burdened by designing a way to get chart information into a database, which would require additional time commitment on their part or the cost of a data extractor. In addition, automated data extraction would eliminate the possibility for any bias that might creep into the information. For example, many referral centers show a tendency to exclude some patients in databases who are sent for the highest level tertiary care, because they tend to bias outcomes negatively. Babies sent for laser surgery for retinopathy of prematurity (ROP), neonates requiring major cardiac or gastrointestinal surgical procedures, and infants with complex congenital malformations all tend to adversely influence outcomes in these NICUs. The hospital stays lengthen with complex issues from care that is rarely straightforward, even in the hands of the finest medical and nursing staff. With intensifying scrutiny being given to outcomes, shouldering the burden for these patients in a database often leads to outcome results that initially appear less than optimal. Consequently, including these types of patients in data sets is often less than ideal. Automated extraction of information, therefore, leads to a much more precise data set, from which sounder conclusions can be drawn.

When attempting this sort of data extraction, several issues become apparent. Each practice must be intimately aware of evolving outcomes. Often, when viewing this information initially, one is often left with a sense of disbelief. Most physicians believe that they perform optimally, and therefore their outcomes must, of course, be second to none. Unfortunately, this view is rarely supported by the actual data, and when viewing the data for the first time, a complex emotional process frequently must be negotiated. Dan Ellsbury, MD, the Pediatrix Director of Quality Improvement, describes humorously (but accurately), with apologies to Elizabeth Kübler-Ross, the five stages of "data grieving":

- Denial: These data can't be right! You must have made a mistake.
- Anger: Why are you picking on me? Don't I have enough to do already?
- Bargaining: My patients must be sicker than everyone else's; my NICU is different; I don't agree with those data definitions.
- Depression: I can't do anything about it anyway....
- Acceptance: OK...what can I do to improve the outcomes in my NICU?

The goals of Pediatrix Medical Group, therefore, have been to help physicians confront their data and move through these stages as quickly as possible so that they can ultimately focus on their outcomes and work toward improvement, which is the primary reason for providing them with this information.

Furthermore, the decision was made to present these data in the form of a graphic report, rather than a table, to provide a more visually and mentally indelible impression. Therefore, many months of inpatient hospital data sometimes had to be rapidly scanned and processed to create certain reports. In addition, developers believed that looking at outcome data in the abstract would not be meaningful, and the data had to have some basis for comparison. In a company of this size, the obvious comparison would be with the remaining patient population in Pediatrix Medical Group, at least as an initial starting point. Each report, therefore, would have to present outcomes from not only the individual practice but also all other Pediatrix practices to provide summary comparative data. These outcomes had to be provided in an easily viewable format so that the practitioner was not overwhelmed by a report that required a significant investment of time to interpret.

Because outcome data were going to be used in a comparative manner throughout Pediatrix Medical Group, the CDW had to be HIPAA (Health Insurance and Portability and Accountability Act of 1996) compliant. Moving data from the consolidated data set required eliminating all patient-identifying information. Although a practice could look at its own outcome data in summary form, it could determine the origin of any patient when viewing other practices' results. Therefore, all identifying information that could be used to trace a patient back to a source had to be methodically eliminated. To accomplish this result, data "cleansing" excludes information such as day, month, and year of birth; date of admission; date of discharge; date of specific therapy initiation; addresses; and free text fields. All events are therefore recorded as days since birth to eliminate any possibility of discovery.

Research use of the de-identified data set is approved annually by the Western Institutional Review Board (IRB). One of the original goals was to use the CDW for novel research observations involving large patient populations, and this IRB certification of HIPAA compliance permits it to be used as a research tool. IRB approval is also required from any institution, company, or university whose investigators wish to query the CDW. During the past decade various groups have published more than 50 peer-reviewed papers using information from the CDW. Some of these papers appear in the reference list.

Elimination of selection bias was also important because practices tend to avoid taking credit for patients who might have adverse outcomes, especially in transport situations. Through collecting data on all patients and allowing comparisons between inborn and outborn patient populations and NICUs of similar size, controls were built into the CDW to avoid situations in which large referral institutions were somewhat unfairly penalized for accepting the most difficult cases in transport. Although some databases either risk-adjust or assign severity indices to outcomes, the developers believed that presenting the actual real data, with selection of appropriate comparison groups, was a preferable way to examine outcomes. Accumulation of these more complex clinical cases often leads to outcomes in tertiary institutions that initially appear far worse on the surface than those in community hospitals, which rarely care for these infants. Finally, to examine any regional variations in outcomes that might be of interest, the CDW also allows grouping of all hospitals covered by an individual practice to allow comparison with other groups within the state or a region of the country.

BABYSTEPS DATA WAREHOUSE REPORTS

The CDW is constantly evolving to provide practicing physicians with the most current data possible, and as many report types as is practical for managing patients in their NICU. By responding to clinician feedback, the CDW has become an increasingly useful tool for meaningful assessment of outcomes and quality improvement initiatives. Data within the CDW is refreshed on a weekly basis to retain currency.

Box 3 lists currently available CDW reports. Reports are categorized into several types: activity reports, which indicate basic demographic types of information; management reports, which reflect decision-making processes in patient care; morbidity and mortality reports, which document a variety of common outcomes of greatest interest in NICU patients; and summary reports, which provide a selected one-page snapshot of outcomes for a specific NICU, or network trends in various outcomes that are constantly tracked.

Summary Reports were developed as a request from the regional management teams, who are each responsible for approximately 40 to 70 practices in one of six regions of the country. To provide a sense of the quality of care being delivered

Box 3
Current Pediatrix Clinical Data Warehouse reports

Activity Reports

- Types of discharges (eg, home, transfer, in-hospital)
- Admissions by gestational age
- Admissions by birth weight
- Length of stay
- Average daily census
- Type of delivery (vaginal vs cesarean section)

Morbidity and Mortality Reports

- Mortality
- Survival
- Oxygen at 28 days of life (bronchopulmonary dysplasia [BPD])
- Oxygen at 36 weeks' gestational age (BPD)
- Intraventricular hemorrhage (IVH)
- Late-onset sepsis, necrotizing enterocolitis
- Patent ductus arteriosus
- Periventricular leukomalacia
- Respiratory distress syndrome and surfactant use
- ROP
- Severe IVH
- Severe ROP
- Pneumothorax

Management Reports

- Maximal ventilator support
- Median ventilator days
- Temperature from delivery room to NICU
- Types of lines inserted and duration of use
- Median daily weight gain during the first 28 days
- Hepatitis B immunization rates
- Percent of infants breastfeeding at discharge
- Bilirubin reports
- Late-onset sepsis rates

Infection reports

- Percent of NICU admissions treated with antibiotics
- Median days of antibiotic therapy with negative cultures
- Use of cefotaxime
- Percent of patients treated without cultures
- Nosocomial/line sepsis: infections/1000 catheter days (in testing)

Medication reports

- All commonly-used medications in the NICU
- Frequency of use

Summary Dashboard Report

Annual quality gauge report

Network trends report

in an individual unit, or all units within the region, the Summary Report was developed to present a snapshot picture of overall outcomes, and is shown in **Fig. 2**. The Summary Report is flexible, in that it can be altered to follow NICU trends of greatest interest at any time. For example, the use of dexamethasone postnatally is included as a medication-related report, because the use of this drug remains controversial. It would be easy, however, to replace dexamethasone with another medication should that be desired, because the CDW tracks the use of most of the important medications used in the NICU. Overall, Summary Reports provide an instant snapshot of a year's general outcome measures that can be evaluated within minutes. Observers desiring more data could reference the more detailed reporting levels available.

A typical CDW report is illustrated in **Fig. 3**. Reports can be viewed for yearly, quarterly, or monthly periods. Many morbidities, even in large NICUs, occur so infrequently that annual reports often work best, but clinicians at least have the option to examine an outcome during various time frames, which is very helpful in quality improvement projects.

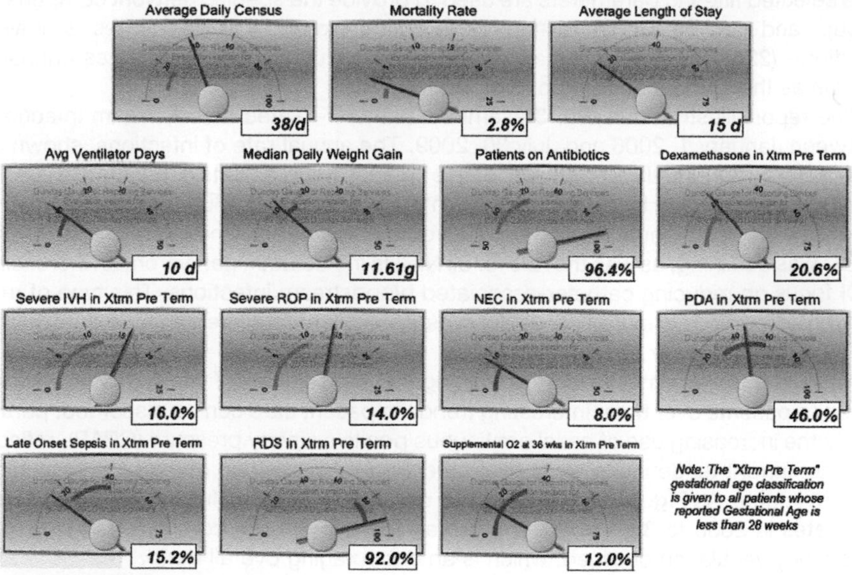

Fig. 2. Annual summary report for an individual NICU from the Clinical Data Warehouse with selected indicators in 14 different areas. The gray bars on each gauge represent the 33rd to 66th outcome percentiles (middle third) for all Pediatrix Medical Group neonatal intensive care units.

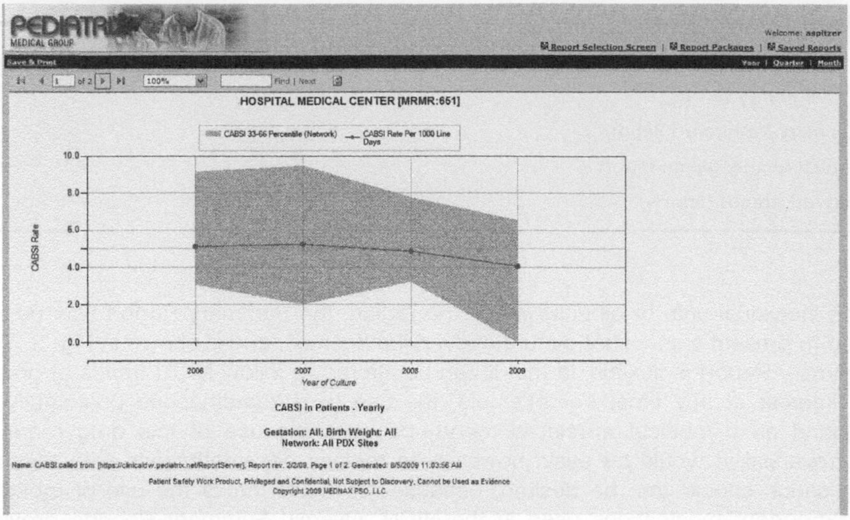

Fig. 3. A typical Clinical Data Warehouse report for an individual NICU. The rate of catheter-associated blood stream infections is shown as connected dots between 2006 and 2009. Rate is shown as number of infections per 1000 catheter line days. The gray background shading represents the 33rd to 66th percentile for all Pediatrix Medical Group neonatal intensive care units.

Clinicians may filter report results using multiple combinations of birth weight and gestational age selections to facilitate detailed "drill down" for various outcomes. Results can also be filtered using admission status - inborn, outborn, or combined. The selected filtering parameters are used to provide the specific network comparison group, and can be further refined by selecting high- (>450 discharges annually), medium- (225–450 discharges annually), or low-volume (<225 discharges annually) NICUs as the comparison group (**Fig. 4**).

The report illustrated in **Fig. 3** examines catheter-related blood stream infections between January 1, 2006 and July 30, 2009. The annual rate of infections, shown as the rate per 1000 line days, is shown for this specific NICU as dots connected by a solid line from year to year. In the background in gray is the 33rd to 66th percentile for all of Pediatrix Medical Group. As can be seen during this period, the infection rate in this NICU was declining, as was the rate for all NICUs in Pediatrix, partly from an increasing CQI focus on reducing catheter-associated bloodstream infections. This type of run-chart methodology is extremely useful in assessing whether interventions in a specific NICU have value over time.

Fig. 5 is a management report examining the highest level of ventilatory assistance given to patients over time. Interesting trends in patient care can be discerned, particularly the increasing use of nasal continuous positive airway pressure (CPAP), reflecting the current tendency to try to avoid mechanical ventilation of extremely low birth weight infants. As **Fig. 5** indicates, the use of nasal CPAP rose from 13% of ventilated neonates in 2006 to 33% in 2009, whereas the use of both conventional and high-frequency ventilation declined, which is an encouraging overall trend.

Some reports cannot be provided easily in graphic form in the CDW, but still have great value for patient care and quality improvement. The medication report is an example of a report in tabular format, again allowing clinicians to examine the use of many of the most common neonatal medications in their NICU, while

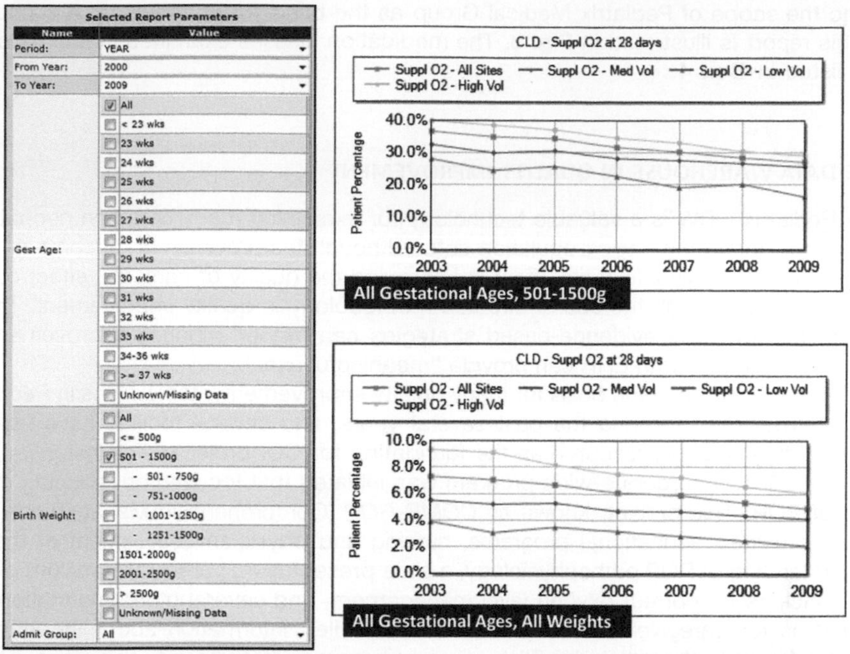

Fig. 4. The panel on the left shows multiple weight and gestational age options that may be selected to filter reports. Admission status (inborn or outborn) is available as an additional filter. The comparison network group may be selected based on annual neonatal intensive care unit (NICU) volume and/or specific region or state (see panels on right for examples of network variation based on NICU volume).

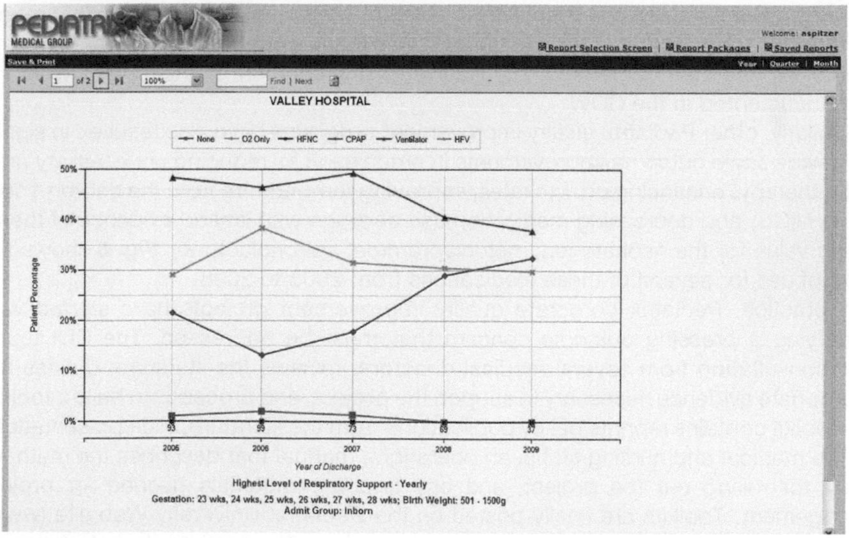

Fig. 5. Clinical Data Warehouse report from an individual neonatal intensive care unit (NICU) showing the changing patterns of ventilator support between 2005 and 2009. *Y* axis shows percentage of NICU admissions treated with each modality. O2, oxygen only; CPAP, continuous positive airway pressure; HFNC, high flow nasal cannula; Ventilator, standard mechanical ventilation; HFV, high frequency ventilation.

using the scope of Pediatrix Medical Group as the basis for comparison. A section of this report is illustrated in **Fig. 6**. The medication classes examined in this report are listed in **Box 4**.

THE DATA WAREHOUSE IN QUALITY IMPROVEMENT

The Pediatrix CDW is a valuable technology for examining many common neonatal outcomes and some basic population data. Although the provision of outcome data can have a strongly influential effect in improving the quality of care, the effect can be magnified through the use of directed methodology in quality improvement. The application of these evidence-based strategies can further enhance improvement, truly illustrating how an EHR can provide "meaningful use."

The CDW has been the basis for many quality improvement interventions in Pediatrix Medical Group during the past several years, and several toolkits have been devised that use this resource as the foundation for CQI projects. For instance, in 2004 to 2005, a corporate-wide program was initiated that focused on reducing the rate of ROP. This project, known as *COMP-ROP* (Comprehensive Management of ROP), provided educational programs, nursing and physician assessment of their understanding of ROP pathophysiology, a slide presentation, parent information, isolette stickers for correct oxygen level management, and several other informational programs for caregivers and parents. More detailed information about this effort can be found in the article by Ellsbury and Ursprung, elsewhere in this issue. The CDW was the tool used to follow ROP rates, which have improved markedly since that time. From 2003 to 2008 a striking decrease in severe ROP (stage 3, 4, or 5, or surgical) was seen in the Pediatrix Network. In infants with birth weights of 400 to 1500 g, severe ROP dropped from 11% in 2003 to 5.8% in 2008 (**Fig. 7**). Given the fact that Pediatrix Medical Group admits 25,000 to 30,000 extremely and very low birth weight infants annually, the reduction in rates of severe ROP unquestionably represents an important public health initiative. Over this 6-year period, several thousand infants experienced decreased morbidity and preservation of their sight, which is well documented in the CDW.

Similarly, other Pediatrix quality improvement programs have also resulted in significant wide scale outcome improvements in areas such as reducing unnecessary antibiotic therapy, enhancing growth rates, improving temperature from the delivery room to the NICU, and decreasing medication use of drugs with limited evidence of therapeutic value for the neonate (eg, metoclopramide, spironolactone). **Fig. 8** shows the rates of use for several of these medications from 2003 to 2008.

In practice, Pediatrix corporate quality improvement projects have started with identifying a pressing outcome concern that must be addressed. The CQI team, with consultation from several medical directors, reviews the literature, defines the appropriate evidence necessary to support the project, and proceeds to build a toolkit. The toolkit contains reprints of key publications from the literature, slide presentations for the medical and nursing staffs, an operations manual that describes the methodology for rolling out the project, and any ancillary materials needed for project management. Toolkits are finally posted on the Pediatrix University Web site (www.pediatrixu.com) for participating practices to review. The toolkits do not represent specific recommendations on how to practice, but rather provide a series of alternate approaches that may be valuable for certain NICUs looking to enhance their outcomes. Each practice has the ability to modify and tailor the toolkit to their particular unit's needs. Timelines are then established for projects, and enrollment is

Antifungal

	Amphotericin			Fluconazole		
	n	%	Netw	n	%	Netw
Year: 2003 | 789 pats.	13	1.6%	1.0%	6	0.8%	0.8%
Year: 2004 | 710pats.	15	2.1%	1.0%	3	0.4%	0.8%
Year: 2005 | 730 pats.	15	2.1%	1.0%	6	0.8%	1.2%
Year: 2006 | 794 pats.	14	1.8%	0.8%	7	0.9%	1.4%
Year: 2007 | 780 pats.	18	2.3%	0.8%	14	1.8%	1.5%
Year: 2008 | 787 pats.	10	1.3%	0.7%	9	1.1%	1.4%

Antibiotics

	Antibiotic-Aminoglycosides			Cefotaxime			Ceftazidime			Ceftriaxone			Nafcillin			Vancomycin		
	n	%	Netw	n	%	Netw	n	%	Netw	n	%	Netw	n	%	Netw	n	%	Netw
Year: 2003 | 789 pats.	663	84.0%	59.9%	87	11.0%	11.3%	7	0.9%	1.5%	3	0.4%	0.2%	0	0.0%	0.7%	64	8.1%	9.1%
Year: 2004 | 710pats.	663	84.4%	61.1%	67	9.4%	9.8%	5	0.7%	1.3%	6	0.8%	0.2%	0	0.0%	0.9%	56	7.9%	8.8%
Year: 2005 | 730 pats.	676	92.6%	64.1%	59	8.1%	5.4%	1	0.1%	1.5%	9	1.2%	0.2%	0	0.0%	0.9%	70	9.6%	8.5%
Year: 2006 | 794 pats.	749	94.3%	63.0%	68	8.6%	3.9%	3	0.4%	1.2%	3	0.4%	0.2%	0	0.0%	0.7%	83	10.5%	8.0%
Year: 2007 | 780 pats.	710	91.0%	63.2%	78	10.0%	3.5%	7	0.9%	1.0%	5	0.4%	0.2%	0	0.0%	0.8%	80	10.3%	8.1%
Year: 2008 | 787 pats.	713	90.6%	62.5%	60	7.6%	2.8%	1	0.1%	0.9%	2	0.3%	0.1%	0	0.1%	0.8%	67	8.5%	7.6%

Fig. 6. Medication usage report. Table of yearly medication use for certain drugs between 2003 and 2008 in the Clinical Data Warehouse. Table shows individual neonatal intensive care unit use (NICU) and comparison with other NICUs.

Box 4
Medication classes examined in the medication report

- Antifungal agents
  - Amphotericin
  - Fluconazole
- Antibiotics
  - Aminoglycosides
  - Ampicillin
  - Cefotaxime
  - Ceftazidime
  - Ceftriaxone
  - Nafcillin
  - Vancomycin
- Antiviral drugs
  - Acyclovir
- Diuretics
  - Furosemide
  - Spironolactone
  - Thiazides
- Erythropoiesis stimulating
  - Erythropoietin
- Gastrointestinal medications
  - H_2blockers
  - Metoclopramide
  - Proton pump inhibitors
- Ibuprofen
- Indomethacin
- Inhalational agents
  - Albuterol
  - Steroids
- Methylxanthines
  - Aminophylline
  - Caffeine
- Steroids
  - Antenatal
  - Postnatal
- Surfactants (by type)
- Vasoactive agents
  - Epinephrine
  - Dopamine

Dobutamine

Milrinone

Vitamins

Access to this type of information allows physicians to better understand many of the decisions made in the care of the neonate, and the long-term implications of practice choices with respect to neonatal outcomes.

initiated for units desiring to participate. The CDW then serves as the primary method of following outcome data.

As can be seen from these data extracted from the CDW, having a tool at this level of sophistication allows truly meaningful health care improvement and cost savings. The scope of cost reduction can be gathered from **Fig. 9**. From 2003 to 2009, when Pediatrix Medical Group intensified its quality improvement efforts, length of stay in the company declined from a mean of 15.9 to 14.2 days. With nearly 90,000 NICU admissions per year and an approximate overall daily cost of care (hospital and physician) during this time period of $2200, this shortened length of stay could potentially result in more than $330,000,000 of health care savings this year in participating NICUs. This saving has not occurred from the more traditional use management approach, in which outliers are identified and an effort is made to discharge them from the hospital. It has instead come about through the application of thoughtful application of evidence-based medicine, leading to reduced hospital use from decreased morbidity and mortality, which also adds immeasurably to parent satisfaction.

THE QUALITY IMPROVEMENT PROJECT SYSTEM (QUALITYSTEPS)

In recognizing the value of data-driven applications in health care, Pediatrix Medical Group has also noted a growing need exists for other applications for measuring patient outcomes. Ideally, these applications should allow simplified data entry, extraction of summarized information, and generation of annotated run charts that would enable users to follow targeted outcomes over time. Furthermore, this system should enable comparisons with other databases, yet be flexible enough to allow modifications for various quality tracking projects. For example, although the CDW

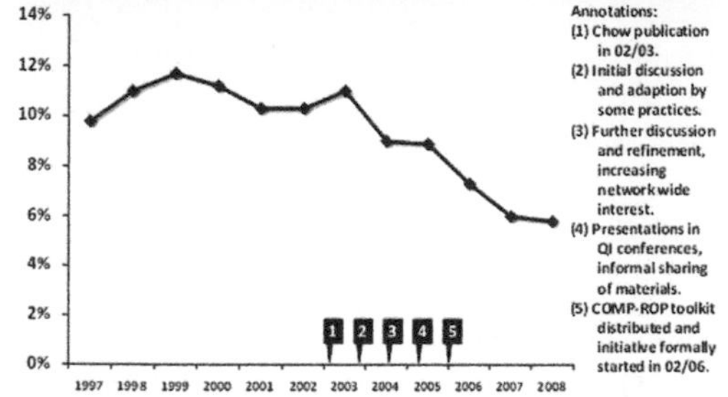

Fig. 7. Network trend reports between 2003 and 2008 for severe retinopathy for prematurity, stages 3 through 5 and surgical.

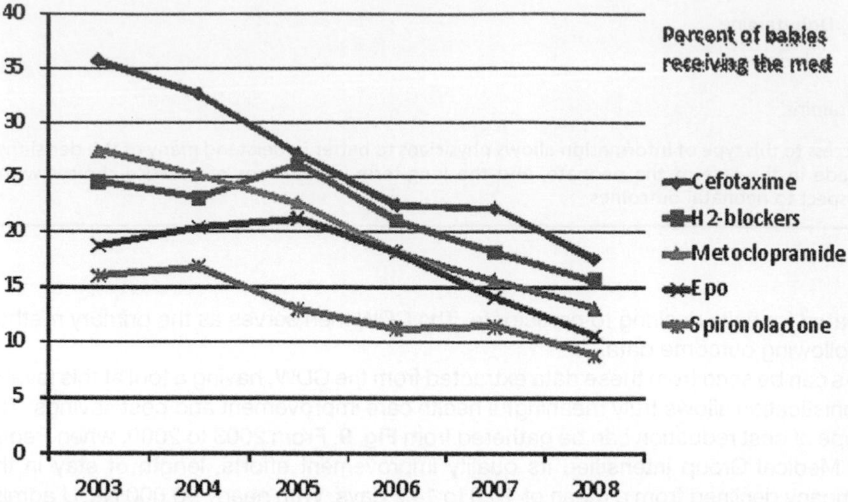

Fig. 8. Declining use of several drugs in the neonatal intensive care unit between 2003 and 2008. *Y* axis represents percentage of patients treated with these medications. *X* axis shows the individual years. Epo, erythropoietin.

facilitates tracking of many outcome variables, some projects of great value and interest might not normally be captured in the daily progress note that forms the basis of the CDW. Safety projects, evaluation of hand hygiene, and similar measures require an alternative tracking mechanism. To meet this demand, the group developed the Quality Improvement Project System, or QualitySteps.

QualitySteps was initially devised to assist Pediatrix Medical Group physicians in creating annotated run charts for CQI projects. Data can easily be extracted from the BabySteps EHR and inserted into QualitySteps for use in quality assessment. The welcoming screen for QualitySteps is shown in **Fig. 10**.

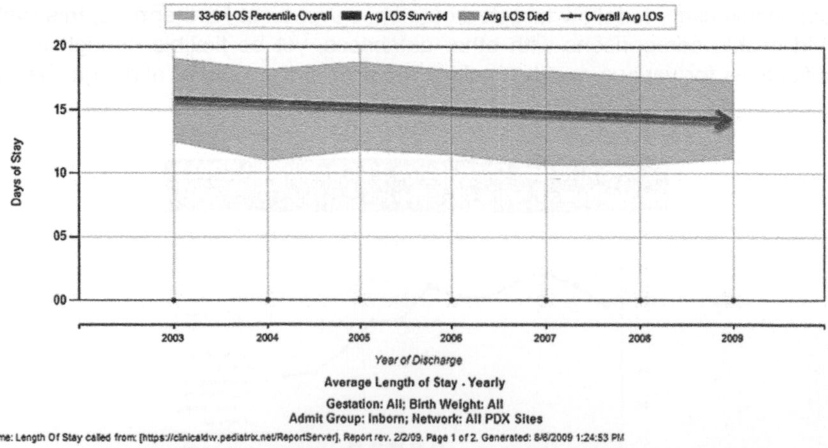

Fig. 9. Length of stay (LOS) report from the Clinical Data Warehouse between 2003 and 2009. Arrow indicates decline in LOS from 15.9 to 14.2 days for all Pediatrix neonatal intensive care units on average.

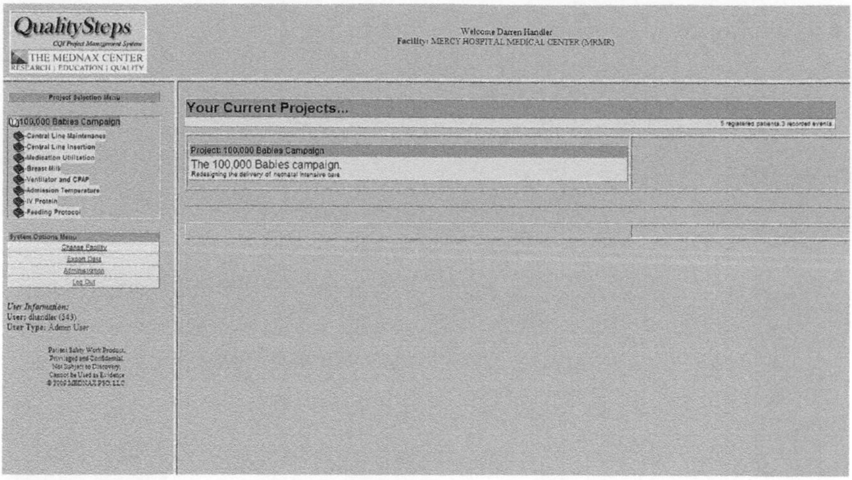

Fig. 10. QualitySteps system welcoming screen.

Projects can be designated and worksheets readily created that allow data entry on a selected patient population. Each facility or practice using QualitySteps has one or more administrators who are responsible for designing the project and devising the appropriate questions to be answered by participants in the module. The administrator's screen is shown in **Fig. 11**. Ultimately, a panel of questions about a specific issue can be designed. Answering the questions allows a run chart to be generated. This process is shown in **Figs. 12** and **13**. On the run chart, annotations can be placed as indicated, along with comments that outline the types of interventions that were initiated on the specific dates. Communication among CQI participants can also occur in the form of text messages left on the Web site, so that all members of the project are always up-to-date with the project status. In addition, administrators can include supporting documentation (eg, published papers, manuscripts) to ensure that the background evidence necessary to support the initiative is available to everyone.

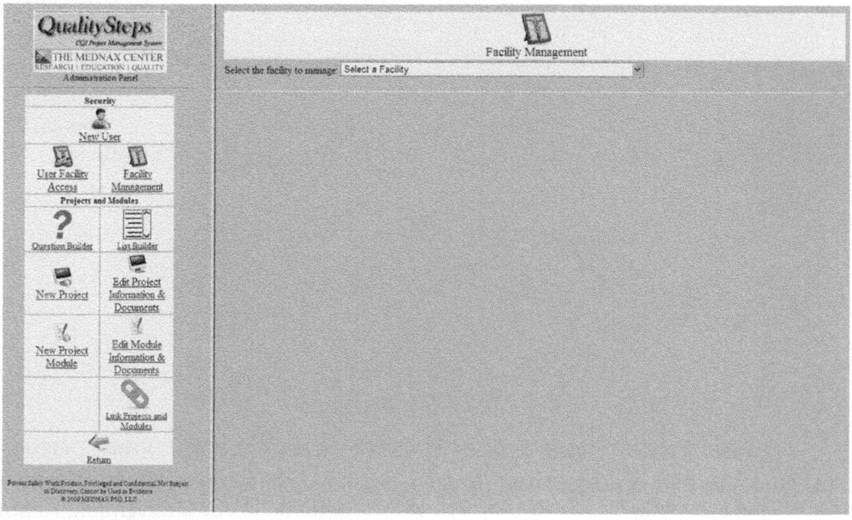

Fig. 11. QualitySteps administrator screen.

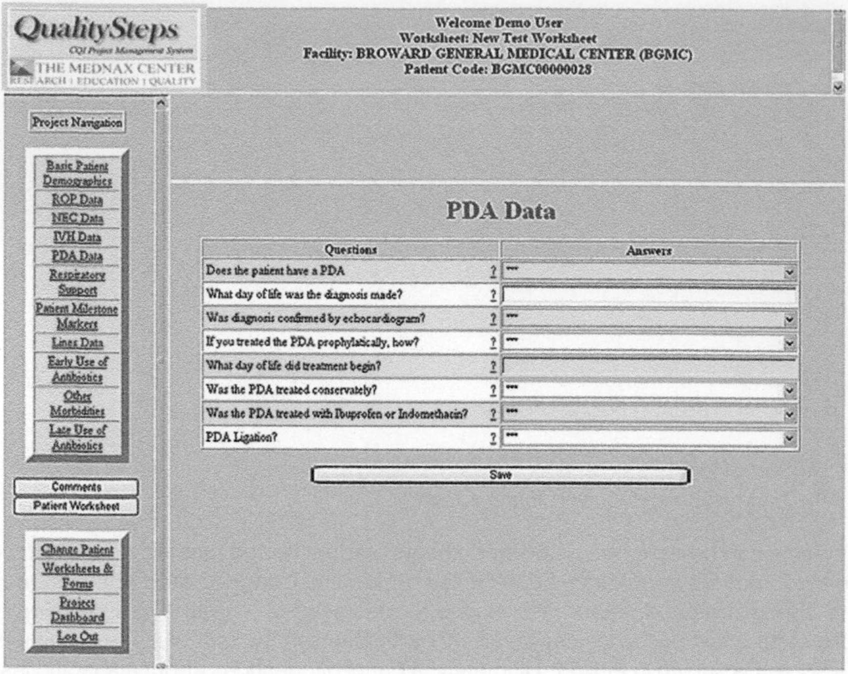

Fig. 12. QualitySteps module screen related to ductus arteriosus management. Other accessible modules are noted in the left-hand column.

Although **Fig. 12** indicates a series of questions related to the presence of the ductus arteriosus, the flexibility of the system permits administrators to devise a module and questions on any topic desired, not only those related to neonatal medicine. As a result, QualitySteps is a very flexible, easy-to-use tool that can be applied in any field of medicine to track a quality improvement initiative.

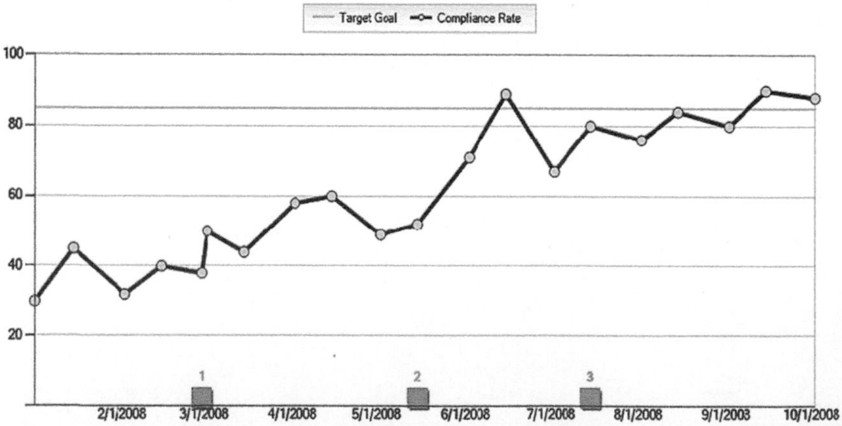

Fig. 13. Run chart tracking outcome of hand hygiene intervention program. Goal line is set at 85% compliance. Three boxes resting on *x* axis indicate points of intervention. Annotations for these interventions are noted elsewhere in the program.

The BabySteps Research Data Warehouse

The clinical value of the CDW is immediately apparent in terms of neonatal outcomes and quality improvement, especially in the areas noted. Furthermore, Pediatrix has attempted to be responsive to the requests of its practicing physicians, and many of the clinical reports that have been developed were designed to meet their needs in providing optimal patient care. Given the fact, however, that the BabySteps record is scoured daily for 563 data fields, when combined with the extraordinary volume of patients in this database (now >600,000), the potential for novel research observations cannot be overlooked. In fact, the CDW has been queried by the NIH and the NICHD Neonatal Network, the FDA, several major universities, and private corporations, all of whom have sought data that are not available elsewhere.

As an example of the usefulness of the CDW, the FDA contacted Pediatrix in 2005 because it was interested in knowing the 30 most commonly used medications in the NICU. These data were furnished to the FDA and published in Pediatrics.[7] On further examination of these data, the FDA noted that three of the five most commonly used medications were antibiotics: ampicillin, gentamicin, and cefotaxime. Because the most common neonatal admission to the NICU is suspected septicemia, these drugs clearly represented the two most common antibiotic regimens used for suspected sepsis, namely ampicillin and gentamicin, and ampicillin and cefotaxime. These two approaches were believed to be equivalent, with equal outcomes and equal risks. Cefotaxime had the advantage of greater central nervous system penetration than gentamicin, and blood levels of cefotaxime did not need to be measured during treatment.

When Pediatrix examined the outcomes in the CDW in more detail, however, they discovered that the use of cefotaxime had nearly a twofold (100%) greater association with mortality at certain gestational ages than gentamicin in this patient population of more than 128,000 infants diagnosed with suspected sepsis.[8] (**Fig. 14**) Extensive attempts to eliminate confounding variables through the use of logistic regression analysis strongly suggested that this finding was correct. Because of this risk, the use of cefotaxime for early-onset suspected septicemia can no longer be supported. Use of this medication has fallen to an extremely low rate in participating NICUs across the country.

This type of observation, which otherwise might have gone unnoticed, became apparent only when sufficient numbers of patients could be evaluated. Many of the

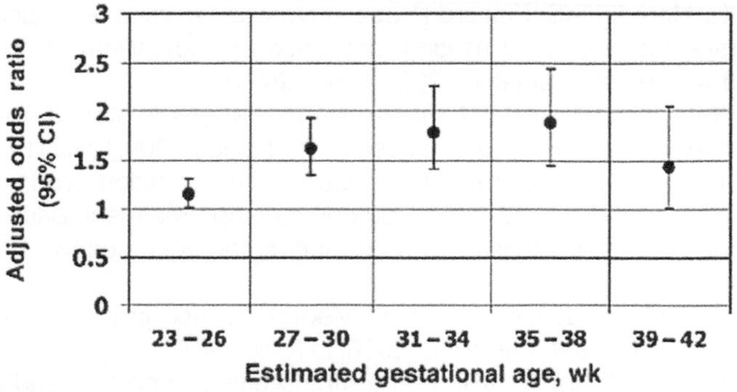

Fig. 14. Adjusted odds ratios for mortality rate of ampicillin and cefotaxime compared with ampicillin and gentamicin; 95% confidence intervals are indicated. (*From* Clark RH, Bloom BT, Spitzer AR, et al. Empiric use of ampicillin and cefotaxime, compared with ampicillin and gentamicin, for neonates at risk for sepsis is associated with an increased risk of neonatal death. Pediatrics 2006;117:67–74; with permission.)

data warehouse observational studies now consist of similar large populations of patients. A more recent publication examining rates of meconium aspiration syndrome and persistent pulmonary hypertension in neonates during the past decade among 162,075 term neonates showed a continuing level of these problems had not changed during this interval, despite what many people believed.[9]

Pediatrix continues to expand the data warehouse capabilities for research, and constantly invites inquiries for its use. This type of database not only provides answers to many outcome questions but also can provide a model for prospective trials and studies in which targeted data collection is required. Much more information can continue to be extracted and evaluated that will have additional significant benefits for the practice of newborn medicine.

SUMMARY

The Pediatrix BabySteps CDW is a rich and novel tool allowing unbiased extraction of information from an entire neonatal population care by physicians and advanced practice nurses in Pediatrix Medical Group. Because it represents the practice of newborn medicine ranging from small community intensive care units to some of the largest NICUs in the United States, it is highly representative of scope of practice in this country. Its value in defining outcome measures, quality improvement projects, and research continues to grow annually. Now coupled with the BabySteps QualitySteps program for defined CQI projects, it represents a robust methodology for meaningful use of an EHR, as designated during this era of health care reform. Continued growth of the CDW should result in continued important observations and improvements in neonatal care.

REFERENCES

1. DHHS.gov News Release, June 16, 2009.
2. Health IT. Policy council recommendations to national coordinator for defining meaningful use final. Available at: http://www.hhs.gov/news/press/2009pres/12/20091230a.html. Accessed January 23, 2009.
3. Clark RH, Bloom BT, Spitzer AR, et al. Medication use in the NICU: data from a large national data set. Pediatrics 2006;117:1979–87.
4. Abrams ME, Meredith KS, Kinnard P, et al. Hydrops fetalis: a retrospective review of cases reported to a large national database and identification of risk factors associated with death. Pediatrics 2007;120(1):84–9.
5. Clark RH, Yoder BA, Harrison M. Time-related changes in steroid use and bronchopulmonary dysplasia in preterm infants. Pediatrics 2009;124(2):673–9.
6. Clark RH, Powers RJ, Spitzer AR, et al. Meconium aspiration syndrome remains a significant problem in the NICU: outcomes and treatment patterns in term neonates admitted for intensive care during a ten-year period. 1. J Perinatol 2009;29(7):497–503.
7. Clark RH, Bloom BT, Spitzer AR, et al. Medication use in the NICU: data from a large National data set. Pediatrics 2006;117:1979–87.
8. Clark RH, Bloom BT, Spitzer AR, et al. Empiric use of ampicillin and cefotaxime, compared with ampicillin and gentamicin, for neonates at risk for sepsis is associated with an increased risk of neonatal death. Pediatrics 2006;117:67–74.
9. Singh BS, Clark RH, Powers RJ, et al. Meconium aspiration syndrome remains a significant problem in the NICU: outcomes and treatment patterns in term

neonates admitted for intensive care during a ten year period. J Perinatol 2009;29: 497–504.

FURTHER READINGS

Abrams ME, Meredith KS, Kinnard P, et al. Hydrops fetalis: a retrospective review of cases reported to a large national database and identification of risk factors associated with death. Pediatrics 2007;120:84–9.

Arnold C, Clark R, Bosco J, et al. Variability in vancomycin use in newborn intensive care units determined from data in an electronic medical record. Infect Control Hosp Epidemiol 2008;29:667–70.

Attridge JT, Clark R, Walker MW, et al. New insights into spontaneous intestinal perforation using a national data set: (2) two populations of patients with perforations. J Perinatol 2006;26:185–8.

Attridge JT, Clark R, Gordon PV. New insights into spontaneous intestinal perforation using a national data set (3): antenatal steroids have no adverse association with spontaneous intestinal perforation. J Perinatol 2006;26:667–70.

Benjamin DK Jr, DeLong ER, Steinbach WJ, et al. Empirical therapy for neonatal candidemia in very low birth weight infants. Pediatrics 2003;112:543–7.

Benjamin DK Jr, DeLong ER, Cotten CM, et al. Postconception age and other risk factors associated with mortality following Gram-negative rod bacteremia. J Perinatol 2004;24:169–74.

Benjamin DK, DeLong E, Cotten CM, et al. Mortality following blood culture in premature infants: increased with Gram-negative bacteremia and candidemia, but not Gram-positive bacteremia. J Perinatol 2004;24:175–80.

Bloom BT, Mulligan J, Arnold C, et al. Improving growth of very low birth weight infants in the first 28 days. Pediatrics 2003;112:8–14.

Bloom BT, Clark RH. Comparison of Infasurf (calfactant) and Survanta (beractant) in the prevention and treatment of respiratory distress syndrome. Pediatrics 2005; 116:392–9.

Clark RH, Auten RL, Peabody J. A comparison of the outcomes of neonates treated with two different natural surfactants. J Pediatr 2001;139:828–31.

Clark RH, Thomas P, Peabody J. Extrauterine growth restriction remains a serious problem in prematurely born neonates. Pediatrics 2003;111:986–90.

Clark RH. Interneonatal intensive care unit variation in growth rates and feeding practices in healthy moderately premature infants. J Perinatol 2005;25:437–9.

Clark RH, Walker MW, Gauderer MW. Prevalence of gastroschisis and associated hospital time continue to rise in neonates who are admitted for intensive care. J Pediatr Surg 2009;44:1108–12.

Garite TJ, Clark R, Thorp JA. Intrauterine growth restriction increases morbidity and mortality among premature neonates. Am J Obstet Gynecol 2004;191: 481–7.

Garite TJ, Clark RH, Elliott JP, et al. Twins and triplets: the effect of plurality and growth on neonatal outcome compared with singleton infants. Am J Obstet Gynecol 2004;191:700–7.

Garges HP, Moody MA, Cotten CM, et al. Neonatal meningitis: what is the correlation among cerebrospinal fluid cultures, blood cultures, and cerebrospinal fluid parameters? Pediatrics 2006;117:1094–100.

Gordon PV, Swanson JR, Clark R. Antenatal indomethacin is more likely associated with spontaneous intestinal perforation rather than NEC. Am J Obstet Gynecol 2008;198:725–6.

Greenberg RG, Smith PB, Cotten CM, et al. Traumatic lumbar punctures in neonates: test performance of the cerebrospinal fluid white blood cell count. Pediatr Infect Dis J 2008;27:1047–51.

Guthrie SO, Gordon PV, Thomas V, et al. Necrotizing enterocolitis among neonates in the United States. J Perinatol 2003;23:278–85.

Laughon M, Meyer R, Bose C, et al. Rising birth prevalence of gastroschisis. J Perinatol 2003;23:291–3.

Laughon M, Bose C, Clark R. Treatment strategies to prevent or close a patent ductus arteriosus in preterm infants and outcomes. J Perinatol 2007;27:164–70.

Lenfestey RW, Smith PB, Moody MA, et al. Predictive value of cerebrospinal fluid parameters in neonates with intraventricular drainage devices. J Neurosurg 2007;107:209–12.

Smith PB, Garges HP, Cotton CM, et al. Meningitis in preterm neonates: importance of cerebrospinal fluid parameters. Am J Perinatol 2008;25:421–6.

Thomas P, Peabody J, Turnier V, et al. A new look at intrauterine growth and the impact of race, altitude, and gender. Pediatrics 2000;106:E21.

Yoder BA, Harrison M, Clark RH. Time-related changes in steroid use and bronchopulmonary dysplasia in preterm infants. Pediatrics 2009;124:673–9.

The Role of Regional Collaboratives: The California Perinatal Quality Care Collaborative Model

Jeffrey B. Gould, MD, MPH

KEYWORDS

- Perinatal quality improvement • Neonatal intensive care unit
- Regional collaborative • California

THE CASE FOR A REGIONAL APPROACH TO PERINATAL QUALITY IMPROVEMENT

Improving the outcome of the infants cared for in one's neonatal intensive care unit (NICU) is the main objective of improvement projects that are pursued independently or as a member of a national collaborative. While improving the outcome of patients is a key motivator for NICUs that are members of a regional perinatal quality improvement collaborative, the very nature of the regional enterprise encourages each member to also take on the responsibility of improving the care and outcomes for the entire population of the region's mothers and infants. Because of the scope of the members' commitment, regional quality improvement collaborations represent the intersection of hospital-based and community-based medicine offering the possibility of coordinated improvement efforts conducted at both the hospital and community level. Let us consider what might drive such a coordinated approach. When clearly presented, data are often a key motivator for quality improvement. **Fig. 1** shows the familiar comparison of an outcome across NICUs, a portrayal that often serves as a strong motivator for action among NICUs. Using the same data source, which includes the rates of antenatal steroid (ANS) administration to eligible mothers collected on the NICU dataset as well as the mothers' residential zip codes (which in California is linked to the NICU dataset), one is able to map ANS use across the region served by the collaborative, creating potential motivators to action at the community level (**Fig. 2**). Regional quality improvement collaboratives enable envisioning a future where member teams will come from both the hospital and the

Division of Neonatal and Developmental Medicine, California Perinatal Quality Care Collaborative, Perinatal Epidemiology and Health Outcomes Research Unit, Stanford University Medical Center, 750 Welch Road, Suite 315, Palo Alto, CA 94304, USA
E-mail address: jbgould@stanford.edu

Clin Perinatol 37 (2010) 71–86
doi:10.1016/j.clp.2010.01.004 perinatology.theclinics.com
0095-5108/10/$ – see front matter

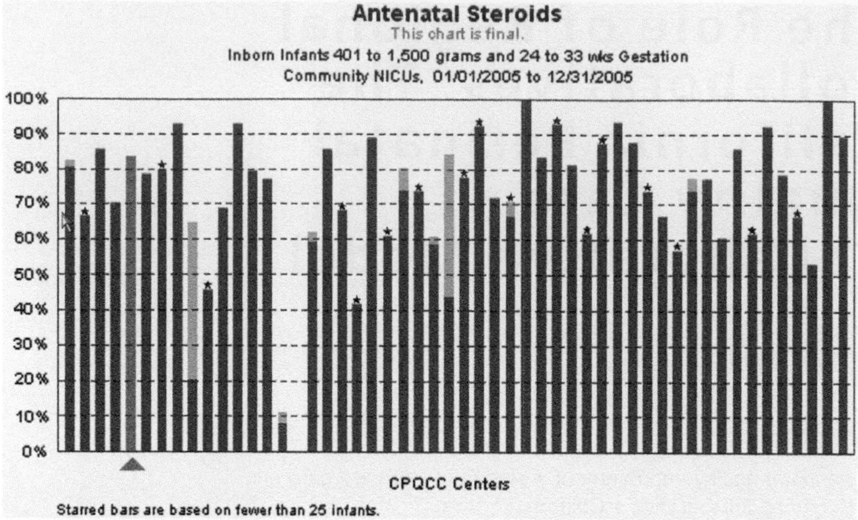

Fig. 1. The distribution of antenatal steroid use in qualifying mothers giving birth in CPQCC Hospitals with community NICUs in 2005. (*Courtesy of* California Perinatal Quality Care Collaborative; with permission.)

community and where improvement bundles are developed that address hospital root causes, community root causes, and root causes that emerge at the interface between hospital and NICU care. Because data are a key motivator for improvement, an important goal for the California Perinatal Quality Care Collaborative (CPQCC) has been to construct a single database that can be used to inform process and outcomes improvement at both the hospital (see **Fig. 1**) and community level (see **Fig. 2**).

Although being a member of a national perinatal quality improvement organization or initiative may provide the tools for effective quality improvement, the shape of these tools is largely independent of the health care context within which the individual NICUs exist. An important potential offered by membership in a regional collaborative is that of understanding the nature of one's regional network of perinatal care. In 2008, 41% of NICU admissions in California were acute, outborn neonatal transports. Given the large number of outborn admissions, a regional collaborative has the ability to provide a platform for quality improvement initiatives that can be directed not only to individual NICUs but also to quality improvement teams that are composed of health care providers from both the referral NICU and several of its major referring hospitals. The value of the network approach to quality improvement is based on the premise that ideal care often represents a continuum that extends from the care provided at the birth hospital and its nursery or NICU to the care provided at the referral NICU. For example, ideal initiatives developed to maximize the improvement of respiratory, nutritional, or severe asphyxia management must identify and create improvement bundles to address the cascade of root causes that emerge at the birth hospital, during transport, and at the referral NICU. While certain components of these bundles may be specific to each location, ideally they are designed and refined by a team from all 3 locations. Although the author knows of no current integrated projects, the interhospital collaborations that are nurtured within regional collaboratives create a milieu for their emergence.

A third important aspect of a regional quality care collaborative is that to a large extent, the activities and operations of all of its members are influenced, facilitated, and constrained by the region's economic, sociodemographic, regulatory, payer, and geophysical context. In addition, the treatment style and its level of effectiveness appear to differ across regions. By taking these local factors into account, regional collaboratives are able to optimize the design and implementation of their improvement initiatives. A further advantage is that members of a regional collaborative are able to compare their performance to hospitals that are operating within a similar demographic, economic, and health services context. Benchmark performance becomes an even more meaningful and powerful motivator as it represents performance that has been achieved locally by one's peers. The members of a regional quality improvement initiative represent a community of change. As a community, they share their approaches to overcoming obstacles to improvement. Whereas many of these obstacles are universal, many of them or their solutions are influenced by the regional context. Members of a regional collaborative have the advantage of being able to share the approaches that were found to work well within their region. In summary, while quality improvement initiatives conducted by individual NICUs and by membership in national collaboratives are important ways to improve care, regional quality improvement collaboratives offer many potential advantages.

THE NATURE OF A REGIONAL PERINATAL QUALITY CARE COLLABORATIVE

At its heart, a regional quality improvement collaborative is a complex organization with multiple stakeholders. A major challenge to the creation of a regional quality improvement collaborative is how to pull these stakeholders together when many of these stakeholders hold very differing opinions as to how health care should work and what should be its most immediate quality issues. For example, a consumer organization may be primarily concerned with creating regional report cards that allow the public to choose hospitals that have demonstrated the best results, and may not consider the investment of the enormous energy required to help hospitals improve their outcomes to be part of their mandate. On the other hand, physicians may be less enamored of public reporting, but willing to invest great energy in quality improvement efforts to improve the clinical outcomes of their patients. It is not unusual for the key stakeholders to have long-standing differences that must be addressed if they are to work together effectively. Bringing disparate stakeholders together requires (1) the identification of a highly valued, common goal and (2) an organizational structure that provides value and minimizes risk for each stakeholder. In the author's experience, these are not easy tasks to accomplish and can be greatly facilitated by enlisting the aid of an experienced consultant in organizational development.

In the mid 1990s there was a great deal of payer activity to promote health performance report carding in California. In this environment, 4 major stakeholders saw the need for a California Quality Care Collaborative: (1) the California Association of Neonatologists (CAN), whose initial concern was with fair comparisons; (2) the State of California, Maternal and Child Health Branch (CA-MCH), which wanted to extend their analysis of risk-adjusted, neonatal mortality in California's approximately 350 birthing hospitals to include risk-adjusted measures of neonatal morbidity; (3) California Children's Services (CCS), one of the state's largest payers of NICU care, which wanted an analysis of the quality of the care it was paying for; and (4) the David and Lucile Packard Foundation, which had supported the Vermont Oxford Network (VON) nationally and wanted to extend and promote the benefits of membership in this organization to its home state of California. A fifth key player was VON whose expertise, input, and support were essential components of the build. These champions met, sketched out a potential mission statement, identified key stakeholders,

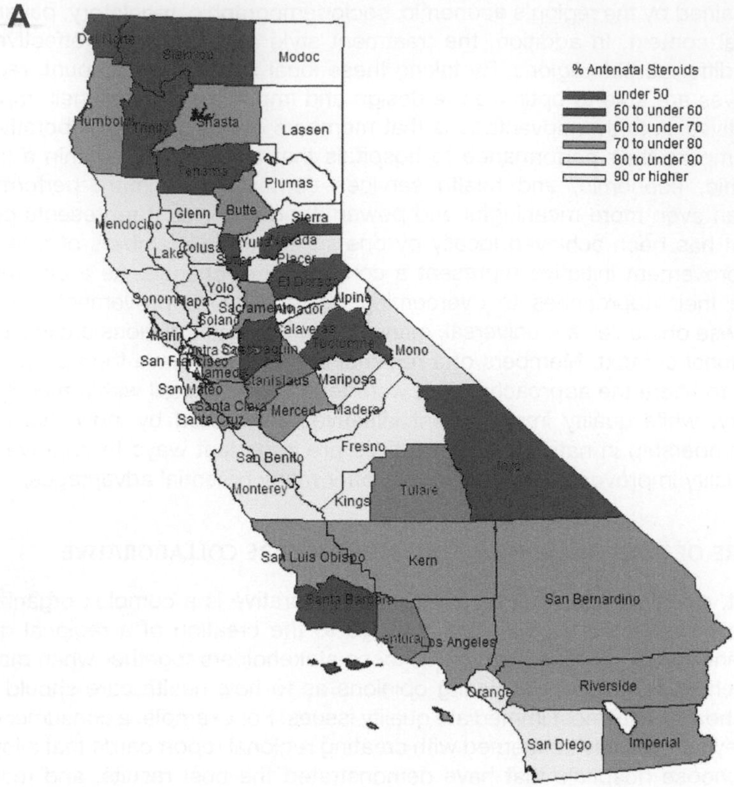

Fig. 2. (*A*) Antenatal steroid percentages for eligible infants of 24 to 33 completed weeks' gestation, California, 2005. Only infants 400 to 1500 g are included in the calculations for this map. (*B*) Antenatal steroid percentages for eligible infants 401 to 1500 g by zip code, Los Angeles County, 2005. Infants 401 to 1500 g and 24 to 33 weeks of gestation are included in the analysis. (*Courtesy of* California Perinatal Quality Care Collaborative; with permission.)

and began the assessment of the potential benefits and risks for each stakeholder's participation. Over the course of a year, CPQCC leadership met with each potential stakeholder individually to ascertain their reaction to the collaborative's proposed mission and to explore how the collaborative might be structured to maximize the value and minimize the risk of each stakeholders' membership. Significant efforts were made to engage the most senior representative of each stakeholder, which required not only the influence of the core project champions and a great deal of networking but also a careful consideration and succinct presentation of how membership in the collaborative could bring value to the stakeholder. Once key stakeholders had been engaged individually, pairs of stakeholders, whose histories suggested that they might have difficulty collaborating, were brought together to discuss the potential values and risks of pursuing common quality improvement goals. **Boxes 1** and **2** list the core CPQCC stakeholders and the potential value that membership could bring. The major stakeholders who were essential to CPQCC's creation and

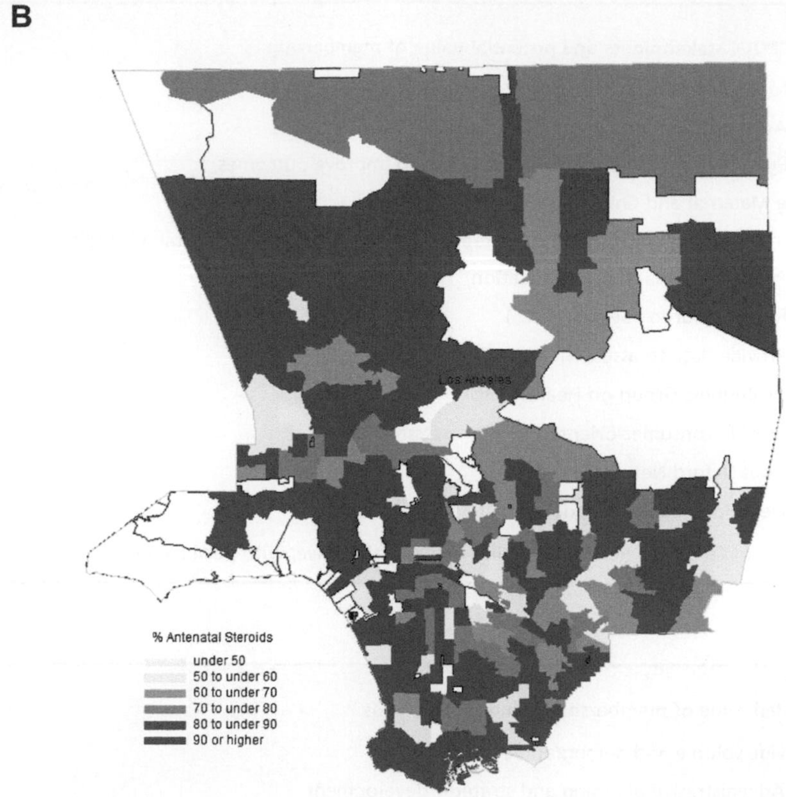

Fig. 2. *(continued)*

development are listed in **Box 3**. Although these individual and paired stakeholder meetings took almost a year to accomplish, these efforts were critical to the successful launching of CPQCC. By the time the initial CPQCC Executive Committee meeting was held, the major interstakeholder issues that could have been major stumbling blocks to CPQCC's development had been already addressed, and the group was keen to get on with the work of creating the collaborative. During the course of these preliminary meetings with the potential stakeholders, there emerged not only a refinement in the mission of the collaborative but also an organizational philosophy that was formally addressed at the first Executive Committee meeting.

ROLE OF THE MISSION STATEMENT AND DEFINITION OF ORGANIZATIONAL PHILOSOPHY

Although the general goal of any quality improvement collaborative is to improve quality, exactly what is meant by quality improvement and specifically how one will go about achieving it has many interpretations. Because of these many interpretations, creating a mission statement is an essential step in building any collaborative enterprise. In essence, the mission statement addresses who you are, your overarching goal, and how you intend to achieve this goal. Although the collaborative may be made up of stakeholders and stakeholder factions with diverse positions,

Box 1
Core CPQCC stakeholders and potential value of membership

- California Association of Neonatologists (CAN)
  - Advocate for fair report cards with malleable outcomes
  - Provide quality improvement initiatives to improve outcomes
- State Maternal and Child Health Branch (CA-MCH)
  - Improve perinatal outcomes by reporting on risk-adjusted neonatal morbidity
  - Promote perinatal regionalization
- California Children's Services (CCS)
  - Provide data to assess NICU medical quality of care
- Pacific Business Group on Health (PBGH)
  - Provide consumer-oriented quality assessment
- Vermont Oxford Network (VON)
  - Develop a regional model of VON

Courtesy of California Perinatal Quality Care Collaborative; with permission.

Box 2
Potential value of membership to individual NICUs

- Provide volume and demographic data
  - Administrative planning and strategic development
- Provide process and risk-adjusted outcomes data
  - Guide quality improvement activities, meet payers' quality improvement requirements, contracting
  - Provide quality improvement support (workshops, toolkits, webcasts)
- Prepare mandated California Children's Services Report
  - Analysis of match between an NICU's infants needs and its capacity
  - Matching a NICU's quality improvement activities to its outcomes
- Facilitate the California Hospital Assessment and Reporting Mandate (CHART)
  - Advocate for malleable quality indicators
  - Prepare risk-adjusted measures for release to CHART
- Develop and manage mandated California Infant Transport Database
  - Facilitate improving system to benefit both referring and receiving hospitals
- Develop and manage High-Risk Infant Follow-Up Database
  - Provide risk-adjusted, 3 year outcomes, including coverage, completion and barriers to care
- Provide participating physicians the opportunity to meet the American Board of Pediatrics (ABP) Maintenance of Certification, Part 4 quality improvement requirement

Courtesy of California Perinatal Quality Care Collaborative; with permission.

Box 3
Major stakeholders who were instrumental to CPQCC's creation and serve as members of the CPQCC executive committee

- Perinatal Practitioner Organizations
  - California Association of Neonatologists
  - California Chapter Academy of Pediatrics
  - American College of Obstetricians and Gynecologists
- State of California
  - Maternal, Child, and Adolescent Health Branch
  - California Children's Services (CCS)
  - Office of Vital Records
  - Office of Statewide Health Planning and Development
- Private Organizations
  - March of Dimes
  - Pacific Business Group on Health
  - California Hospital Council
  - David and Lucile Packard Foundation
  - Vermont Oxford Network, Inc (VON)

the mission statement's goal(s) and operational approach to achieving those goals become the common ground that all of the stakeholders must agree to and value highly. Although a draft mission statement can be formulated and a rough plan of operations achieved fairly rapidly, it is critical that the individual collaborative members themselves have the freedom to hammer out and agree on who they are, the goals that they all value, and their agreed-upon path to achieving this goal, which can take several long sessions. Engaging an experienced expert in organizational development to conduct these meetings will greatly facilitate the creation of the collaborative's foundation. In business organizations, the mission statement serves to succinctly state what the enterprise is about and is often posted prominently on walls, writing tablets, computer screens, and so forth, to constantly reinforce the "who we are, what we want to achieve, and how we go about it" message. In quality improvement collaboratives, the mission statement can often be used to resolve impasses that emerge due to stakeholder differences by reminding them that they are all trying to move toward a common, highly valued, and agreed-upon goal. As CPQCC grew and developed, all stakeholders were in agreement that the mission of CPQCC was "to optimize the health and outcomes of California's pregnant women and their infants by developing a collaborative network of public and private, obstetric and neonatal providers, insurers, public health professionals and business groups to support self assessment, bench marking, and performance improvement activities for perinatal care."

In addition to a mission statement, it is important to develop an organizational philosophy, which is a set of key principles that guide the structure, operations, and growth of the Collaborative. The main features of CPQCC's organizational philosophy are that: (1) quality improvement is a worthwhile endeavor; (2) participating in the design and conduct of quality improvement initiatives is professionally rewarding;

(3) CPQCC should be a bottom-up or grass roots organization; and (4) CPQCC should strive to optimize the value that it brings to its members and its stakeholders.

OVERVIEW OF CPQCC AND ITS ORGANIZATIONAL STRUCTURE

The CPQCC is a consortium of NICUs that cares for, collects, and stores clinical data on more than 90% of all neonates who receive neonatal intensive care in California. The CPQCC was initiated in 1997 by the California Association of Neonatologists, with the goal of blending academic and private neonatology into a common body politic to partner with various private and public institutions that share the common goal of improving health care outcomes for mothers and babies in California. Building on the VON and its data system, CPQCC became the first regional application of the Vermont Oxford Neonatal Network. The organizational authority for CPQCC comes from the California Association of Neonatology (CAN) and Stanford University serves as its fiscal intermediary. Although one could consider CPQCC a grass roots, physician-based organization, such a narrow view would miss the importance of the organization as also representing a true collaborative effort of multiple key stakeholders, all of whom guide CPQCC's direction as members of its Executive Committee. Using CCS definitions, its 129 member Hospitals include 22 regional-level, 72 community-level, 25 intermediate-level, and 10 undesignated NICUs. (CCS is a state "HMS" program that sets the standards of care and outcomes for California's NICUs, provides on-site classification and monitoring, and approves payment from public payers.) In 2008, CPQCC members cared for 18,671 infants, 64% (11,994) of whom were high-morbidity infants greater than 1500 g and 36% (6677) of whom were very low birth weight (VLBW). Forty-one percent (7638) of the infants were acutely transported during the neonatal period.

Leading CPQCC's organizational structure is an Executive Committee that develops, prioritizes, and oversees the collaborative's strategic plan. An Executive Steering Committee, made up of the project Principal Investigator, Administrative Director, Data Center Director, and Director of Quality Improvement, is responsible for the collaborative's day-to-day operation as performed by 3 arms: the Data Arm, the Quality Improvement Arm, and the Research Arm.

The Executive Committee is made up of the key stakeholders (see **Box 3**). Because of the many sectors that make up neonatology in California, it was crucial that there was appropriate representation from across the state. In addition to membership of the current Chair of CAN and of the American Academy of Pediatrics (AAP), Perinatal Section, District IX, the Executive Committee (as well as all major committees) have balanced representation from Northern California, Southern California, and Academic, Private, and Medical System neonatology groups.

One of the first major decisions of the Executive Committee was to select increasing the rate of antenatal steroid (ANS) administration use as the first topic for quality improvement. A Perinatal Quality Improvement Panel was created under the Quality Improvement Arm to develop the toolkit, conduct workshops, and design the initiative. At the same time, it was felt to be essential that the Executive Committee establish a Data Release Subcommittee to develop a position with respect to public release of data that was in keeping with the collaborative's approach to quality improvement. CPQCC's fundamental position is that the goal of quality improvement is not to identify the few units that are particularly challenged, but rather to increase the performance of all the participating units. Operationally, it was believed that a successful quality improvement initiative should increase a desired outcomes mean and decrease its variation across the participating NICUs. **Fig. 3** illustrates this achievement. Because

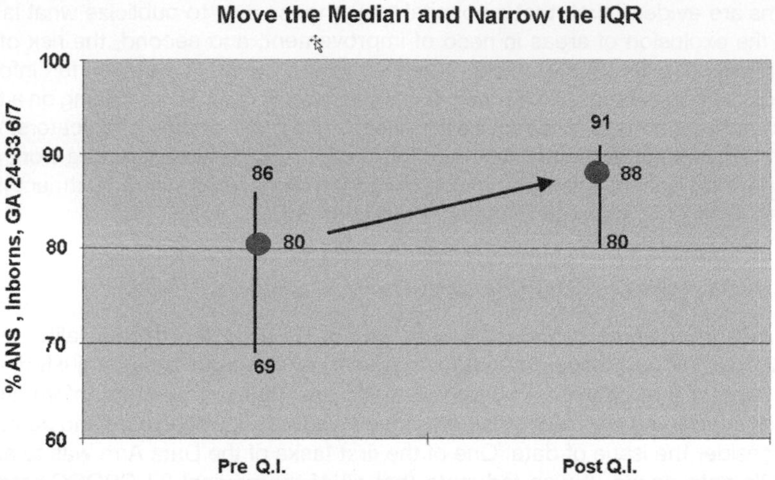

Fig. 3. The goal of the CPQCC Quality Improvement Program is to move the group's mean and reduce its variability, as is seen in the results for the Antenatal Steroid Quality Improvement Initiative. (*Courtesy of* California Perinatal Quality Care Collaborative; with permission.)

the results of this project were to be publicly released on the Pacific Business Group on Health's Web site, the Data Release Subcommittee spent a great deal of time formulating a public description of the project that would fairly portray what could be inferred from this data. It was also decided that if, after reviewing its data, a Hospital did not want it to be publicly released, this was acceptable but would be noted on the public release site. In keeping with CPQCC's fundamental position, it was decided that in any releases by the collaborative, only the names of the participating hospitals and their achievement as a group would be presented. A more complete description of this project is available.[1]

The CPQCC's approach of working together with a commitment to improving the performance of the group, rather than focusing on the identification and remediation of hospitals whose performance is below expectation, has helped to firmly establish CPQCC as a collaborative working together to improve outcomes in all members for the benefit of all of the mothers and infants across California. In keeping with this philosophy, hospitals performing below expectation are not viewed as "bad apples to be weeded out," but rather as colleagues who are challenged in a specific area of care. Operating under the perspective that only by investing in quality improvement can clinicians be assured that their patients will have access to high-quality care in the future, the role of the CPQCC is to give them the tools and support to overcome these challenges. While physicians and hospitals easily accept this position, it may not fit the agenda of consumer advocacy members who may see the value of performance reporting as a tool for smart buying rather than as a motivator and guide for quality improvement. One of the dynamics of a collaborative is to strike a balance between these two positions.

The Data Release Subcommittee also established the policy that CPQCC members were not allowed to publicly release their confidential data nor use it for marketing purposes, with violation of this rule resulting in loss of membership in the collaborative. The recent increase in the need for transparency, however, especially from hospital leadership, has once again brought the issue of public release to the forefront. Two concerns are evident: first, that a hospital may choose only to publicize what is does well to the exclusion of areas in need of improvement, and second, the risk of data being released without the background information that is needed for informed nonmedical interpretation. To address the first concern, CPQCC is working on a transparency approach that would require the release of a panel of quality indicators. When the components of the panel have been finalized, the committee will then work on an accompanying patient-oriented description of the items, their risk-adjustment limitations, and any other caveats to their interpretation.

THE QUALITY IMPROVEMENT CHALLENGE

The quality improvement challenge is threefold: (1) to collect high-quality, reliable data; (2) to transform these data into information by developing risk-adjusted, confidential reports that inform and organize work; and (3) to move from information to action by supporting perinatal providers in their work of improving care and outcomes. First, consider the issue of data. One of the first tasks of the Data Arm was to assess CPQCC's data needs. It was fortunate that all of the original 27 CPQCC members were also members of the VON, collected VLBW infant data using VON definitions/specifications, and received standard VON reports in which each NICU was compared with VON national metrics. Although the VON database was considered to adequately capture VLBW infants, it was deemed crucial that reports were created to provide comparisons and metrics that were specific to CPQCC members (the special group analysis is now a standard feature available from VON) and that collection of data on high-acuity infants of weight greater than 1500 g was begun. The CPQCC Data Committee recommended that a CPQCC Data Center be established to achieve these two goals as one of its first operational priorities. The goal was to create a portrait of each NICU's activity with respect to who was cared for, what was done for them, and how well it was done. CPQCC-specific data forms were developed that could be scanned into a computer with the resulting data tapes being sent to VON. VON was then able to produce their standard reports, while CPQCC retained the ability to produce CPQCC-specific reports. Having collected the data, the next task was to develop reports that inform and organize the work of quality improvement. CPQCC's approach was to develop an Internet-based, real-time data entry, data management, and report-on-demand information system (http://www.cpqccreport.org, logon 0000, password test to access a sample "real" report). The reports are structured so that they can be readily cut and pasted into spreadsheets for local analysis or powerpoint presentations. To increase accessibility to users who are uncomfortable with numbers, cartoon displays of one's position with respect to the interquartile range of the comparison group (**Fig. 4**) were developed. Choice of comparison groups include (1) all infants, (2) only inborn infants, and (3) only outborn infants, across: (1) all CPQCC NICUs, (2) only NICUs of the same level of care, or (3) all NICUs in any of 11 Perinatal Regions of California. All major processes and outcomes are risk adjusted and reporting is specific to the location of the event. To aid interpretation, any significant result is automatically highlighted in blue by the system.

In 2007, an Acute Infant Transport Database was developed and added to the system. The database was specifically designed to collect information that would guide 5 specific issues that had been identified by focus groups as priority areas for improvement: (1) underutilization of maternal transport, (2) delayed decision to transport, (3) difficulty in obtaining a transport, (4) too long a wait for the team to arrive, and (5) variability in transport team competency. **Fig. 5** shows the resulting 36-item transport form. Every item included on the form is essential to addressing 1 or more of the

RESPIRATORY DIAGNOSES, INTERNVENTIONS, AND OUTCOMES

All Infants 401 to 1,500 grams or 22 to 29 weeks of Gestation born between 01/01/2008 and 12/31/2008

This report is final.

California Perinatal Quality Care Collaborative (CPQCC)

CENTER ID: 0000

	Center (N = 54)			CPQCC (N Centers = 127)			Center-Network Comparison
	N	%	Last Year %	% Median	% Lower Quartile	% Upper Quartile	
Diagnoses							
Respiratory Distress Syndrome	41	75.9	68.5	74	63	85	
Meconium Aspiration Syndrome	0	0.0	0.0	0	0	0	
Pneumothorax	3	5.6	0.0	2	0	5	
Pneumothorax at This Center #	2	3.7	NA	2	0	4	
CLD - VON Def 1 *	13	39.4	28.3	25	10	39	
CLD - VON Def 2 *	13	26.0	21.3	17	7	28	
CLD - VON Def 3 *	12	26.1	22.4	17	7	29	
Interventions							
Use of Ventilation *	39	72.2	65.8	72	63	82	
Oxygen	39	100.0	97.9	100	100	100	
CPAP	28	71.8	50.0	60	31	74	
Conventional Ventilation	38	97.4	91.7	97	92	100	
HiFi Ventilation	12	30.8	41.7	28	10	42	
ECMO	0	0.0	0.0	0	0	0	
Inhaled Nitric Oxide	2	3.7	2.7	0	0	3	
Surfactant at any Time	33	61.1	61.6	66	57	77	
Supplemental Oxygen on Day 28	22	52.4	51.9	46	30	59	
Supplemental Oxygen at 36 Wks AGA	13	39.4	28.3	25	10	39	
Postnatal Steroids	9	16.7	15.1	11	3	19	
Chronic Lung Disease (CLD)	3	33.3	0.0	33	8	56	
Extubation	4	44.4	0.0	20	0	44	
Blood Pressure	5	55.6	90.9	48	11	62	
Other Reason	0	0.0	18.2	0	0	11	
Steroids for CLD - VON Def 1 *	2	15.4	0.0	13	0	28	
Steroids for CLD - VON Def 2 *	2	15.4	0.0	13	0	25	
Steroids for CLD - VON Def 3 *	2	16.7	0.0	13	0	25	
Outcomes							
Discharged Home	40	74.1	72.6	72	60	83	
... on Oxygen	6	15.0	5.7	9	0	16	
... on Apnea or Cardio Respiratory Monitor	6	15.0	9.4	10	2	20	
... on Mechanical Suction Device	1	2.5	0.0	0	0	3	
... Home on Other Respiratory Support Device	0	0.0	0.0	0	0	0	
Transferred to Other Hospital	13	24.1	11.0	26	15	42	
... on Oxygen	7	53.8	75.0	60	35	83	
... on Apnea or Cardio Respiratory Monitor	9	69.2	87.5	83	50	100	
... on Mechanical Suction Device	4	30.8	50.0	40	12	67	
... on Other Respiratory Support Device	1	8.3	0.0	0	0	10	
Died	4	7.4	16.4	7	2	11	

Fig. 4. Example of CPQCC data report with cartoons showing the NICU's position on the networks interquartile range. (*Courtesy of* California Perinatal Quality Care Collaborative; with permission.)

5 priority issues identified. In 2008, data was collected on more than 7000 acute neonatal transports.

Beginning in 2009, CPQCC instituted a Quality Improvement Database for California's statewide High-Risk Infant Follow-up program. The program follows high-risk infants from 28 days until age 3 years and will provide important outcome data for the NICUs that cared for these infants. In addition to long-term neurodevelopmental outcomes and autism screening, the database will assess rates of successful enrollment and program completion, as well as the medical and social needs of these infants and the extent to which they have been met at the individual program, regional, and state level.

CORE CPeTS ACUTE INTER-FACILITY- NEONATAL TRANSPORT FORM - 2009

REFERRAL		
C.1 Transport type ☐ Requested Delivery Attendance ☐ Emergent ☐ Urgent ☐ Scheduled ☐ Other		
C.2 Indication ☐ Medical Services ☐ Surgery ☐ Insurance ☐ Bed Availability		
PATIENT IDENTIFICATION/HISTORY:		
C.3 Birth weight ___ ___ ___ ___ grams **C.4** Gestational Age ___ ___weeks___ days **C.5** ☐ Male ☐ Female ☐ Unknown		
C.6 Prenatally Diagnosed Congenital Anomalies ☐ Yes ☐ No ☐ Unknown Describe:		
C.7 Maternal Gravida	**C. 8** Steroids ☐ Yes ☐ No ☐ Unknown	
C.9 Surfactant Given ☐ Yes ☐ No ☐ Unknown ☐ Delivery Room ☐ Nursery		
TIME SEQUENCE	**Date**	**Time**
C.10 Maternal Admission to Perinatal Unit or Labor & Delivery		
C.11 Last Antenatal Steroid Administration (last dose)		
C.12 Infant Birth		
C.13 Surfactant (first dose)		
C.14 Referral (and Referring Hospital Evaluation)		
C.15 Acceptance		
C.16 Transport Team Departure from Transport Team Office/NICU for Referring Hospital		
C.17 Arrival of Team at Referring Hospital/Patient Bedside and Initial Transport Evaluation		
C.18 Initial Transport Team Evaluation		
C.19 Arrival at Receiving NICU and Initial Evaluation		

INFANT CONDITION				**REFERRAL PROCESS**
Modified TRIPS Score: to be recorded on referral, within 15 minutes of arrival at referring hospital and admit to NICU.				**C.30** Referring Hospital Name
	Referral	Initial Transport	NICU Admit	**C.31** Previously Transported? ☐ Yes ☐ No From:
Time (24 hour)	**C.14**	**C.18**	**C.19**	**C.32** Birth Hospital Name
C.20 Responsiveness✪				**C.33** Transport Team On-Site Leader ☐ Sub-specialist Physician ☐ Pediatrician ☐ Other Physician/Resident ☐ Neonatal Nurse Practitioner ☐ Transport Specialist ☐ Nurse
C.21 Temperature C°				
C.22 Heart Rate				**C.34** Team From ☐ Receiving Hospital ☐ Referring Hospital ☐ Contract Service
C.23 Respiratory Rate				
C.24 Oxygen Saturation				**C.35** Mode ☐ Ground ☐ Helicopter ☐ Fixed Wing
C.25 Respiratory Status✱				Death ☐ No ☐ Yes ☐ Prior to Team Arrival ☐ Prior to Departure from Referring Hospital ☐ Prior to Arrival at Receiving NICU
C.26 FiO_2				**For all deaths prior to Receiving NICU admission fax form to the Data Center at (650) 721-5751.**
C.27 Respiratory Support ☈				Comments
C.28 Blood Pressure Systolic/ Diastolic, Mean				
C.29 Pressors	☐Y ☐N	☐Y ☐N	☐Y ☐N	RN Signature
✪Responsiveness: 0=Death 1=None, Seizure, Muscle Relaxant 2=Lethargic, no cry 3=Vigorously withdraws, cry ✱Respiratory Status: 1=Respirator 2= Severe (apnea, gasping, intubated but not on respirator) 3=Other ☈Respiratory Support: 0 = None, 1 = Hood/Nasal Cannula. 2 = Nasal Continuous Positive Airway Pressure, 3 = Endotracheal Tube				Patient Identification Stamp

Fig. 5. Acute neonatal transport form. (*Courtesy of* California Perinatal Quality Care Collaborative; with permission.)

An important goal of the CPQCC data system is to provide information that can guide quality improvement activities at both the community and hospital level. To this end, with the sponsorship of the California March of Dimes, CPQCC has developed an All-California, Perinatal Data Resource that links the NICU clinical data with birth certificate, census, and infant and maternal hospital administrative discharge data. The dataset's first projects include: (1) the identification of communities whose qualifying mothers have lower than expected ANS rates, and (2) the identification of geographic areas whose mothers have higher than expected elective early term deliveries. As regional collaboratives emerge, the linking of NICU data to local databases will be an important feature and will play a critical role in the development of coordinated community-hospital quality improvement initiatives.

The databases described here allow a region and its individual member NICUs to assess and prioritize potential areas for quality improvement. In addition they can be used to assess, in a global sense, the gains made as a result of a quality improvement initiative and, of major importance, the extent to which these gains are being maintained over time. Although accurate data are essential, these functions may not require high levels of granularity. Experience has shown that the selection, recording, and careful analysis of key process, outcomes, and balancing measures require the construction of a project-specific database, report structures (control charts), and metrics (such as time since last event) that are uniquely sensitive to tracking changes over short periods of time. However, an important step in the evolution of regional databases will be to identify those items that will facilitate tracking and maintenance of quality improvement gains, and incorporate these items into the core NICU database.

How one assures data quality remains an important issue. Initially, on-site data audits were conducted. While these were very informative, the time and expense made them prohibitive. A possible consideration for the future is a directed self-audit in which, following a data entry session, a few important items are asked to be reentered for confirmation. At present, the CPQCC employs logic and range checks at the time of data entry, as well as obtaining confirmation of records that exceed a threshold for missing or unobtainable items. Using a linked patient dataset, the consistency of items when an infant is transferred across member NICUs is also tracked. However, CPQCC's major strategy is to address the needs of the data abstractors. The Data Contact Advisory Committee was one of CPQCC's first committees, considered essential to any regional collaborative. This committee is made up of data abstractors from a wide range of data settings, from the night nurse who abstracts and enters data between his or her various clinical duties to staff whose sole job is data abstraction and entry. The Data Center Advisory Committee reviews and must approve all data manuals for clarity of definition, all data items for ease of abstraction, and all data entry screens and forms for ease of completion before implementation. Their input and final approval is essential because some items that neonatologists believe are readily available and clearly defined may be very difficult to abstract. A key CPQCC strategy has been to address the data quality horse before it leaves the barn. To this end, it conducts annual training for data abstractors throughout California. In 2009, 4 data training sessions representing 103 hospitals and including 156 participants were held. Though labor intensive, these meetings are an effective way to promote data quality.

QUALITY IMPROVEMENT

The Perinatal Quality Improvement Panel (PQIP) is a permanent subcommittee that began with the inception of CPQCC in 1997. Its aim is to support perinatal providers in California in their efforts to continuously improve perinatal outcomes and neonatal care. Important to PQIP's success is its membership and their commitment. The panel is made up of neonatologists, maternal fetal medicine specialists, epidemiologists, and representatives from the CA-MCH, CCS, and Regional Perinatal Programs of California (RPPC). PQIP members volunteer their time and expertise to analyze CPQCC data, review current, relevant publications, and address local and national priority areas for quality improvement. Using this information, PQIP defines indicators and benchmarks, recommends quality improvement objectives, provides models for performance improvement, and assists providers in a multistep transformation of data into improved patient care. PQIP's approach is to create, initiate, and complete quality and research projects through the evaluation and application of evidence based care.

A major challenge confronting any quality improvement organization is how to address the needs of all the NICUs in one's region. Two issues arise: (1) developing an approach that would be accessible to the large number of sites within the region, and (2) aligning regional quality improvement priorities with those of the individual member hospitals. Initially, PQIP developed an inventory of toolkits addressing topics that were selected as being of high priority and supported these toolkits with academic presentations, workshops, and webcasts. This approach was extremely effective in building across California's NICUs what Jeffery Horbar of VON refers to as the "Habit for Change." Each year, CPQCC rolled out 1 to 2 toolkits at the yearly CAN meeting. This highly attended meeting provided the venue for presenting the academic findings and rationale for the improvement topic as plenary presentations, often by highly visible, nationally recognized experts. On a pré-meeting day, workshops were conducted that included a review of pre-workshop evaluations and mini root cause analyses. Participants included teams from the NICUs who brought completed pre-workshop analyses with them. The workshops addressed aspects of quality improvement with formal presentations, as well as discussions of root causes and approaches to overcoming them. The toolkits were very extensive, addressing fundamentals of quality improvement, potential best practices, the rationales supporting these best practices, typical root causes, and possible solutions. The workshop was followed up with a combination of workshops and webcasts. These toolkits are freely available (http://www.cpqcc.org) and include Antenatal Steroids Administration, Postnatal Steroids, Hospital Acquired Infection Prevention, Improving Initial Lung Function, Nutritional Support of the VLBW Infant, Perinatal Group B Streptococcus Prevention, Hyperbilirubinemia Prevention, Perinatal HIV Prevention, Delivery Room Management of the VLBW Infant, and Late Preterm Infant Management. Although it is clear that several of these initiatives have been effective in improving outcomes in participating units,[1,2] the success of this approach in involving a major segment of the 129 member hospitals, or in effectively meeting their various quality improvement needs, is as yet uncertain.

Beginning in 2007, an evaluation and restructuring of PQIP's functions and responsibilities was undertaken, and PQIP activities were broadened to include 4 foci: Quality Improvement Infrastructure, Education, Analysis, and Research. The skill set requirements for each focus has been identified and additional recruitment among clinicians and stakeholders is under way. During this time, the overall effectiveness of the standard "Toolkit-Workshop" approach to implementing quality improvement strategies was also called into question. Although early initiatives did not have an integrated evaluation component and had demonstrated some success with toolkit/workshops, the "community of learning" approach developed by the Institute for Healthcare Improvement (IHI) was emerging as not only highly effective but also suitable for statewide initiatives.[3] This model, with its emphasis on the control chart and monthly reporting of process, outcome, and balancing measures, also meets the American Board of Pediatrics (ABP) Maintenance of Certification, Part 4 requirements. CPQCC's first experience with this model was as a supporting partner in a collaborative to reduce catheter-related infections that eventually enrolled all of the Regional NICUs in California (see the article by Powers and Wirtschafter elsewhere in this issue). This collaboration, led by CCS and the California Children's Hospital Association, began in late 2006 and was extremely successful, lending further support to PQIP's decision to move from the "Toolkit-Workshop" approach to the IHI "Community of Change" approach. The first CPQCC-sponsored initiative using the IHI approach addressed health care associated infections (HAI), with the aim of decreasing catheter-associated blood stream infection (CABSI) rates by 25% to 50% in participating California, community-level NICUs. Between the baseline (September 1, 2007 through February 29, 2008) and intervention (March 1, 2008 through December 31, 2008), crude CABSI rates decreased by 56.1%. CPQCC's second collaborative, Breast Milk Nutrition, is currently under way with the goal of increasing the percentage of infants born at birth weights less than 1500 g who receive breast milk at discharge. In addition to the standard 3 learning sessions, collaborative members participate in monthly conference calls, which include data reports and strategy sessions, as well as a "Hold the Gains" meeting scheduled 6 to 8 months after the third (final) learning session. During all of these sessions, member hospitals participate in a free exchange of ideas, share strategies that have worked to overcome obstacles (which minimizes duplication of effort by each NICU to rediscover an effective solution), and experience the incentive of tacit competition. Unlike the open-ended, multiple strategies, toolkit approach, the IHI model uses an agreed-upon change bundle.

Even with the commitment to roll out an IHI-style collaborative every 18 months, there remains the formidable challenge of how to facilitate quality improvement at the individual hospital level in a way that is effective, documented, and qualifies participants for ABP recognition. As a result, CPQCC has begun developing a "QI-Lite" approach. In this context, "Lite" refers to the extent of the operational input from CPQCC during the course of the NICU's quality improvement project, not to the extent of the NICU's Quality Improvement commitment or activity. This approach will be more directed then previous Toolkit-Workshop strategies in that it will specify: (1) the elements that could be incorporated into a change bundle, (2) a selection of candidate outcome, process, and balancing measures, and (3) basic control chart and reporting templates. To meet the ABP requirements of participating in a valid and effective initiative, "QI-Lite" will also require a quality improvement mentor approved by CPQCC and a final report from the NICU that includes the monthly outcome, process, and balancing measures. Over the next year, the CPQCC plans to establish "QI-Lite" as a robust quality improvement support structure for California NICUs unable to participate in the current CPQCC regional quality improvement initiative due to a variety of potential reasons (their need to address a "local" higher priority quality improvement topic, the timing of the regional initiative, or the cost of participating in the CPQCC-sponsored IHI initiative, which currently ranges from $5000 to $7000 per project).

RESEARCH

Because the main activities of the CPQCC over the last decade have been focused on building the collaborative and conducting quality improvement initiatives, research has not been a major priority. Moving forward, the goal is to build the research base in the areas of epidemiology/health services research and quality improvement science. One of several CPQCC databases, the All-California Perinatal Quality Improvement Data Resource, links an infant's (1) maternal residential, sociodemographic, census data; (2) birth certificate data; (3) acute infant transport data; (4) NICU clinical data; (5) maternal and infant hospital charges and ICD9 data; and (6) high-risk infant follow-up data to age 3 years, providing a strong foundation for research. This dataset has been used to investigate the extent of postnatal steroid use,[4] the relationship between hypothermia (as defined by the World Health Organization) and neonatal mortality and morbidity,[5] and an analysis of the characteristics, morbidity, and mortality of high-acuity, non-VLBW, NICU admissions.[6] Studies investigating (1) the strength of relationship between NICU measures of process and outcome, (2) the geographic distribution of antenatal steroid use, (3) the rate and characteristics of infants discharged home who are readmitted for exchange transfusion or bilirubin greater than 25 mg/dL, and (4) an analysis of the medical and social needs of high-risk follow-up infants at the time of their first follow-up visit are being actively pursued.

The CPQCC quality improvement science research agenda is still in the formative stage. In general, members have been pleased with the effectiveness and efficiency of the IHI model, especially with respect to the free exchange of ideas on overcoming obstacles, minimizing duplication, and the motivation provided by the structure's "tacit competition." A formal evaluation component has been built into these initiatives with the hope of identifying best approaches that could be formally tested in the future. While it is clear that the IHI approach is extremely effective over its initiation period, developing effective approaches to hold these gains will be a high priority research goal for CPQCC.

ON COLLABORATION

In this brief review the author has tried to present a picture of the aspirations, workings, and achievements of CPQCC, a regional collaboration to improve perinatal care. While it is never easy to align the often differing fundamental positions held by the various member factions and stakeholder groups, the common overarching goal of a universally agreed-upon mission statement can act as a magnet drawing the various components together. Moreover, rapid development of a first quality improvement initiative is an effective strategy to engage the participants in a way that allows them to demonstrate, share, and build on their individual expertise, and provides them a strong sense of professional accomplishment. The success of one's first regional quality improvement initiative will not be recognized as solely the success of the participating NICUs, but as the success of all those who have contributed to creating, maintaining, and building the collaborative. Successful collaboration, while never easy, builds on itself.

REFERENCES

1. Wirtschafter DD, Danielson BH, Main EK, et al. Promoting antenatal steroid use for fetal maturation—results from the California Perinatal Quality Care Collaborative (CPQCC). J Pediatr 2006;148(5):606–12.
2. Wirtschafter DD, Powers RJ. Organizing regional perinatal quality improvement: global considerations and local implementation. NeoReviews 2004;5:e50.
3. Pronovost P, Needham D, Berenholtz S, et al. An intervention to decrease catheter-related bloodstream infections in the ICU. N Engl J Med 2006;355:2725–32.
4. Finer NN, Powers RJ, Ou CS, et al. Prospective evaluation of postnatal steroid administration—a one year experience from the California Perinatal Quality Care Collaborative. Pediatrics 2006;117(3):704–13.
5. Miller S, Lee HC, Gould JB. Hypothermia in very low birth weight infants—incidence and risk factors. 2007 Pediatric Academic Societies' Meeting. Toronto, Ontario, May 5–8, 2007. PAS 2007:6280.31.
6. Zlotnik PJ, Palmon M, Gould JB. Attributes of high acuity infants greater than 1500 grams admitted to NICU. Poster presentation at the 2006 Pediatric Academic Societies' Annual Meeting in San Francisco, CA, April 29 to May 2, 2006.

A Primer on Quality Improvement Methodology in Neonatology

Dan L. Ellsbury, MD*, Robert Ursprung, MD, MMSc

KEYWORDS

• Change • Model for Improvement • NICU
• Quality improvement

This article provides a pragmatic approach to quality improvement (QI) in the neonatal intensive care unit (NICU) setting. The "model for improvement," as described by Langley and coworkers[1] and heavily used by the Institute for Healthcare Improvement, serves as the foundation for the approach. The model for improvement is based on three core questions, followed by cycles of testing: What is one trying to accomplish? How will one know that a change represents an improvement? What changes can be made that will result in continuous improvement?

In the practical use of the model for improvement, the authors have found it useful to modify it in the format of "seven questions to consider when designing a QI project."

1. Which problem should one select?
2. Who will be on the project team?
3. What is the goal?
4. What will one measure?
5. How will one analyze the measurements?
6. What changes will one make to create an improvement?
7. How will one test the changes?

This format can serve as a template for virtually any QI project. In the remainder of this article these questions are reviewed in detail and specific examples are provided to highlight the practical use of this methodology.

WHICH PROBLEM SHOULD ONE SELECT?

To start, review the NICU's outcome data, focusing on mortality and the morbidities most commonly encountered in the NICU. In addition to standard NICU databases

Center for Research, Education, and Quality, Pediatrix Medical Group, 1301 Concord Terrace, Sunrise, FL 33323, USA
* Corresponding author.
E-mail address: dan_ellsbury@pediatrix.com

Clin Perinatol 37 (2010) 87–99
doi:10.1016/j.clp.2010.01.005 perinatology.theclinics.com

(eg, Pediatrix Medical Group, Vermont Oxford Network, California Perinatal Quality Care Collaborative), many hospitals collect a variety of data on nosocomial infections, breast-feeding, mortality, length of stay, and other outcomes. When possible, benchmark the center's outcomes to both a national data set and to your own center's historical outcomes. If available, compare your center's outcomes with other centers providing the same level of care (eg, a level II NICU should compare outcomes with other level II NICUs and avoid comparisons with level IIIC NICUs).[2] Identify a problem area for your center that is clinically important and amenable to modification.[3] Modifiable problems characteristically demonstrate large center-to-center variability, and are responsive to current evidence-based interventions.

An Example of a Good Project

As an example, consider reducing catheter-associated bloodstream infection (CABSI). On review of data one notes the baseline CABSI rate is fairly high compared with network data and has not been improving. CABSIs are clinically very important and are modifiable by improvements in the process of inserting and maintaining central lines. This is an excellent project for a QI team to pursue.

An Example of a Poor Project

Another example is reducing periventricular leukomalacia (PVL). A review of the center's baseline PVL rate shows it is low compared with network benchmarks. Of note, there seems to be little numerical difference between the best and worst performing network NICUs. Although PVL is clinically important, the incidence in the center is relatively low, and there are few evidence-based interventions available to impact its incidence. Essentially, PVL does not seem to be a major problem in this NICU, and one cannot do much beyond standard clinical care to reduce it. As a result, PVL is a poor project for most QI teams to pursue.

WHO SHOULD BE ON THE PROJECT TEAM?

NICU care involves a large number of personnel who interact with an infant in a variety of ways; the sine qua non of an effective QI team is its multidisciplinary composition. The specific make-up of the team depends on the project and the goals for success. Ideally, teams should be of modest size, approximately 5 to 7 people, to facilitate communication and promote "ownership" of the project. Smaller teams may not be sufficiently multidisciplinary, nor have enough people to carry out the work. Too large a team can make it difficult to keep all members effectively involved.[4,5] Different problems require different team compositions. Three elements should be considered when selecting the QI team: system leadership, clinical technical expertise, and day-to-day leadership.

System Leadership

At least one individual should have enough authority to affect changes in the specific target area. It is difficult to improve if the team does not have the authoritative leadership to implement change.

Clinical Technical Expertise

Include people who have expert knowledge of the key processes involved in the project. Lack of knowledge regarding key project processes may result in faulty analysis and flawed improvement approaches. Include personnel with basic QI training to keep the team focused while following standard QI methodology.

Day-To-Day Leadership: Project Champion

Every project needs a spark. It is critical to include a team member who drives the day-to-day progress of the project. Often this person is someone who is highly invested in the targeted outcome. The enthusiasm and momentum that this "project champion" brings to the team is crucial. Many projects do not get past the talking stage without this type of person on the team.[6]

Team Flexibility

Each team should be constructed to fit the specific problem. If specialized information is needed for certain aspects of a project, ad hoc committees can be added and used in a focused fashion. A common ad hoc group is a parent committee or council that can be consulted for a family perspective on various issues on various projects.

EXAMPLES OF EFFECTIVE TEAM COMPOSITION

Project: Improving Nasal Continuous Positive Airway Pressure Use to Decrease Bronchopulmonary Dysplasia

The QI team might include a respiratory therapist, physician, nurse practitioner, nurse, and nurse educator. The team would have the background and authority to introduce new equipment and expertise to train the NICU staff.

Project: Reducing Medication Errors by Use of Standardized Order Sets

The QI team might include a physician, nurse practitioner, pharmacist, information technology specialist, and nurse. This team composition would provide the background and authority to develop and introduce new standardized order sets.

What is the Goal?

The QI project team must write a goal statement. To be useful, the goal statement should be realistic and specific, and include numerical targets for specific measures. Further, the goal statement should include a time frame for the project. Without a clear goal, teamwork may be impaired. Many projects are plagued by goals that are too optimistic and vaguely defined.[1,5]

Examples of goal definition

The goal statement "we will eliminate bronchopulmonary dysplasia (BPD)" lacks a timeline and is neither specific nor tangible. This approach sets the team up for failure. The following goal statement is clear, specific, and realistic: "through the improved use of continuous positive airway pressure, we will decrease BPD, as defined as a room air oxygen saturation of less than 90% at 36 weeks postmenstrual age, in babies less than 1500 g, from our baseline of 40% to 30% within 9 months."

What Will One Measure?

Measurement for QI is often misunderstood. Many individuals desire to implement research measurement methodology in their QI projects. This concept is understandable, because most neonatologists have participated in research at some point in their careers and read the research literature on a regular basis. Unfortunately, this bias can slow improvement, waste resources, and cause confusion when developing measures for QI projects.

Key point: QI is not clinical research

Measurement for QI is different from measurement for clinical research. QI typically is focused on the implementation of current knowledge, not the creation of new knowledge. QI uses sequential small tests, is not blinded, is not randomized, and uses a small set of measures for multiple short cycles of change (**Table 1**).[7] Measurement for QI is ideally built around data that are already being collected at the facility.

Additional measurement may be appropriate for some projects, but it should be kept to a minimum because extra resources are rarely available to enable extensive data collection. "Measurement burden" is a major impediment to productive QI. Years can be spent acquiring consensus on measures and seeking funding to hire data abstractors and create databases. The time, energy, and resources that could have been spent using simple and available measures for effective improvement activities are wasted, with little or no demonstrated patient improvement.[3,5]

Key point: measurement is not a substitute for doing QI

The mere possession of outcome measures for the NICU does not improve quality. Many NICUs have access to detailed outcome reports containing risk-adjusted clinical outcomes. Unfortunately, this knowledge is often not acted on to facilitate improvement.

Three types of measures are commonly used in QI projects: (1) outcome, (2) process, and (3) balancing.[1] Outcome measures refers to the primary outcome of the project, the indicator that changes have resulted in improvement. It may sometimes be viewed as the long-term outcome. An example is that in a project focused on reducing BPD, the BPD rate is the primary outcome measure.

Process measures are those that indicate if one has successfully made the desired changes in a targeted process; they may be considered the short-term measures of the success of a project. An example is that in a BPD reduction project, if the interventions planned included use of prophylactic surfactant and vitamin A, then the process measures might include the rates of prophylactic surfactant and vitamin A usage.

Balancing measures are those that indicate if other parts of the system have been disrupted by the changes (adverse effects). These measures are often difficult to define. In general, surveillance of all of the basic morbidities is sufficient to observe for unintended consequences. Sometimes specific adverse effects can be anticipated. An example is that in a project focused on improving growth by early and aggressive enteral feeding and maximized and prolonged use of parenteral nutrition, the rates of necrotizing enterocolitis and CABSIs are reasonable potential balancing measures.

Whenever a measure is considered for a QI project, it is important to create a "standard operational definition" of the measure. The definition is a clear, quantifiable description of what the measure is and how it is measured. Seemingly subtle

Table 1
Contrast between measurement for improvement and measurement for research[a]

	Measurement for Improvement	Measurement for Research
Purpose	Implement current knowledge	Discover new knowledge
Tests	Sequential small observational tests	One tightly controlled test
Biases	Try to stabilize bias from test to test	Maximally controlled
Data	Gather "just enough" data to learn from	Gather "as much data as possible"
Duration	Multiple short test cycles	Months or years

[a] Measurement for improvement is pragmatic and focused on implementation of current knowledge. In contrast, measurement for research is tightly controlled and intended for the discovery of new knowledge.

alterations in definitions can have a dramatic impact on the measurement.[1,3,5,8] An example is where mortality is defined as the death of any baby less than 1500 g. Compare this with the example where mortality is defined as the death of any baby with a birth weight of less than 1500 g, limited to inborn infants, who receive nonpalliative care. The mortality calculation is then the deaths of infants who meet this criteria divided by all infants with this criteria, during a specific time interval, as gathered from the NICU admission log.

How Will One Analyze the Measurements?

NICU outcome data often report yearly rates (eg, BPD rate of 25% in 2008, necrotizing enterocolitis rate of 6% in 2008). These annualized data, although useful in providing a perspective on performance relative to other NICUs, are best used as "judgment data." They can help answer the questions "Do we have a problem?" and "How big is the problem?" Unfortunately, annualized data do not provide timely feedback for doing improvement work. Trends within the data can be hidden, leading to false interpretations of the data (**Figs. 1–3**). Additionally, many process measures (central line insertion bundle compliance, hand hygiene, oximeter alarm audits, and so forth) are not routinely collected for standard neonatal databases.

Dynamic data displays, such as run charts, provide immediate feedback on measures and are simple to construct. The measurement is plotted on the y-axis, and the date on the x-axis. Annotations can be made to the run chart to identify when specific changes were made, allowing temporal correlation between interventions and changes in the measure (**Fig. 4**). Simple run chart interpretation rules allow useful extraction of information from the charts, and can be productively used for most QI work. If enough data points are available (>20), additional analysis may be pursued by the use of statistical process control charts (discussed elsewhere in this issue).[1,3,5,9–12]

What Changes Will One Make to Create an Improvement?

Deciding what changes to make to create an improvement can be a challenging task. Once a specific outcome is targeted for improvement, the first step is an evidence-based review of the interventions that are currently available to improve the outcome. Often, this aspect of the project is very simple; the interventions are well known for many common problems. The more important question then becomes, "How do we effectively implement these strategies in our center?"

As an example, there is general consensus in the neonatology community that breast milk is the optimal nutrition for premature infants. Its use is associated with improved neurodevelopmental outcome and a reduced incidence of necrotizing enterocolitis and nosocomial infections.[13] Despite this knowledge, less than half of very low birth weight infants are receiving breast milk at the time of discharge from the NICU, and many never receive any breast milk. The problem is not "the knowing" what is right; the problem is "the doing" of what is right.

How can this knowing-doing gap be bridged? How can one successfully implement evidence-based therapies to improve outcomes for patients? Answering this question requires an understanding of the complex adaptive system of the NICU. Each NICU is unique, with its own history, culture, and workflow.[5]

A useful early step for many QI projects is to determine the attitudes and beliefs of the staff regarding the therapies of interest. Surveys provide an important initial step in assessing "knowledge gaps" in the NICU. Educational efforts that address these gaps are an effective and important part of QI project implementation. An example is a breast milk survey. A survey of the NICU staff regarding breast milk use may reveal

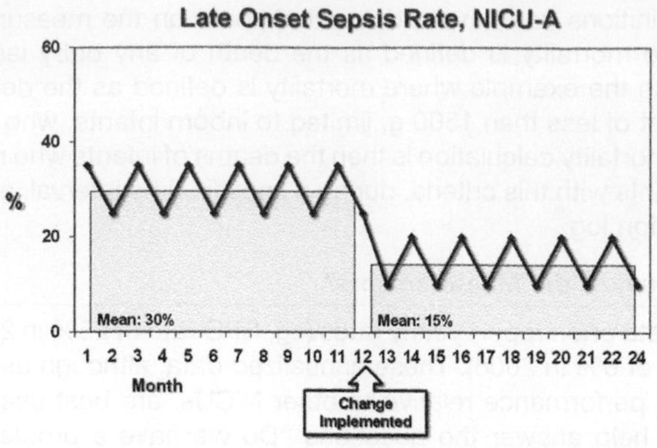

Fig. 1. Stable rate of late-onset sepsis in the first year. Following implementation of the change the rate decreased in the second year. Yearly data are representative of the monthly trends.

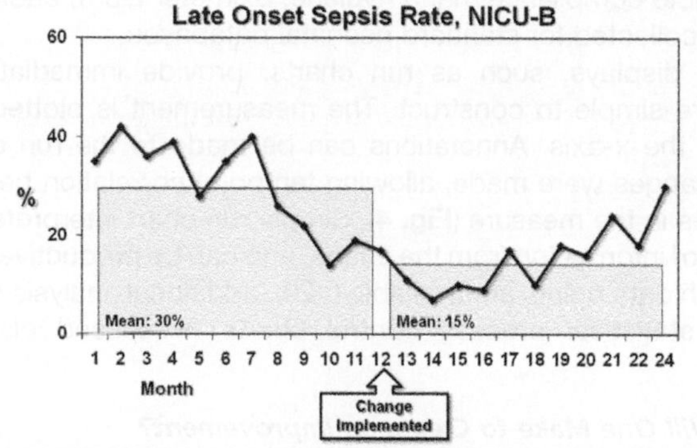

Fig. 2. Sepsis rate decreased in the first year. Following implementation of the change, the rate decreased slightly, then increased in the second year. The change may have worsened the outcome. Despite the mean rate for the second year being half the first year, the monthly trend is showing worsening sepsis rates. Yearly data alone miss this important trend.

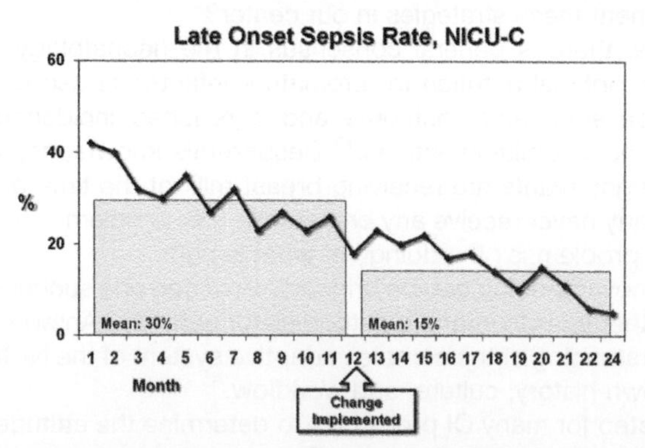

Fig. 3. Sepsis rate decreased steadily in the first year. Following implementation of the change, the rate continued to steadily decrease. It is unclear if the change was effective, because the outcome was already improving, and continued to improve after the change. Yearly data, used alone, could lead to an overestimation of the effectiveness of the change.

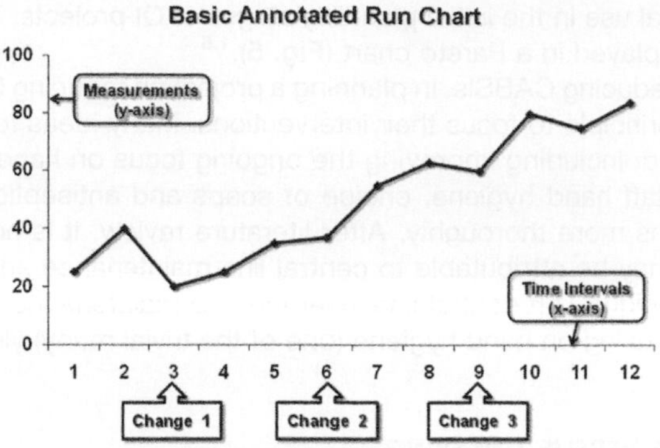

Fig. 4. To construct an annotated run chart, plot the date on the x-axis and the measurement on the y-axis. When changes are implemented, annotate the chart to enable a temporal link between changes and measurement.

that the staff generally views breast milk and formula as equivalent and they fear "making moms feel guilty" if they push mothers toward providing breast milk. If this thinking is common among the NICU staff, it is very difficult to improve breast milk use. Use of the survey enables targeted educational intervention to address the knowledge gaps that contribute to low breast milk usage rates.

PROCESS MAPPING

Another very useful technique is process mapping. Process maps (flow charts) are graphic representations of a series of steps that define a process. These maps are very useful for clarifying how a process works and identifying "leverage points," critical points in the process where change or standardization may lead to improvement.

Process maps require participation of individuals who know the process in detail. The mapping may initially be done at a macro level, with a detailed "drill down" into the specifics as needed. Often, as teams attempt to create a process map, they discover there is not a defined process in the unit. Each staff member "does his or her own thing." Some degree of standardization of process may be the primary intervention needed.[1,5]

An example is improving the rate of prophylactic surfactant administration. The project team, composed of individuals who commonly attend deliveries, creates a process map for delivery room administration of surfactant. They find that the team has clear criteria for surfactant administration and the needed equipment is generally available. The current process, however, requires that surfactant must be ordered from the pharmacy before the delivery. Often the time of delivery cannot be predicted or anticipated, resulting in delays in surfactant availability. This rate-limiting step in providing surfactant was identified through the process map and was resolved by establishing a small ward stock of surfactant that is immediately available when needed.

PARETO CHARTS

The Pareto principle (also known as the "80–20 rule") states that, for many events, roughly 80% of the effects come from 20% of the causes. Identifying and targeting the "vital few" causes rather than the "trivial many" causes of a problem is of enormous practical use in the initial planning stages of QI projects. This concept can be graphically displayed in a Pareto chart (**Fig. 5**).[1,5]

An example is reducing CABSIs. In planning a project on reducing CABSIs, the team uses the Pareto principle to focus their interventions. Many ideas for reducing infections are proposed, including improving the ongoing focus on hand hygiene for visitors, improving staff hand hygiene, choice of soaps and antiseptic hand rubs, and cleaning the rooms more thoroughly. After literature review, it is noted that 67% of these infections may be attributable to central line maintenance and 20% to central line insertion technique.[14] If central line insertion and maintenance (the vital few) are not optimized, focusing on hand hygiene (one of the trivial many) yields little benefit.

SYSTEM CHANGES VERSUS TINKERING

Two general categories of change are "tinkering" and "system change." Tinkering (also known as "first-order change") generally refers to simple changes that are focused on individuals "trying harder" or "being more careful." These effort-based changes are unlikely to yield significant or sustained improvement. System change (also known as "second-order change") refers to redesign of the system to always produce the desired outcome. Additional individual effort is generally not required. Over time, system changes are more likely to yield meaningful, sustained improvements in the desired outcome.[1]

An example is poor handwriting of medication orders resulting in medication errors. Tinkering is to encourage physicians to write more legibly. A system change is to use preprinted order sheets to minimize the amount of handwriting necessary. Alternatively, one could introduce a computerized physician order entry system.

CHANGE CONCEPTS

Change concepts are general ideas or approaches to change that have been useful in a variety of settings to improve system design and create improvements. Examples of change concepts include using affordances, decreasing handoffs, removing bottlenecks, standardization, eliminating multiple entries, removing intermediaries, and using checklists.[1,5]

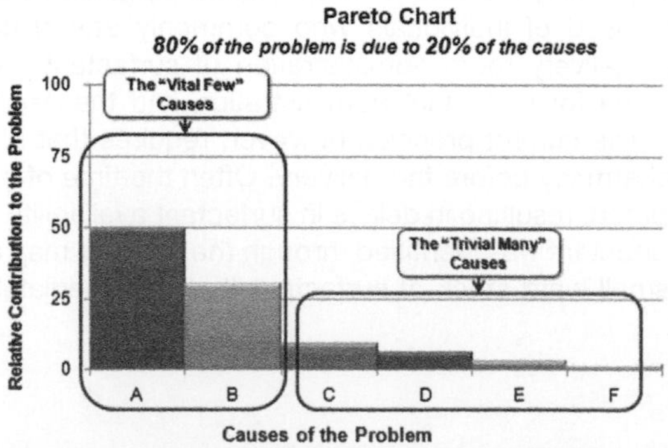

Fig. 5. The Pareto chart is used to evaluate the relative contribution of various causes for a problem. Quality improvement efforts can then be focused on the "vital few" causes of the problem, without wasting energy and resources on the "trivial many" causes.

Example: Checklists

A simple and very effective change concept is use of a checklist (**Box 1**). A central line insertion checklist provides a simple list of key elements of appropriate central line insertion. An observer monitoring the insertion of the central line uses the checklist to ensure that all of the appropriate components are successfully performed during the procedure. If a deviation occurs, the observer halts the procedure until the problem is corrected. This simple change concept has been widely and successfully used to decrease central line infections.[15,16]

CHANGE PACKAGES

Change packages are groups of interventions or implementation techniques that can be used together to improve an outcome. These templates or toolkits provide a useful starting point for many QI projects and build on the successes others have achieved with their own projects.[1,5]

BUNDLES

A QI bundle is a collection of interventions that when used together improve an outcome. The key phrase in this case is "when used together." The bundle should be viewed as one intervention with several synergistic components. A very common error that is made is the implementation of some aspects of the bundle, but not all of them, resulting in suboptimal improvement.[17]

An example is that the central line checklist described previously contains the elements of the central line insertion bundle (**Table 2**). A decision to use all of the elements, except the use of sterile gloves, renders the rest of the bundle useless.

How Will One Test Changes?

All improvement requires making changes, but not all changes result in improvement. Changes must be tested in the actual environment of the individual NICU, regardless

Box 1
A representative central line insertion checklist

The checklist should be completed by an observer, not the person performing the insertion.

Before the procedure, did the inserter

Yes No* Perform hand hygiene before the procedure?

Yes No* Put on a cap, mask, sterile gown and sterile gloves?

Yes No* Prepare the insertion site per protocol?

Yes No* Cover the patient and procedural field with a large sterile drape?

During the procedure

Yes No* Was a sterile field maintained at all times?

Yes No* Was an observer present?

Yes No* Did any staff within 3 ft of the sterile field wear a cap and mask?

* If "No" for any of the above:
Yes No Was the procedure stopped (if nonemergent) and corrective action taken?
Any "No" responses, without corrective action taken, are considered "noncompliance with the central line insertion bundle"
Date: Line Type (circle): UAC – UVC – PICC – PAL – Other:

Table 2
A representative central line insertion bundle

Required Bundle Elements	Comments
Maximal barrier precautions used during the entire procedure	Cap, mask, sterile gown and gloves, large sterile drape; hat and mask required for other staff when within 3 ft of the sterile field
Hand hygiene before the procedure	Inserter must do this immediately before the procedure
Sterile preparation of the insertion site	Cover adequate surface area, allow for appropriate drying time
Observer monitoring the entire procedure	Observer completes the insertion bundle checklist, is required to stop the procedure if there is a breach in technique

of how insightful the suggested change seems. Generally, the changes are tested on a small scale, results are reviewed, and adjustments are made until the change is considered effective and ready for wide-scale implementation within the NICU. The changes are sometimes quite obvious and need little refinement, allowing rapid wide-scale implementation. Other changes are not so certain and require small-scale testing and further refinement (**Table 3**).[1,5]

Testing change is the purpose of the "plan-do-study-act" (PDSA) cycle. This simple feedback cycle has a long history of successful use in improvement activities in industry and many other fields.[1,5,10,18,19]

PLAN: State the objective of the cycle, make predictions of the intervention's effect, develop the plan to implement the interventions, and measure its effect.
DO: Implement the intervention and measure the effect.
STUDY: Complete analyses, compare data with predictions, and summarize what was learned.

Table 3
Framework for determining the scale of testing[a]

Determining the Scale of Testing Changes		Staff Readiness for the Change: Not Ready	Unsure	Ready
Uncertain if the change will lead to improvement	Cost of failure is large	Very small-scale testing	Small-scale testing	Small-scale testing
	Cost of failure is small	Small-scale testing	Small-scale testing	Medium-scale testing
Confident that the change will lead to improvement	Cost of failure is large	Small-scale testing	Medium-scale testing	Large-scale testing
	Cost of failure is small	Medium-scale testing	Large-scale testing	Implement

[a] Rapid large-scale implementation of a change can be costly and ineffective if the staff is resistant or if it is uncertain the change will be successful. Smaller-scale tests of change allow for refinement of a change before widespread implementation. This matrix provides a framework for determining the scale of testing.

ACT: Determine what changes to make. What is the next cycle?"

The authors' observation, after teaching the PDSA cycle to health care providers, is that the PDSA model is not intuitive to many with a medical mindset. An alternative approach that is more familiar to the analytical and problem solving mindset used by most physicians is the "assessment and plan" (AP) cycle.

ASSESSMENT: What is the problem? How can we modify systems or processes to improve the effectiveness of care?"

PLAN: State the implementation and measurement plan and carry these out.

The AP cycle is representative of how a physician typically provides daily NICU care. For example, consider the familiar scenario of a premature infant with hypotension:

A: The infant is hypotensive, hypoperfused, tachycardic, and oliguric. We assess the baby as symptomatically hypotensive, possibly related to volume depletion or sepsis.

P: Give a normal saline bolus and reassess. Do a septic work-up and start antibiotics.

A: No improvement in hemodynamic status. Severe neutropenia is now present, metabolic acidosis has developed. Probable septic shock.

P: Give dopamine, continue antibiotics, give crystalloid and reassess.

Using this same model, consider CABSIs:

A: CABSI rate is high in my NICU. I am uncertain if central line insertion technique is contributing to CABSI.

P: Observe the next three central line insertions, assessing for adherence to basic sterile technique as described in the Centers for Disease Control and Prevention guideline.

A: Observed three insertions, with three different individuals doing the insertions. Hand hygiene was not done immediately before any insertions. Gown, glove, cap, and mask were used by all. The sterile drape was small and did not cover the infant. The procedure cart did not contain all of the needed equipment. One might suspect that all of these factors may be contributing to the CABSI rate.

P: Convene the insertion team to agree on the use of a basic central line insertion checklist.

A: The team meets, and the checklist is approved. An observer will be used to document compliance with checklist items.

P: Observers will document checklist compliance for the next five insertions and report back at the next scheduled team meeting.

A: Difficulty in obtaining observers was reported. Observers reported they felt intimidated and did not want to point out variances.

P: Re-educate the insertion team on the importance of their role and value of the observer. Establish a small group of specifically trained observers.

The AP or PDSA cycles are simply multiple feedback loops that are used to perfect a change and attain the desired improvements. Cycles are repeated until the desired result is obtained and maintained. Recording the AP or PDSA cycles as a type of "QI progress note" enables an ongoing analytic approach to documenting and learning from each step in the QI project. This information can be used to annotate run charts of any data that are being collected for the project.

MAINTAINING THE GAIN

It is common to see initial, often striking improvements fail to stick. Within a year or two of initiating the project the outcome is back to its previous undesirable baseline. Why does this failure to maintain previous gains occur? Commonly, it is because the changes were not system focused. Although "tinkering" might be effective in improving an outcome, the effect is typically less robust than system-focused change and is often short lived, given the enormous extra energy and motivation required to keep people "trying harder." System changes are essential to enable sustainable improvement.[1,5,10,20]

Another cause of failure to maintain a gain is a change in the overall system. If there has been a major system change in the NICU, a ripple effect may occur and affect other NICU subsystems. An example is oxygen management for reducing retinopathy of prematurity. A small NICU successfully introduces an oxygen management approach to avoid hyperoxia. Retinopathy of prematurity rates decrease. The NICU becomes progressively busy and overcrowded over the next year, resulting in a move to a very large facility with individual patient rooms. Retinopathy of prematurity rates increase. No change has been made in the oxygen management approach, so why has the increase occurred? The underlying NICU system has been changed, with busier nurses and greater distance between babies, creating delays in getting to the baby to answer alarms and adjust oxygen. This alteration in the NICU system has diminished the effectiveness of the previous oxygen management approach. The specific complexities of the new NICU environment need to be considered in a revision of the oxygen management approach.

SUMMARY

Despite the complexity of the NICU environment, significant improvements in outcome can be accomplished by use of basic QI methodology. Start by finding a clinically important and modifiable outcome to target for improvement. Assemble a small team with knowledge of the problem and the authority to effect system-based changes specific to this problem. Establish a specific and tangible goal for the team; determine basic outcome, process, and balancing measures. Collect the fewest possible measures needed to allow determination of the effect of the intervention. Display and analyze data with annotated run charts. Use established evidence and change concepts to make system changes and improve outcomes. Test changes to determine their effectiveness and modify them as indicated until the goals are achieved and success is maintained. Continuously review outcomes and system status to maintain improvements.

ACKNOWLEDGMENT

The authors thank Robert Lloyd and Sandra Murray of the Institute for Healthcare Improvement's Improvement Advisor Professional Development Program for their continued contributions to education in quality improvement methodology, which heavily influenced the contents of this article.

REFERENCES

1. Langley G, Nolan K, Nolan T, et al. The improvement guide: a practical approach to enhancing organizational performance. San Francisco (CA): Jossey-Bass; 2009.
2. Stark AR. American Academy of Pediatrics Committee on Fetus and Newborn. Levels of neonatal care. Pediatrics 2004;114(5):1341–7.
3. Nelson EC, Splaine ME, Plume SK, et al. Good measurement for good improvement work. Qual Manag Health Care 2004;13(1):1–16.

4. Harkins SG. Social loafing: allocating effort or taking it easy? J Exp Soc Psychol 1980;16(5):457–65.
5. Nelson EC, Batalden PB, Godfrey MM. Quality by design: a clinical microsystems approach. San Francisco (CA): Jossey-Bass; 2007.
6. Damschroder LJ, Banaszak-Holl J, Kowalski CP, et al. The role of the champion in infection prevention: results from a multisite qualitative study. Qual Saf Health Care 2009;18(6):434–40.
7. Solberg LI, Mosser G, McDonald S. The three faces of performance measurement: improvement, accountability, and research. Jt Comm J Qual Improv 1997;23(3):135–47.
8. Braun BI, Kritchevsky SB, Kusek L, et al. Evaluation of Processes and Indicators in Infection Control (EPIC) Study Group. Comparing bloodstream infection rates: the effect of indicator specifications in the evaluation of processes and indicators in infection control (EPIC) study. Infect Control Hosp Epidemiol 2006;27(1):14–22.
9. Nelson EC, Splaine ME, Batalden PB, et al. Building measurement and data collection into medical practice. Ann Intern Med 1998;128(6):460–6.
10. Plsek PE. Quality improvement methods in clinical medicine. Pediatrics 1999; 103(1 Suppl E):203–14.
11. Lloyd R. Quality health care: a guide to developing and using indicators. Boston: Jones & Bartlett Publishers; 2004.
12. Carey RG, Lloyd RC. Measuring quality improvement in healthcare: a guide to statistical process control applications. Wisconsin: Quality Press; 2001.
13. Gartner LM, Morton J, Lawrence RA, et al. American Academy of Pediatrics Section on Breastfeeding. Breastfeeding and the use of human milk. Pediatrics 2005;115(2):496–506.
14. Garland JS, Alex CP, Sevallius JM, et al. Cohort study of the pathogenesis and molecular epidemiology of catheter-related bloodstream infection in neonates with peripherally inserted central venous catheters. Infect Control Hosp Epidemiol 2008;29(3):243–9.
15. Pronovost P, Needham D, Berenholtz S, et al. An intervention to decrease catheter-related bloodstream infections in the ICU. N Engl J Med 2006;355(26): 2725–32.
16. Hales BM, Pronovost PJ. The checklist: a tool for error management and performance improvement. J Crit Care 2006;21(3):231–5.
17. Institute for Healthcare Improvement. Available at: http://www.ihi.org. Accessed November 20, 2009.
18. Deming WE. The new economics for industry, government, education. 2nd edition. Cambridge (MA): Massachusetts Institute of Technology; 2000.
19. Deming WE. Out of the crisis. Cambridge (MA): Massachusetts Institute of Technology; 2000.
20. Plsek P. Redesigning healthcare with insights from the science of complex adaptive systems. Institute of Medicine. Crossing the quality chasm: a new health system for the 21st century. Washington, DC: National Academy Press; 2001. p. 309–22.

Navigating in the Turbulent Sea of Data: The Quality Measurement Journey

Robert C. Lloyd, PhD

KEYWORDS

- Quality measurement • Statistical process control
- Improvement sequence

WHERE AWAY AND WHY ALONE?

In 1892, Captain Eben Pierce offered his friend Joshua Slocum (1844–1909) a ship that "wants some repairs." Slocum went to Fairhaven, Massachusetts, to find that the ship was a rotting, old, 37-foot, oyster sloop propped up in a field. It was known as the *Spray*. Slocum spent 13 months repairing this vessel and on April 24, 1895, at the age of 51 years, he cast off from Gloucester, Massachusetts, in the *Spray*. As he was about to set off on his voyage a group of people called out to him, "Where away and why alone?"

Slocum covered 46,000 miles during his solo journey and landed back in Newport, Rhode Island, on June 27, 1898. His account of this journey, *Sailing alone around the world,* was published by the Century Co in 1900.[1] On November 14, 1909, at the age of 65 years, he set out from Martha's Vineyard on another lone voyage to South America, but was never heard from again.

Like Joshua Slocum, we are also on a journey. We are not battling 30-foot waves, howling winds, or pirates. But we are facing pressures and challenges that test our knowledge, experience, and our abilities. The primary question is this: Do you have a plan to guide your quality journey? Or are you adrift in a turbulent sea of data, hoping that your numbers meet the internal and external demands that are constantly testing your navigational skills? Or are you headed in the wrong direction and feeling a little like Joshua Slocum, adrift alone in a turbulent sea? "Where away and why alone?"

WHY ARE YOU MEASURING?

In 1997, Solberg and colleagues[2] described what they called the 3 faces of performance measurement. They wrote:

Institute for Healthcare Improvement, 20 University Road, 7th Floor, Cambridge, MA 02138, USA
E-mail address: rlloyd@IHI.org

Clin Perinatol 37 (2010) 101–122
doi:10.1016/j.clp.2010.01.006 perinatology.theclinics.com
0095-5108/10/$ – see front matter

We are increasingly realizing not only how critical measurement is to the quality improvement we seek but also how counterproductive it can be to mix measurement for accountability or research with measurement for improvement.

The investigators describe in detail various characteristics of performance measurement for accountability (what many today call data for judgment), research, and improvement. These characteristics are summarized in **Table 1**. The authors' distinctions between the various aspects of the measurement journey help us quickly realize that not all measurement is the same. Yet many health care professionals do not think about why they are actually measuring. You will hear managers or frontline workers say, for example, "Look, we need to submit some data on our progress related to ventilator-associated pneumonias in the neonatal intensive care unit, so find some recent numbers and send them in." Frequently this means the data submitted may not be the most recent data, defined in the same way they were defined when they were first submitted or stratified according to the same criteria used the previous year. Furthermore, the data may be presented in a manner that works when accountability questions are driving the inquiry, but they may be inadequate for questions related to quality and safety or conducting randomized control trials (RCTs).

Brook and colleagues[3] have also helped to clarify the performance measurement journey. They point out that research (ie, RCTs) designed to determine the efficacy

Table 1
The 3 faces of performance measurement

Aspect	Improvement	Accountability	Research
Aim	Improvement of care	Comparison, choice, reassurance, spur for change	New knowledge
Methods			
• Test observability	Test observable	No test, evaluate current performance	Test blinded or controlled
• Bias	Accept consistent bias	Measure and adjust to reduce bias	Design to eliminate bias
• Sample size	Just enough data, small sequential samples	Obtain 100% of available, relevant data	Just in case data
• Flexibility of hypothesis	Hypothesis flexible, changes as learning takes place	No hypothesis	Fixed hypothesis
• Testing strategy	Sequential tests	No tests	One large test
• Determining if a change is an improvement	Run charts or Shewhart control charts	No change focus	Hypothesis, statistical tests (*t* test, F test, χ^2), *P* values
• Confidentiality of the data	Data used only by those involved with improvement	Data available for public consumption and review	Research subjects identities protected

of a drug, procedure, or treatment is designed to answer questions about efficacy. Quality improvement research, on the other hand, is directed at improving the efficiency or effectiveness of processes and their related outcomes.

Anyone engaged in performance measurement needs to be clear about the reasons for collecting and analyzing data. As shown in **Table 1**, each of the 3 faces uses different methods and different statistical techniques to derive conclusions from the data. If an organization is genuinely interested in leading the way for quality and safety then it needs to be clear about the reasons for measurement. All too often organizations say they are focused on quality and safety. Then they discover that their approach to performance measurement is based primarily on data for accountability or judgment. This observation is not to suggest that 1 of the 3 faces is more correct than the other. All 3 faces of performance measurement can be useful. A problem arises, however, when organizations attempt to mix the 3 faces. This error is what Solberg and colleagues[2] indicate leads to the development of counterproductive performance measurement systems.

THE QUALITY MEASUREMENT JOURNEY

Aim

The milestones in the quality measurement journey (QMJ) are outlined by Lloyd[4] and summarized in **Fig. 1**. The first milestone in this journey requires clarity about the aim of measurement. Measurement should be directly and overtly connected to the organization's mission, aims, and objectives. One can easily determine how connected a team is to the organization's strategic objectives. The next time you are involved with a pediatrics improvement team, just pose the following question: "Can anyone tell me how this team's work fits with the organization's strategic objectives?" After a period of silence, some brave soul might respond, "I have no idea. We were told by our boss to improve this process." If the employees of an organization do not understand and internalize how their work fits into the organization's overall strategy for quality and safety, they will end up going through the motions and think they are "doing quality." They will fail to connect their work to the organization's purpose and objectives, and they will go through the motions but never connect the dots. Aims help answer the question "Why are you measuring?"

Concepts

Concepts, the next milestone in the QMJ, stem from clarity around the high-level aims. Yet the concepts do not represent measurement. They are essentially an intermediate step designed to help a team set the boundaries for measurement and data collection.

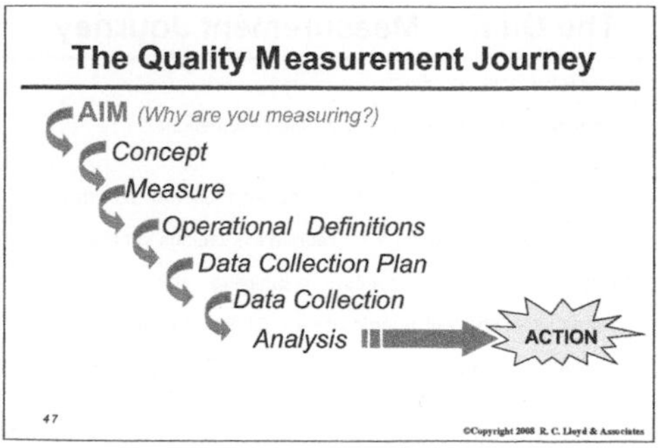

Fig. 1. Milestones in the QMJ. (*Courtesy of* R.C. Lloyd & Associates.)

For example, in **Fig. 2** the aim is to have freedom from harm. This type of statement will be found frequently in an organization's mission statement. From this aim emerge various concepts that address different aspects of harm. In **Fig. 2**, the example is reducing neonatal unplanned extubations of endotracheal tubes (ETTs). We have become more specific by saying that we want to reduce unplanned extubation as a form of harm but this is still not measurement. Reducing unplanned extubation is a desired outcome. It is not until you move to identifying a specific way to measure unplanned extubation that you can take the first steps toward reducing it.

Measures

There are numerous options to consider as we move from a concept to a measure. The first one is deciding which measure to select out of all the potential measures.[5] Using the concept of unplanned extubations we might consider the following measures:

- We could count merely the number of unplanned extubations in a defined period of time (eg, during a shift, during a week, or for the entire month). What does this give us? Is a count of the number of unplanned extubations the most appropriate way to measure the concept? This month we had 21 unplanned extubations. Last month we had 13. What does this tell us? It becomes even more challenging if you want to compare your performance to that of another hospital in your area or system. Hospital A's neonatal intensive care unit (NICU) and B's NICU each had 19 unplanned extubations this month. Which one is better? You really cannot decide which is better or worse in this situation because you have no context for the absolute numbers. If you are told, however, that hospital A is a large urban teaching hospital with 50 isolettes and hospital B is a community hospital with only 10 isolettes, you now have a context and would most likely say that it is not fair to compare the two because of differences in size, volume, location, and so forth.
- Next, we could consider computing the percentage of neonates who have an unplanned extubation. In this case, we would need to define a denominator (ie, all neonates who could possibly have an unplanned extubation). The numerator would then be all the neonates who did experience an unplanned extubation during their stay in the NICU aggregated for the defined period of time (eg, a week or a month). With these 2 numbers we could compute the percentage of neonates with an unplanned extubation during the defined time period. Because an unplanned extubation could happen more than once during a stay in an NICU, however, the percentage would not capture the multiple unplanned

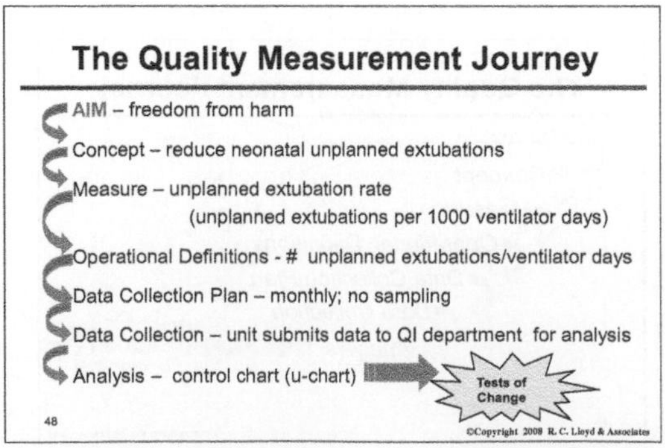

Fig. 2. Example of a QMJ. Reducing undesired or accidental extubations in neonates.

extubations. A percentage is based on a binomial distribution. Measuring unplanned extubations with a percentage, therefore, means that the team is not concerned with the specific number of times a baby experienced an unplanned extubation, but rather if the patient had an unplanned extubation once or more. The question is simply, "Did this baby experience an unplanned extubation, yes or no?"

- This question leads us to the third option for measuring an unplanned extubation, a rate. Like a percentage a rate is calculated by having a numerator and a denominator but they are different from the ones defined for a percentage. An unplanned extubation rate would have as the numerator the total number of unplanned extubations, including multiples for 1 baby, during a defined period of time (eg, a shift, a day, a week, or a month). The denominator would then be the total number of ventilator days in the defined period of time. These calculations would produce an unplanned extubation rate (eg, 18 unplanned extubations per 1000 ventilator days). A rate-based statistic has a different measure in the numerator and the denominator (eg, extubations over days). A percentage has the same measure in the numerator and denominator but they are merely different classes of the same variable (neonates experiencing an unplanned extubation over total neonates on an ETT). Examples of potential measures for various health care concepts can be found in Lloyd.[4]

Operational Definitions

Once a team has decided what to measure, they can proceed to the next milestone in the QMJ, namely building operational definitions. This task is 1 of the most interesting stops along your journey because it addresses the lack of precision in human language. According to Deming,[6] "An operational definition puts communicable meaning to a concept. Adjectives like good, reliable, uniform, round, tired, safe, unsafe, unemployed have no communicable meaning until they are expressed in operational terms of sampling, test, and criterion. The concept of a definition is ineffable: It cannot be communicated to someone else. An operational definition is one that reasonable men can agree on."

Operational definitions are not universal truths. They are merely ways to describe, in quantifiable terms, what to measure and the specific steps needed to measure it consistently. A good operational definition has the following characteristics:

- It gives communicable meaning to a concept or idea
- It is clear and unambiguous
- It specifies the measurement method, procedures, and equipment (when appropriate)
- It provides decision-making criteria when necessary
- It enables consistency in data collection.

Again, using the concept of an unplanned extubation, it is necessary to ask, "What is the operational definition of an unplanned extubation?" All unplanned extubations are not the same. There could be a partial extubation or a complete extubation. What is the difference between a partial extubation and a complete extubation? What if the tape holding the ETT came loose and the tubing sags a little on 1 side? Is this a partial extubation? Do we all agree on the characteristics of a partial versus a complete extubation? If we sent out 3 people to collect data on unplanned extubations would they all define a partial extubation in the same way? Would the data be valid and reliable? Could we combine the data from the 3 people and have confidence that we were comparing apples with apples? If our operational definition of a partial extubation met the 5 criteria listed earlier for a good operational definition, our data would most likely be consistent from person to person. If, on the other hand, the 3 people did not use consistent operational definitions, you would end up with fruit salad rather than apples compared with apples. Additional detail on the critical role of operational definitions plus examples can be found in Lloyd[4] and Provost and Murray.[7]

Data Collection

After reaching consensus on the operational definitions for your measures the next milestone in the QMJ (see **Fig. 1**) is to develop a data collection plan and then go out and gather the data. These 2 steps in the QMJ frequently run into roadblocks because team members or improvement advisors are not well trained in the methods and tools of data collection. The major speed bump at this point in your journey, however, is that most people wait until it is time to collect the data before they start thinking about it. A well-developed data collection plan saves you time, effort, and money. A few key questions to consider at this junction are as follows[4]:

- What is the rationale for collecting these data rather than other types of data?
- Will the data add value to your quality improvement efforts?
- Have you discussed the effects of stratification on the measures?
- How often (frequency) and for how long (duration) will you collect the data?
- Will you use sampling? If so, what sampling design have you chosen?
- How will you collect the data? (Will you use data sheets, surveys, focus group discussions, telephone interviews, or some combination of these methods?)
- Who will go out and collect the data? (Most teams ignore this question.)
- What costs (monetary and time costs) will be incurred by collecting these data?
- Will collecting these data have negative effects on patients or employees?
- Do your data collection efforts need to be taken to your organization's institutional review board for approval?
- Do you already have a baseline?
- Do you have targets and goals for the measures?
- How will the data be coded, edited, and verified?
- Will you tabulate and analyze these data by hand or by computer?
- How will these data be used to make a difference?

Besides having a serious dialog about these questions, there are 2 key skills needed during this part of your journey. The first is stratification and the second is sampling.

Stratification is the separation and classification of data into reasonably homogeneous categories. The objective of stratification is to create groupings that are as mutually exclusive as possible. Such groupings are intended to minimize variation between groups and maximize variation within a group of similar patients, procedures, or events. Stratification is also used to uncover patterns that may be suppressed when all of the data are aggregated. Stratification allows understanding of differences in the data that might be caused by:

- Day of the week (Mondays are different from Wednesdays)
- Time of day (turnaround time [TAT] is longer between 9 AM and 10 AM than it is between 3 PM and 4 PM)
- Time of year (we treat more patients with influenza in January than June)
- Shift (the process is different during day shift than during night shift)
- Type of order (short turnaround time [STAT] vs routine)

- Weight of the baby
- Type of machines or equipment.

Stratification is more of a logical issue than a statistical one. It requires talking with people who have subject matter expertise, knowing how the process works, and where pockets of variation may exist.

Returning to our example of unplanned extubation we might ask the following stratification questions:

- Does it matter if the baby is secreting fluids that could affect the tape being used to hold the ETT in place? If so, then we might stratify by mild, moderate, or copious amounts of fluid.
- Does the activity level of the baby affect unplanned extubation? If the answer is yes, then we might consider stratifying by mild, moderate, or high levels of activity, or use an activity index.
- What if a hydrocolloid dressing was placed across the neonate's philtrum before taping the ETT to the infant? Does a hydrocolloid dressing make a difference in unplanned extubations?
- Does the type of tape used to hold the ETT in place matter? If it does, then should we stratify by the type of tape (brand A vs brand B)?
- Finally, does it matter if we apply the tape to the baby's face in an H or Y pattern? If the NICU staff believe that the taping pattern makes a difference, then we should stratify on this characteristic also.

Stratification is critical especially if you think that certain factors may differ depending on the characteristic (or stratum) being used in the measurement. Once the data have been collected, it is usually too late or too time consuming to try to separate the stratification issues that may arise. Further details and examples of stratification can be found in Lloyd[4] and Provost and Murray.[7]

Sampling is the second key skill needed during the data collection stage of your journey. Sampling is an efficient and effective way to gather data when you: (1) do not need all the available data, and (2) do not have unlimited resources (time, effort, and money). First, consider the volume issue. Each day a typical hospital processes hundreds of complete blood counts (CBCs). If you are interested in TAT for CBCs, you do not need to analyze all 293 tests done on Monday each day to get a good picture of the TAT for that day. When you have these many data (ie, 293 tests during 1 day) you might consider stratification into day, afternoon, and night shifts; then stratify further to sort out STAT and routine test requests for each shift. We could then select a stratified random sample from each shift that also lets us know how STAT and routine TATs varied within the shift. In this case, a sample of 15 CBCs would be sufficient to analyze the variation on each day. Analyzing all 293 TATs is not necessary. A well-designed sampling strategy will work well.

The second reason to sample is to conserve resources. Imagine that you wanted to collect data that required 3 staff nurses to record 4 different measures on each baby in the NICU. This effort represents an expensive proposition. Rather than collect the 4 measures on all babies, you might consider developing a sampling plan to select 3 to 5 babies a day, or select a random day of the week on which to gather the data. Sampling provides a parsimonious approach to data collection. The critical question is how to draw appropriate samples.

There are 2 basic major types of sampling: probability and nonprobability. The details on the advantages and disadvantages of the various sampling approaches can be found in Lloyd[4] and Provost and Murray.[7] Also you can find practical discussions of sampling methods in any basic text (old or new) on statistical methods or research designs.

Probability sampling methods are based on a simple principle: within a known population of size n, there is a fixed probability of selecting any single element (n_i). The selection of this observation (and the remaking members of the sample) must be determined by objective statistical means if the process is to be truly random (not affected by judgment, purposeful intent, or convenience). There are 4 basic approaches to probability sampling:

- Systematic sampling, which is achieved by numbering or ordering each element in the population and then selecting every *k*th element. The key point that most people ignore when pulling a systematic sample is that the starting point for selecting every *k*th element should be generated through a random process. For example, if you were evaluating how long it takes to get a newborn baby from the delivery room to the NICU, and you wanted to draw a systematic sample, you would pick a random number between 1 and 10 (eg, 7) and then start observing the time of every *k*th baby after the seventh one. If you said, "Let's start at the first baby and then take every 10th baby to check the time it takes from delivery to the NICU" you would potentially be introducing bias. A random starting point is critical to making systematic sampling a form of probability sampling.
- Simple random sampling is accomplished by giving every element in the population an equal and independent chance of being included in the sample. A random number table or a random number generator in a computer program is usually used to develop a random selection process.
- Stratified random sampling results when stratification is applied to a population; then a random process is used to pull samples from within each stratum. The CBC example presented earlier provides an illustration of this approach.
- Stratified proportional random sampling is more complicated because it requires figuring out what proportion each stratum represents in the total population, then replicating this proportion in the sample that is randomly pulled from each stratum. To successfully use this approach, you need to have sufficiently large populations that can be divided into smaller stratification levels, yet still have enough data from which to draw an appropriate sample. For example, if you stratify all deliveries by age, race, and prior deliveries within the last 30 days, you may have a category of Hispanic women more than 40 years old who had a previous cesarean section that contains only 2 patients. In this case, you have stratified by so many levels that you have reduced the number of patients to a point that sampling does not make sense.

Nonprobability sampling methods are usually used when the researcher is not interested in being able to generalize the findings to a larger population. The basic objective of nonprobability sampling is to select a sample that the researchers believe is typical of the larger population. A chief criticism of these approaches to sampling is that there is no way to factually measure how representative the sample is of the total population under consideration. Samples pulled through nonprobability designs are assumed to be good enough for the people drawing the sample, but the finding should not be generalized to larger populations.

- Convenience sampling is the classic man-on-the-street interview approach to sampling. In this case, a reporter may select 10 people standing on the train platform (who look interesting or approachable) and ask them what they think of the national health care debate and the public option. Although these interviews may provide interesting sound bites, they should not be used to arrive at a conclusion that this is how the general public feels about the issue.

- Quota sampling is frequently used with convenience sampling. When this approach is used, the reporter knows that they need to get a total of 2 sound bites (the quota) for the producer to use. So the reporter focuses on obtaining these 2 interviews as the quota. This technique is used frequently in health care settings, when a quota of *n* charts or *m* patient interviews is set as the desired amount of data. There are steps that can be taken in developing quota samples[8] to ensure reasonably robust data. Most of the time these steps are not followed, and the quota sample represents a weak and biased approach to sampling.
- Judgment sampling is frequently used in quality improvement initiatives. Judgment sampling relies on the knowledge of subject matter experts. These individuals can tell you when the performance of a process varies and when this variation should be observed. For example, if the admitting clerk tells you that patients bunch up between 08:30 and 09:30 AM, and that this is a different process than what she observes between 15:00 and 16:00 PM, then we should consider sampling differently during these 2 time periods. Similarly, if a staff nurse tell you that "Things get crazy around here at 11:00 due to discharge timing," we would want to create a sampling plan for "crazy time" and "noncrazy time." The critical point for judgment sampling is that the person offering the judgment needs to be a subject matter expert on the process and how it works. Otherwise, bias increases dramatically in this form of sampling.

Building knowledge in sampling methods is 1 of the best things that someone can do to enhance data collection processes. Good sampling techniques help to ensure the validity and reliability of the data that are taken to the next milestone in your QMJ analysis.

Analysis

How you analyze your data depends on a critical question: Will you approach data analysis from a static or dynamic perspective? Deming[9] labeled these 2 approaches as enumerative (static) and analytical (dynamic). He pointed out that quality improvement studies are best approached from an analytical perspective. Yet, most health care professions have received statistical training that is grounded solely in static approaches to data analysis.

Static approaches are designed to summarize a characteristic of the data with a single measure that is fixed at a single point in time. The descriptive statistics used include measures of central tendency (mean, median, and mode) and measures of dispersion (minimum, maximum, range, and standard deviation). Once the descriptive statistics have been computed the next step in the static journey is to compare 2 or more data points to find out if they are statistically different. In this example, techniques such as χ^2, Student *t* test, analysis of variance, or correlation/regression analyses are used to determine if 1 data point is different from another. Statistical tests of significance, usually determined by a *P* value, are the standard method to verify differences.

The analytical approach to data analysis stands in contrast to the static approach. Analytical methods are based on statistical process control (SPC) methods. This branch of applied statistics was developed by Dr Walter Shewhart in the early 1920s while he was working at Western Electric Co.[10] The primary SPC tools are the run and control charts. Statistical analysis conducted with SPC methods looks at variation in a process or outcome measures over time, not at a fixed point in time, or compares 2 data points and asks if they are statistically different.

Because variation exists in all processes (eg, consider morning commute time), the use of run charts and Shewhart control charts allows the researcher to analyze data as a continuous stream that has a rhythm and pattern. Statistical tests are used to detect whether the process performance reflects what Shewhart classified as common cause variation or special cause variation. Decisions about improvement strategies and their effects are based on understanding the type of variation that lives in the process, not on whether 1 data point is different from another. SPC charts, therefore, are more like the patterns of vital signs seen on telemetry monitors in the NICU.

Run Charts

A run chart provides a running record of a process over time. It offers a dynamic display of the data and can be used on virtually any type of data (eg, counts of events, percentages, rates, or physiologic measures). **Fig. 3** shows the layout for a typical run chart. The measure of interest is always plotted along the y-axis, whereas the x-axis is reserved for the subgroup or unit of time used to organize the data. Day, week, month, shift, or even patient are typical units that are placed on the x-axis. Because run charts require no complex statistical calculations, such as sigma limits, they can be understood easily by everyone. The major drawback in using run charts, however, is that they can detect some but not all special causes in the data.

The first step in analyzing a run chart is to understand what is meant by a run. A run is defined as 1 or more consecutive data points on the same side of the median. When you are counting runs, you should ignore points that decrease directly on the median. **Fig. 4** shows the number of runs on the chart shown initially in **Fig. 3**. An alternative way to count the number of runs is to examine the number of times the sequence of data points crosses the median and add 1. If you count the number of circled runs, or if you add 1 to the number of times the data cross the median, you get the same number: 14. So, in **Fig. 4**, there are 14 runs.

Once the number of runs is identified, you can then decide if the chart indicates the presence of common cause (random variation) or special cause (nonrandom variation). Four simple run chart rules are used to detect the 2 types of variation. The tests include:

- A shift in the process (6 or more consecutive data points above or below the median)

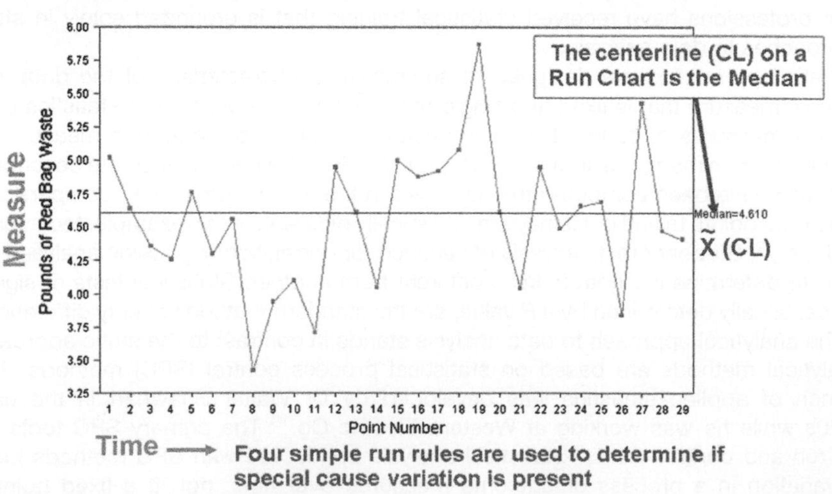

Fig. 3. Elements of a run chart.

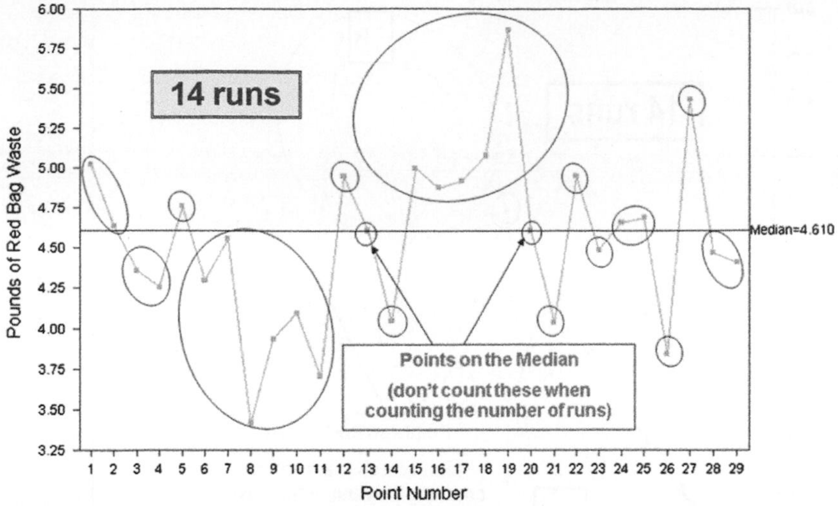

Fig. 4. Determining the number of runs.

- A trend (5 or more consecutive data points constantly going up or down)
- Too many or too few runs (determined by using a table that shows the number of runs expected for a given data set)
- An astronomical data point (this is a judgment call to decide if there is 1 or more data points in the set that seem to have an extreme variation).

Fig. 5 provides a visual display of these 4 run chart rules. The run chart rules are applied to the chart shown in **Fig. 6**.

The box next to **Fig. 6** shows how the run chart would be analyzed. There are 29 total data points on the chart. Two of the data points are on the median so they are not counted. This assessment leaves 27 useful observations (data points not on the median). When you look up 27 useful observations in a table,[11] you will see that the

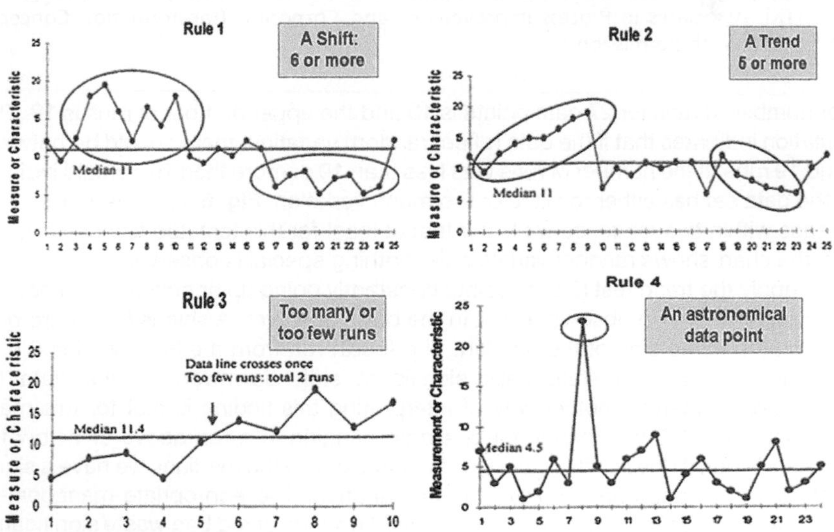

Fig. 5. The 4-run chart rules.

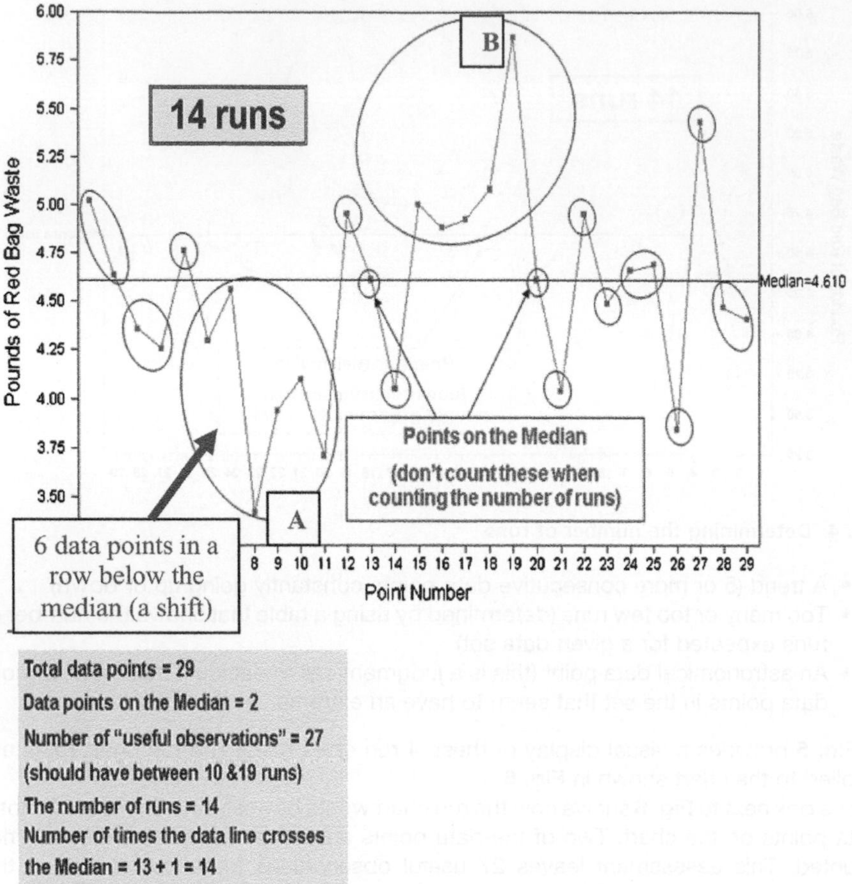

Fig. 6. Applying the run chart rules. (*Adapted from* Provost L, Murray S. The data guide. Austin [TX]: Associates in Process Improvement and Corporate Transformation Concepts; 2007. p. 3–15; with permission.)

lower number of runs for 27 data points is 10 and the upper number of runs is 19. This calculation indicates that if the data reflect random variation, there should be between 10 and 19 runs. If the number of runs was less than 10 or more than 19 it would indicate that the data set has either too little or too much variation. **Fig. 6** contains 14 runs that decrease within this range, so we know that at least for this test (too few or too many runs), the chart shows random variation (ie, nothing special is observed).

If we apply the trend test (5 data points constantly going up or down) we do not find such a pattern. We do observe a shift in the data, however. A shift is 6 or more data points on the same side of the median. The fourth run from the left contains 6 data points and indicates a statistically significant shift downward in the data (ie, a nonrandom pattern). Another way of interpreting this finding is that for this many data points (n = 27) we should not see data hanging in a run above or below the centerline. When it does (in this case 6 data points below the median), we have a signal that the process does not display random variation. The appropriate management decision in this case is to investigate why we had pounds of red bag waste significantly lower than at other points in the data collection period for 6 weeks in a row. Did we have fewer patients? Were fewer procedures performed? Were more staff on vacation during this period? Because the goal is to reduce the amount of red bag waste, we would like the process to function at lower levels. So, what does it take to shift the entire process average (the median in this situation) to a more desirable level? This is an improvement question for a team to investigate.

The last run chart test determines if there are astronomical data points present. Remember that in any given data set, there will be a high and low data point. These points are not necessarily astronomical. Rule 4 in **Fig. 5** shows an astronomical data point. In **Fig. 6**, some might conclude that point A or point B is astronomical. Neither of these points is astronomical because they essentially balance each other out. If you had only point B on the chart and point A was nuzzled in the midst of the rest of the data, then point B might be an astronomical data point. Another way to look at this issue is to imagine that all the data points were pushed to the far right side of the chart to form a distribution. The data in **Fig. 6** would form an almost perfect normal distribution, with points A and B lodged in the outermost tails of the normal curve. In conclusion, the management decision with these data rests on the answers to 2 important questions: (1) Are we comfortable that, on average, about 4.6 pounds of red bag waste is produced each shift (shift is the unit of time across the x-axis)?; and (2) Are we willing to accept the variation in the process? A "No" response to either of these questions would indicate the need for improvement.

Shewhart Charts

Although most people refer to control charts as the primary SPC tool, the appropriate terminology is actually Shewhart charts, in honor of Dr Walter Shewhart, who developed the fundamental aspect of the charts in the early 1900s while he was working at Western Electric Co.[10] In 1931, Shewhart published his classic work, *Economic control of quality of manufactured product*. This book has served as the foundation for all subsequent work in SPC.

Shewhart charts are preferred to run charts because they:

1. Are more sensitive than run charts
   - A run chart cannot detect special causes that are a result of point-to-point variation (the median of the run chart is replaced with the mean on a Shewhart chart)
   - Tests for detecting special causes can be used with control charts, whereas the run charts are able to identify random or nonrandom patterns in the data
2. Have the added feature of control limits, which allow us to determine if the process is stable (common cause variation) or not stable (special cause variation)
3. Can be used to define process capability (which run charts cannot do)
4. Allow us to more accurately predict process behavior and future performance.

Like the run chart, Shewhart charts are plots of data arranged in chronologic order (**Fig. 7**). The mean or average is plotted through the center of the data; then the upper control limit (UCL) and lower control limit (LCL) are calculated from the inherent variation in the data. The control limits are not set by the individual constructing the chart. If appropriate, the individual making the chart can place specification limits or a target on the chart to determine how well the actual variation matches the desired performance of the process.

Shewhart was keenly interested in trying to understand the scientific basis for statistical control. As he observed the world around him, he realized that certain types of variation (common cause variation) were part of the normal function of life. At other times, however, he observed that variation was not normal and random, but a result

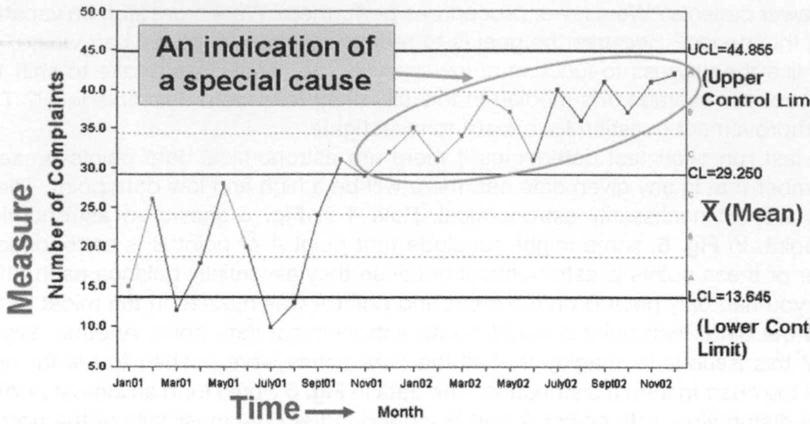

Fig. 7. Elements of a Shewhart chart.

of special or assignable causes. From Shewhart's perspective, the challenge was to distinguish 1 type of variation from the other. In 1931 he wrote:

> *A phenomenon will be said to be controlled when, through the use of past experience, we can predict, at least within limits, how the phenomenon may be expected to vary in the future. Here it is understood that prediction within limits means that we can state, at least approximately, the probability that the observed phenomenon will fall within the given limits.*

This definition provides a verbal description of the purpose of a Shewhart chart: prediction of the future. The question that most people ask at this point, however, is "Okay, I understand what Shewhart is trying to tell us, but I do not understand where these control limits come from." If you are asking this question, it is a sign that you are comfortable with the analytical concept of variation and ready to proceed with some of the more technical aspects of SPC. If, on the other hand, you would like to read more about understanding variation you may want to review Provost and Murray,[7] Lloyd,[4] Wheeler,[12] and Duncan.[13]

The technical aspects related to the Shewhart charts are numerous and too involved for the space limitations of this article. There are, however, several key points that need to be highlighted. The reader can then decide if a deeper dive into the theory and mechanics behind the Shewhart charts is required. Additional details on SPC methods can be found in Refs.[4,7,12,14–19]

The first step in applying Shewhart charts to your work is to decide if your data can be classified as variables or attributes. This consideration is not an issue with run charts because there is only 1 way to make a run chart and you can place any type of data on a run chart without distinguishing whether those data are characterized as a count, a percentage, or a rate. It does make a difference with the Shewhart charts, however, because there are different types of charts for different types of data.

Variables data (sometimes referred to as continuous data) can take on different values on a continuous scale. These data can either be whole numbers, or they can be expressed in as many decimal places as the measuring instrument can read. Examples of continuous data include time in minutes, weight in grams, length of stay, blood sugar levels, total number of procedures, or total number of discharges. Attributes data, on the other hand, are basically counts of events that can be aggregated into discrete categories (eg, acceptable vs not acceptable, infected vs not infected, or late vs on time).

It is helpful to distinguish 2 types of attributes data. The first type involves counting the occurrences and the nonoccurrences of an event and reporting the number or percentage of defectives. An example would be the percentage of neonates who had an unplanned extubation during their stay in the NICU. In this case, you know the occurrences (total number of unplanned extubations) and you know the nonoccurrences (total number of babies with an ETT). The ability to obtain a numerator and a denominator allows you to calculate the percentage of incomplete patient charts.

There are times, however, when you know the occurrences but you do not know the nonoccurrences. At first this may seem like an anomaly, but there are many situations in health care that have this characteristic. For example, on a given day you can count the number of patient falls but you do not know how many "nonfalls" there were. Similarly, you can count the number of needlesticks but you do not know how many "nonneedlesticks" occurred. Counts of this nature are usually regarded as defects, compared with defectives. For many students of SPC this distinction between defectives and defects requires a little soaking time to fully absorb. This may be 1 of the areas that you bookmark for further study and consideration.

Once you know the type of data you have collected, it is time to decide which control chart is most appropriate for your data. There are basically 7 different control charts, as summarized in **Fig. 8**. Note that 3 of the charts relate to variables data, whereas 4 charts are appropriate for attributes data.

The Shewhart decision tree shown in **Fig. 9** provides an algorithm that many find useful when deciding which chart is most appropriate for their data. The successful use of the decision tree requires understanding the following terms: subgroup, observation, and area of opportunity. These terms are defined in **Table 2**. Note that subgroup and observation relate to all the charts, whereas the area of opportunity is pertinent to only the attributes charts.

Of these 7 charts, health care data are most often displayed on 5 of the charts. These include X bar and S chart, XmR chart (individuals chart), the p-chart (percentages or proportions), the c-chart, and the u-chart (rates). Specifically, applications and examples of the use of these charts can be found in Provost and Murray,[7] Lloyd[4]; Carey,[15] and Carey and Lloyd.[16]

Once you have selected and made the appropriate Shewhart chart, it is time to interpret the chart. This process is similar to the one we used for determining if the run chart

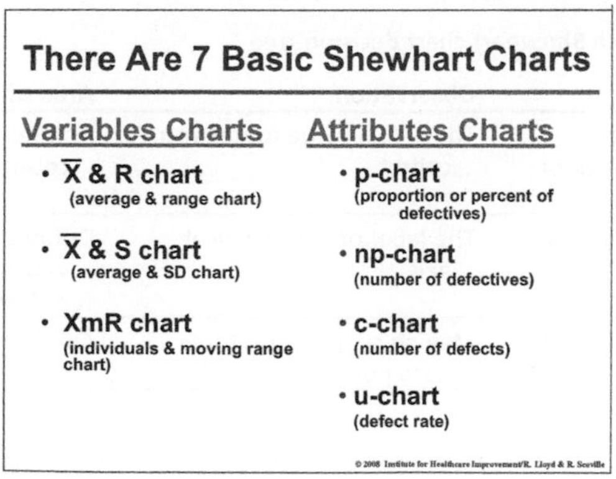

Fig. 8. The basic Shewhart charts. (*Courtesy of* Institute for Health Improvement.)

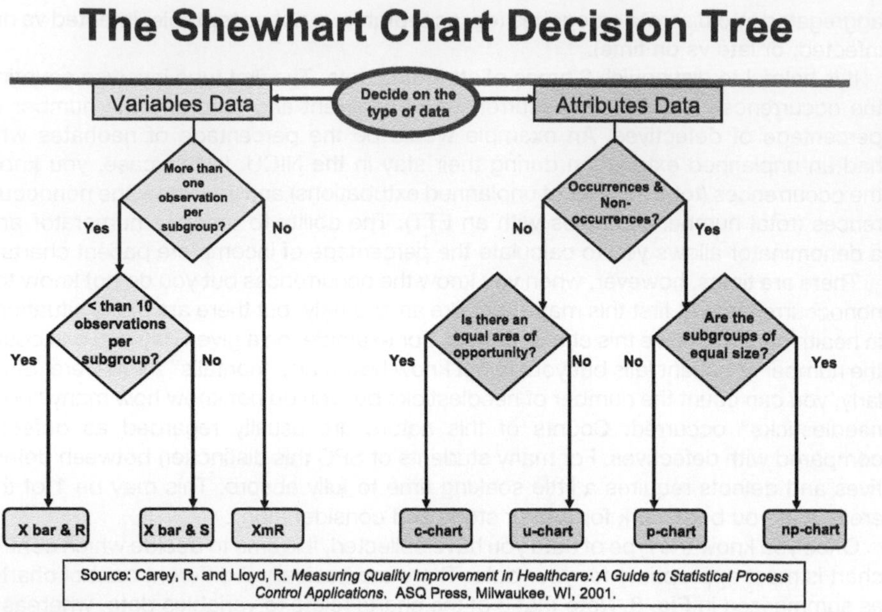

Fig. 9. The Shewhart chart decision tree. (*Courtesy of* Institute for Health Improvement.)

had random or nonrandom data patterns. Because the Shewhart charts perform at a higher level of statistical precision than the run chart, however, the rules to detect common or special causes of variation are more precise. There are rules to identify a shift on a Shewhart chart (8 data points above the centerline rather than 6 on a run chart) and a trend (6 data points constantly going up or down rather than 5 used on the run chart). There are also new rules that the run charts did not have. For example 1 of the rules (called a 3-sigma violation) occurs when a data point exceeds the UCL or LCL. Other rules help to detect what are referred to as abnormal data patterns, and relate to whether the data are bunching toward the outer regions of the chart, or hugging the centerline (ie, too many data clustered in close proximity to the mean). All of these tests are detailed in standard SPC texts.[4,7,17,19] In addition,

Table 2
Key terms in using the Shewhart chart decision tree

Subgroup	Observation	Area of Opportunity
How you organize your data (eg, by day, week or month)	The actual value (data) you collect	Applies to all attributes or counts charts
The label of your horizontal axis	The label of your vertical axis	Defines the area or frame in which a defective or defect can occur
Can be patients in equal or unequal sizes	May be single or multiple data points	Can be of equal or unequal sizes
Can be of equal or unequal sizes	Applies to all the charts	
Applies to all the charts		

SPC software packages automatically mark the presence of special cause variation on a Shewhart chart either by changing the color of the line when a special cause is detected or changing the symbol used to denote a data point on the chart.

In addition to the 7 basic Shewhart charts there are 2 other advanced charts that are appropriate for NICU data. These charts are known as the t-chart and the g-chart.[14] These charts are used when you are faced with 2 conditions. First, when you have small denominators (eg, fewer than 10 observations in the denominator) percentages can become volatile and show extreme swings in variation. For example, 2 out of 4 is 50% but it is not so strong as 50% that is based on 20 out of 40. Small denominators can be 1 reason to use a t- or g-chart. The second reason is that events happen so infrequently that they are considered to be rare. In both these circumstances (small denominators or rare events), the t-chart (plotting time between events) or the g-chart (successful cases between ones considered not successful) provide an alternative to the more traditional p-chart or u-chart. For example, if the unplanned extubation rate which was normally running about 15 per 1000 ventilator days was reduced to 1 or 2 per 100 ventilator days, you should consider moving the measure to a t- or g-chart. In this case we would plot the number of days that went by without an unplanned extubation, or the number of cases that had an ETT and never had an unplanned extubation (ie, a successful application of the ETT during the NICU stay). The goal with either type of chart is to have ever-increasing accumulation of successes without a failure. Every time you have a failure (ie, an unplanned extubation), you start counting the number of days or cases again. This method has been used successfully in manufacturing plants, construction, or the mining industry, where a sign is placed outside the work site stating "147 days without a workplace injury." The next day the sign reads "148 days" and so on, until an injury on the job takes the counter back to zero and the count starts all over again.

SPC Examples Using Perinatology Data

Imagine that you are sitting in a meeting designed to review several quality measures for 2 NICUs within your system. The measures of interest for this meeting include:

- Average ventilator days for all babies with birth weight of 501 to 1500 g
- Catheter-associated bloodstream infections (BSIs) per 1000 line days for infants with a birth weight of 501 to 1500 g for NICU1 and NICU2.

Now imagine 2 scenarios for this meeting:

- Scenario 1: you are given tabular data
- Scenario 2: you are given SPC charts.

Think about how you would guide the group's discussion around these measures if you decided to use scenario 1 and the data shown for average ventilator days shown in **Table 3**. What do you conclude from the tabular data? Is the NICU getting better, staying the same, or getting worse? Do we have any special causes in the data? Are the data performing at or near expectations (target), or are the data demonstrating considerable variation and far from target? The tabular data make it difficult to answer these questions. If, on the other hand, we went into the meeting using scenario 2 and distributed the Shewhart chart shown in **Fig. 10**, we would set up a totally different context for the group's discussion. These data reveal the following:

- There is considerable variation in the average ventilator days. The overall average is 25.4 days; the minimum is 8.2 days and the maximum is 67.3 days. Although

Table 3
Average ventilator days and number of patients by month

Month	Average Ventilator Days	Number of Patients
2003/01	18.9	22
2003/02	8.2	20
2003/03	18.1	29
2003/04	26.6	22
2003/05	28.8	24
2003/06	20	14
2003/07	23.6	13
2003/08	27.6	13
2003/09	13.8	18
2003/10	30.2	28
2003/11	13.5	22
2003/12	32.7	36
2004/01	12.9	18
2004/02	12.7	12
2004/03	22.6	28
2004/04	19.9	28
2004/05	26.2	16
2004/06	19.1	11
2004/07	18.7	17
2004/08	46.5	14
2004/09	36.9	16
2004/10	13.1	22
2004/11	31.4	16
2004/12	18.4	26
2005/01	19	17
2005/02	23.3	29
2005/03	16.1	20
2005/04	19.9	19
2005/05	32.7	23

these summary numbers could be calculated from the tabular data, the Shewhart chart provides a visual running record of the variation over time, which is lost in the tabular data.

- With the exception of the last data point (67.3 days), the variation is essentially common cause.
- The last data point is a special cause (above the UCL) and deserves investigation. Is this a data entry error? If it is accurate, then why is this average so high? Remember this is not 1 baby but the average for all 19 babies on a ventilator for the month of December 2008.
- If a target or other comparative reference data are available, the team could determine how far from the target the current process is performing.

Figs. 11 and **12** show the second measure (catheter-associated BSIs per 1000 line days for infants with a birth weight of 501 to 1500 g for NICU1 and NICU2) as a rate

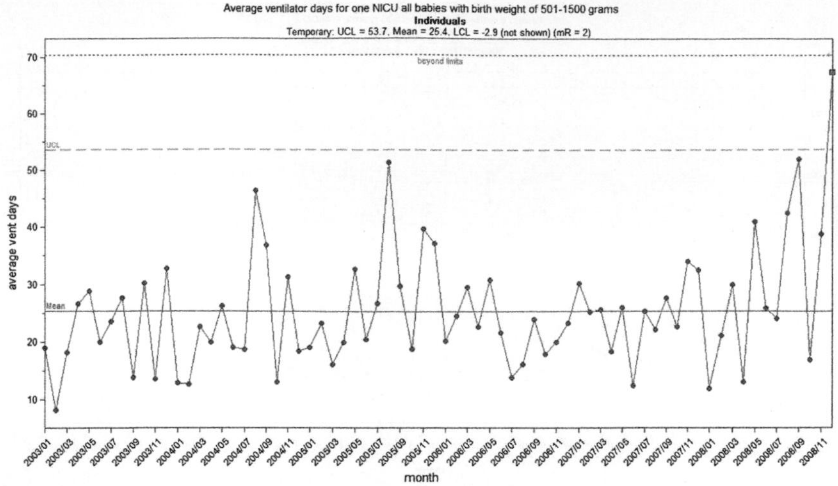

Fig. 10. Average ventilator days for all babies with birth weight of 501 to 1500 g.

(u-chart). Imagine what it would be like trying to make sense out of the tabular data for these 2 NICUs. But at a glance, you can see that the 2 sites have fundamentally different patterns. Questions we can ask include:

- Why does NICU1 have so many rates equal to zero, whereas NICU 2 has few zero points? NICU1 has so many of its data points at zero that this would be a perfect time to move this measure to a t- or g-chart and track the time between BSIs or the cases between BSIs. Note that when you have more than 50% of the data at zero or alternatively at 100%, this observation represents a sign that the t- or g-charts should be considered. The t- and g-charts would not be appropriate for NICU2, however.

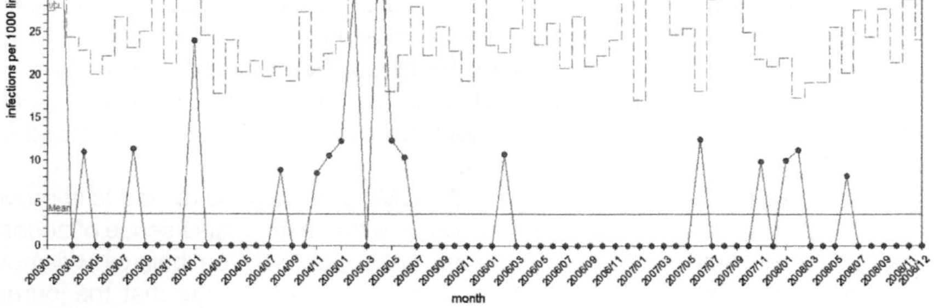

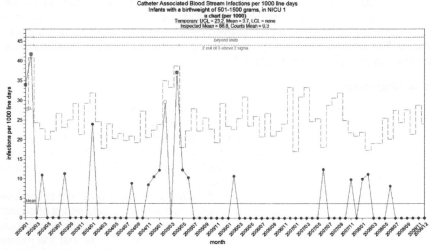

Fig. 11. Catheter-associated BSIs per 1000 line days for infants with a birth weight of 501 to 1500 g for NICU1.

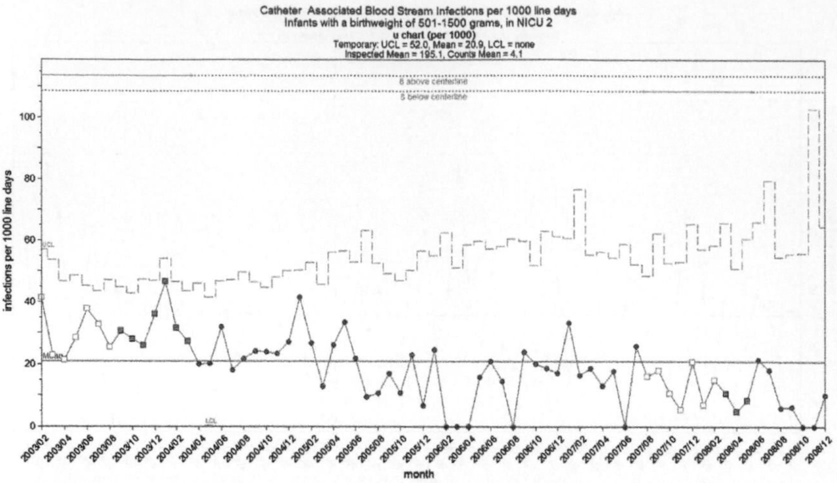

Fig. 12. Catheter-associated BSIs per 1000 line days for infants with a birth weight of 501 to 1500 g for NICU2.

- Note that the average for NICU1 is low, whereas the mean for NICU is considerably higher. Are these units fundamentally different in size, complexity of patients, or types of populations being served?
- The measure has shifted downward at NICU2. This finding signals that improvements may have been put in place. We would want to understand what has caused this downward shift (note the changes in the color of the dots and the connecting lines, which signal special causes in the data). There is also an opportunity to define 2 sets of control limits on the chart. One set would be for the left side of the chart, which is performing at a higher level, and the second set would be used for the data after they shifted downward.

In summary, the Shewhart charts provide a fundamentally different view of the data. The charts should enable dialog and learning. Typically, the tabular data lead the team to engage in shallow levels of learning, boredom, or worse yet, jumping to conclusions. Quality and safety cannot be improved by looking at tabular data and summary statistics. The context for learning comes when you plot data over time and understand the variation in the entire data set.

Linking Measurement to Improvement

Joshua Slocum was well known for keeping detailed diaries and data on his sailing adventures. But he did not collect data and measure his progress just to fill the many lonely hours while circumnavigating the globe. He collected data to help him make better decisions. Slocum was by all accounts a most intriguing yet enigmatic individual. What is clear from reading his diaries, however, is that he understood the linkage between measurement and improvement.

All the preceding milestones and steps in the QMJ are designed to lead to improvement. Data without a context or plan for action give the team a false sense of accomplishment. It is not until you identify change concepts that you believe will move performance in the desired direction and conduct tests of change that the journey becomes complete. All too often health care managers and leaders see data as the beginning and end of the journey. These individuals need to spend a little time with

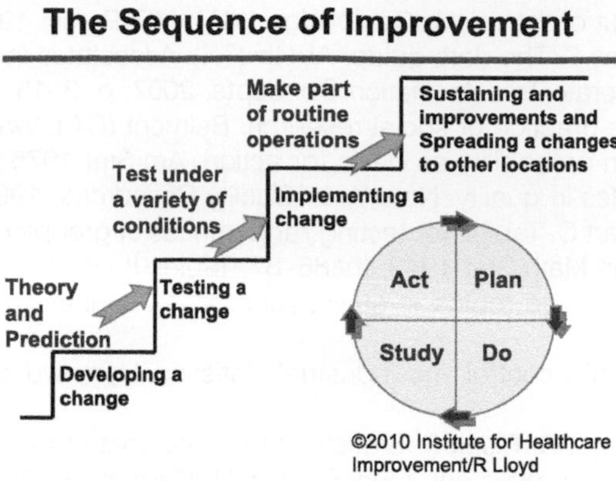

Fig. 13. The sequence for improvement. (*Courtesy of* Institute for Health Improvement.)

Captain Slocum to learn the true value of data collection. Data allow us merely to set the direction of our improvement journey, not define the end of the journey.

The sequence for improvement is shown in **Fig. 13**. Note that although data are used throughout this sequence, the primary objective is to start with small tests of new ideas, build on the success and failures of these tests, and move to testing under different conditions to determine how robust and reliable the new ideas are. When sufficient testing has been accomplished, it is time to implement the new ideas and make them a permanent part of the daily work in the pilot or demonstration area. Once implementation has been successful, it is time to turn your attention to sustaining the gains that have been realized and then start to make plans to spread the improved practices to other locations. Other articles in this issue address the steps in the improvement journey and should be consulted for additional guidance.

ACKNOWLEDGMENTS

The author wishes to acknowledge Dr John Chuo and William Peters for their contributions to this article. Dr Chuo, a neonatologist at Children's Hospital of Philadelphia, provided extensive background information on neonatal unexpected extubations. His willingness to share his knowledge and the planned experiment he has developed to address this issue are greatly appreciated. Peters, an Improvement Advisor and statistician, gave generously of his time to prepare the control charts used in this article.

REFERENCES

1. Teller WM. The voyages of Joshua Slocum. Dobbs Ferry (NY): Sheridan House Inc; 2002.
2. Solberg L, Mosser G, McDonald S. The three faces of performance measurement. Journal on Quality Improvement 1997;23(3):135–47.
3. Brook R, Kamberg C, McGlynn E. Health system reform and quality. JAMA 1996; 276(6):476–80.
4. Lloyd R. Quality health care: a guide to developing and using measures. Sudbury (MA): Jones and Bartlett; 2004.
5. Lloyd R. The search for a few good indicators. In: Ransom S, Joshi M, Nash D, editors. The healthcare quality book: vision, strategy and tools. Chicago (IL): Health Administration Press; 2005. p. 89–116.

6. Deming WE. Out of the crisis. Cambridge (MA): MIT Press; 1992.
7. Provost L, Murray S. The data guide. Austin (TX): Associates in Process Improvement and Corporate Transformation Concepts; 2007. p. 3–15.
8. Babbie ER. The practice of social research. Belmont (CA): Wadsworth; 1979.
9. Deming WE. On probability as basis for action. Am Stat 1975;29(4):146–52.
10. Schultz L. Profiles in quality. New York: Quality Resources; 1994.
11. Swed F, Eisenhart C. Tables for testing randomness of grouping in a sequence of alternatives. Ann Math Stat 1943;XIV:66–87, Tables II and III.
12. Wheeler D. Advanced topics in statistical process control. Knoxville (TN): SPC Press; 1995.
13. Duncan AJ. Quality control and industrial statistics. Homewood (IL): Irwin Press; 1986.
14. Benneyan J, Lloyd R, Plsek P. Statistical process control as a tool for research and health care improvement. Qual Saf Health Care 2003;12:458–64.
15. Carey R. Improving healthcare with control charts. Milwaukee (WI): ASQ Quality Press; 2003.
16. Carey R, Lloyd R. Measuring quality improvement in healthcare: a guide to statistical process control applications. Milwaukee (WI): ASQ Quality Press; 2001.
17. Western Electric Co. Statistical quality control handbook. Indianapolis (IN): AT&T Technologies; 1985.
18. Mohamed MA, Worthington P, Woodall WH. Plotting basic control charts: tutorial notes for healthcare practitioners. Qual Saf Health Care 2008;17:137–45.
19. Wheeler D, Chambers D. Understanding statistical process control. Knoxville (TN): SPC Press; 1992.

Human Factors and Quality Improvement

James Handyside, BSc[a,b,*], Gautham Suresh, MD[c]

KEYWORDS

• Human factors • Quality improvement • Ergonomics

BACKGROUND AND DEFINITION

An important conceptual framework for quality improvement (QI) that was proposed by Donabedian[1] is one of structure, process, and outcome. Outcomes are the final results of interest (eg, the health status of patients). Process refers to the sequence and timing of activities that occur between providers and patients. Structure refers to the physical aspects and the resources of the health care setting in which the patients are cared for. It is important to pay attention to process and to structure in designing and implementing QI and patient safety interventions. A science that can help us understand and enhance the structural dimensions of QI interventions, and improve processes, is that of human factors engineering (HFE). HFE is defined as "The scientific discipline concerned with the understanding of interactions among humans and other elements of a system, and the profession that applies theory, principles, data and methods to design in order to optimize human well-being and overall system performance" (International Ergonomics Association, www.iea.cc). Thus, HFE can be considered 1 of the basic sciences underlying QI.

The terms human factors and ergonomics are used interchangeably by some, whereas others differentiate the 2 terms. In common parlance, ergonomics is often used to describe the physical aspects (shape, dimensions) of work-related equipment and furniture. The scientific discipline itself is much broader, however, and is concerned with the human-system interface in any situation, and is not confined solely to equipment and furniture. The fundamental principle of human factor engineering is to design devices, processes, services, and the work environment based on the users' requirement (user-centered design) that uses scientific principles, so that human performance is optimized.

[a] Improvision Healthcare, RR 2 Lucan, Ontario N0M 2J0, Canada
[b] NICQ Projects, Vermont Oxford Network, 33 Kilburn Street, Burlington, VT 05401, USA
[c] Department of Pediatrics, Children's Hospital at Dartmouth, Rubin 529, Dartmouth-Hitchcock Medical Center, One Medical Center Drive, Lebanon, NH 03756, USA
* Corresponding author. Improvision Healthcare, RR 2 Lucan, Ontario N0M 2J0, Canada.
E-mail address: jim@improvisionhealthcare.com

Clin Perinatol 37 (2010) 123–140
doi:10.1016/j.clp.2010.01.007 perinatology.theclinics.com

HISTORY OF HFE AND ITS USE IN HEALTH CARE

HFE emerged during World War II with the realization that the design of equipment with good displays and controls can prevent operator error, and that good training and adherence to procedures can enhance human performance.[2] The principles of HFE are currently widely applied in planning, design, and operation in diverse fields such as aviation, space exploration, chemical manufacturing, the oil and natural gas industries, nuclear power generation, computer systems, automobile manufacturing, and manufacturing of household devices and personal devices.[3] In health care, HFE has a rich history of application within anesthesia practice.[4,5] In patient safety, the application of human factors and ergonomics to patient safety has become recognized as a vital component of optimal practice.[6] The use of this approach, however, in designing and implementing QI interventions and improving clinical care is not widespread, even though these issues, like patient safety, have concerns about the human-system interface at their core.[7]

The recognition of human user requirements in the design and deployment of QI interventions can ensure the success of such interventions. In particular, the rapid adoption of the electronic health record and the rapidly growing interest in its potential to improve the quality of health care through features such as computerized provider order entry and decision support create a substantial need for the principles of HFE within the health care arena.[8]

APPLICATIONS OF HFE IN IMPROVING HEALTH CARE QUALITY AND SAFETY

Human factors science can be applied to improve the quality of health care through:

- The analysis of errors, near misses, and adverse events, to understand causal and contributory factors better.
- The development of preventive interventions in response to an error or an adverse event, and through design of improved work environments, processes, and equipment.
- Proactive prevention of medical errors.
- Improvement in efficiency, timeliness, and accuracy of work processes in health care, and decrease in stress.
- Implementation of best practices or potentially better practices, and change management during QI projects.

Analysis of Incidents

When a medical error occurs, whether it harms the patient (an adverse event), or not (a near miss), it should be investigated to identify the factors that contributed to its occurrence. An important component of such an investigation is an exploration of the human factors that have contributed to the incident. A systematic inquiry should be made into the exact circumstances surrounding the incident: the lighting; the noise level in the environment; the physical locations of the equipment, the patient, and the involved health professionals; any malfunctioning of equipment; and the level of alertness and fatigue among the health professionals involved in the incident. A list of factors that could potentially have contributed to the occurrence of an incident, and that should be systematically investigated, is provided in **Table 1**.

Development of Interventions to Improve Safety

After the analysis of an incident is completed, the health care team usually develops some hypotheses about why the incident occurred and what factors might have contributed to it. Based on these hypotheses, a review of the literature, and, if

Table 1 **List of potential causal and contributory factors to errors and adverse events**
Use during the investigation of a patient safety incident. Check the items that you believed played a role in the case. Add comments if needed.
Work environment
Staffing levels and skills mix
Workload and shift patterns
Equipment design, availability, maintenance
Ergonomic factors
Administrative and managerial support
Task factors
Task design and clarity of structure
Availability and use of protocols
Individual (staff) factors
Knowledge and skills
Motivation and attitude
Physical and mental health
Emotional state and stress
Rule violations
Institutional factors
Economic and regulatory context
Medicolegal environment
Organization and management
Financial resources and constraints
Safety culture and priorities
Policy standards and goals
Safety culture and priorities
Team factors
Verbal communication
Written communication
Supervision and willingness to seek help
Team structure and leadership
Patient and patient's family factors
Condition (complexity and seriousness)
Language and communication
Personality and social factors

Adapted from Vincent C, Taylor-Adams S, Chapman EJ, et al. How to investigate and analyse clinical incidents: Clinical Risk Unit and Association of Litigation and Risk Management protocol. BMJ 2000;320:777–81.

possible, the experiences of other institutions that have dealt with similar problems, the team usually decides to implement some safety interventions. These interventions should be designed according to the principles of HFE. For example, an investigation into an infusion pump error in a neonatal intensive care unit (NICU) may reveal that the error occurred because of poor lighting in the area where the infusion pump was placed and because the nurse experienced numerous distractions when she was trying to load the infusion tubing into the pump and program the infusion rate into the pump. Therefore, the interventions to be implemented to prevent similar errors in the future should include improved task lighting in the vicinity of the infusion pumps, the use of infusion pumps that have brighter screens that are visible in the dark, and methods to prevent nurses from being distracted when performing critical tasks during their shift.

Proactive Prevention of Medical Errors

Prevention of errors can be accomplished by the application of HFE to the purchase of new equipment, and the design of new facilities, operating rooms, and patient spaces. Sometimes, an existing patient-care area can be altered using HFE principles to enhance efficiency and safety. Processes can also be designed de novo or redesigned using HFE principles. The design of medical devices and surgical and endoscopy instruments requires the use of HFE. The use of heuristic checklists such as the ones described later can help in proactively designing products and processes for efficiency and safety.

Improvement in Efficiency, Timeliness, and Accuracy and Decrease in Stress

Delays can be decreased and efficiency (the amount of work output for a given amount of energy and resources expended) can be improved through the use of HFE. For example, when health professionals perform their work, if the required equipment is within easy reach, fully functional, easy to use, and optimally arranged spatially, work will result in less fatigue, and be accomplished faster and more accurately with fewer errors. For example, when a nurse practitioner is inserting a central venous catheter, the patient's bed (radiant warmer or incubator) should be at the optimal height, there should be adequate lighting at the insertion site, there should be an adequate space (preferably a dedicated procedure table) for the equipment to be laid out, the equipment should be placed close to the operator's dominant arm, a waste receptacle should be available in close proximity, and cognitive aids should be used that eliminate reliance on memory (such as a checklist of required equipment, procedural steps, precautions, and the ideal depth of catheter insertion). Ensuring all these will enable the catheter insertion to be performed quickly, without errors, and with minimal fatigue experienced by the operator.

Implementation of Best Practices or Potentially Better Practices and Change Management

The introduction of potentially better practices based on evidence involves first the development of those practices and then implementation, standardization, and ongoing measurement. Ensuring that unit staff adhere to the desired changes and practices requires more than an in-service training session, a notice at a meeting, or a communication book. Such change must be integrated into the current system in a way such that the operator can easily perform the task, and is reminded or otherwise guided to perform this task. Such is the domain of the behavioral science arm of human factors.

One useful model of HFE in clinical work was proposed by Karsh and colleagues[9] (**Fig. 1**).

Several tools are used in HFE for specific purposes. For example, hierarchical task analysis (HTA) is used to analyze the task requirements necessary to accomplish goals and identify the operator or user demands for successful task completion.[10] Incident reviews and root cause analysis (RCA) (see article by Ursprung and Gray elsewhere in this issue) are used to analyze contributing factors and causes of adverse events. Although there are standards for the inclusion of human factors review in the design

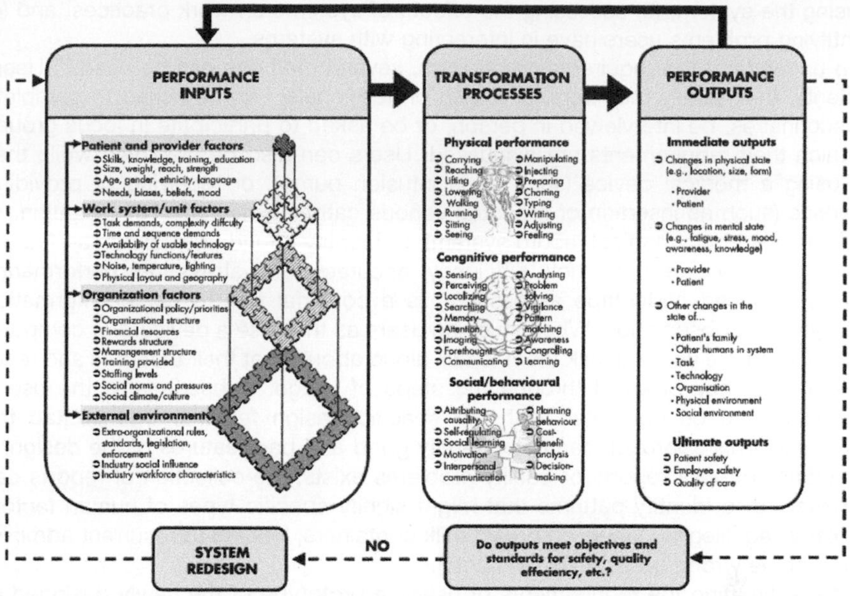

Fig. 1. Input-transformation-output model of health care professional performance. (*From* Karsh BT, Holden RJ, Alper SJ, et al. A human factors engineering paradigm for patient safety: designing to support the performance of the healthcare professional. Qual Saf Health Care 2006;15(Suppl 1):i59–65; with permission.)

and development of medical devices, for instance, there are few regulated or voluntarily accepted standards.[11] The clinical team is thus charged with the integration and operational issues that come with such variation.[7]

In applying the principles of HFE to improving safety and quality, the 4 key questions to be asked are:

1. Are the requirements of the users (patients, their families, health care providers, and other participants involved in this effort) understood?
2. Does the design of the process/device/service/workplace meet the anticipated needs of the users?
3. Does the design facilitate efficient, accurate, and error-free performance by the users?
4. Does the design achieve the best compromise between efficiency, effort, accuracy, safety, and costs for that specific situation?

UNDERSTANDING USER REQUIREMENTS

The capacity of a system to allow users to perform their tasks safely, effectively, efficiently, and enjoyably is known as usability.[12] Usability engineering is the application of scientific methods for improving system development, and such methods are currently widely used in systems that involve human-computer interaction.[13,14] Similar methods can also be used for the design and improvement of devices, work processes, and physical environments in health care.

The methods of usability engineering[15] consist of: (1) characterizing how easily a user can carry out a task using the system, (2) assessing how users attain mastery in using the system, (3) assessing the effects of systems on work practices, and (4) identifying problems users have in interacting with systems.

To understand the requirements of users, several methods can be used.[15] Users (patients, their family members, or health professionals) can be asked to complete questionnaires, be interviewed in person, or be asked to participate in focus groups in which their requirements are discussed. Users can also be observed while they are using a medical device (such as in infusion pump), or receiving or providing a service (such as insertion of a central venous catheter, neonatal resuscitation, or using an electronic medical record system), to identify if fundamental human factors principles are violated and how efficiency, accuracy, and stress-free performance can be achieved. Videotape assessment is a powerful tool to gather information through direct observation. When studying users as they use a device or a computer system, it can be useful to ask them to talk aloud about what their thoughts and reactions are as they proceed through the steps of usage. Subsequently, the users' comments can be correlated with the specific design features that elicited the comments. This approach can help identify good and bad features of the design. If a database of error reports or quality problems exists, the collection of reports can be reviewed to identify patterns that might signify specific types of human factors problems (eg, illegible labels on breast milk containers, leading to recurrent administration of the wrong breast milk to infants).

After estimating the requirements of users, a prototype of the newly designed or altered work process or device can be provided to users, and reactions to the prototype can be assessed in the ways listed earlier. For example, if the NICU QI team is working on the prevention of nosocomial infection, and they observe that alcohol gel dispensers in their unit are placed in locations that are not convenient for their nurses, they might develop a prototype of a method to provide alcohol gel dispensers in locations immediately adjacent to incubators (eg, mounting the dispensers on the bedside poles on which intravenous infusions are hung). In testing prototypes of such work processes, the reactions of the users can be assessed and measures can be obtained of efficiency, accuracy, and effectiveness (time taken to perform a task, the frequency of errors, successful completion of a task). This information will provide guidance about how the prototype can be redesigned and refined.

In all methods of testing users' experiences so that the findings can inform design and redesign, users should be selected so that they are representative of the ultimate target population of users, and the context of the testing should be as realistic as possible. As far as possible, user observations should be carried out in the actual clinical environment of the NICU in which improvements are planned.

EXAMPLES OF APPLICATION OF HFE PRINCIPLES IN THE NICU

Neonatal intensive care is complex and involves many technological systems and subsystems, whose reliability is, in part, determined by natural limitations in human performance. Therefore, neonatal intensive care provides numerous opportunities for the application of the principles of HFE, particularly to minimize the potential for human error. Since 2002, through the Vermont Oxford Network's collaborative project to improve the quality and safety of neonatal care, Neonatal Intensive Care Quality (NIC/Q), the authors have been promoting the use of human factors science to improve patient care. As part of the NIC/Q project, the NICU Human Factors Checklist Series[16] (described in detail in **Table 2**) was developed. These checklists allow NICUs to proactively assess, using HFE principles, whether or not their systems of care are optimally designed and to identify opportunities for

Table 2
Vermont Oxford network NIC/Q human factors checklist series

Checklist Topic	NICU Examples	Key Human Factors
Clinical alarms	Pulse oximeter, monitors, intravenous pumps, ventilators	Parameter setting and response behavior
Labels and displays	Drugs, breast milk, monitors	Image characteristics, size, color
Procedure following	Daily care, line insertion and care	Omission affordances, reminders, checklists
Device usability	Medical devices and equipment	Usability heuristics and testing
Alertness	Hours of work, fatigue effects	Fatigue countermeasures, awareness
Warnings	Signs, stickers, labels	Design, placement, content
Paper forms	Orders, charts	Process guide and communication
Team performance	Crisis response, obstetrics/perinatal	Performance shaping factors, communication pattern
Unit design	Bedspace, headwalls, single-patient rooms	Process and proximity, communication
Physical ergonomics	Posture, layout, visual demand	Adjustability, visibility, maintenance

improvement. They also enable NICUs to make changes that reduce the potential for error, thus improving patient safety. A secondary purpose was to educate users on human factors and help to build a culture that focuses on system reliability. These checklists are based on a method called heuristic evaluation,[14] a usability inspection method in which the system is evaluated from well-tested design principles such as visibility of system status, user control and freedom, consistency and standards, flexibility, and efficiency of use.

Ideally, the checklists should be administered by a small multidisciplinary team of people from the NICU and from other relevant disciplines (such as biomedical engineering, purchasing, environmental services). The team can conduct a walk-through in the NICU and perform assessments using the checklists. After a discussion among the team members, each item on the checklist is assigned a grade based on the best judgment of the team.

A. This characteristic is adequate at this time.
B. This characteristic is being modified or changed.
C. This characteristic requires further investigation.
D. This characteristic is not adequate.

In addition, for each of the items on the checklist, the team should reflect on and review any adverse incidents or near misses in their unit related to that checklist item.

Efforts can then be made to correct those characteristics that are not adequate, by modifying the design of the device or the process, or by replacement with a new device or process. An example of the complete checklist for labels and displays in the NICU is provided in Appendix 1.

Clinical Alarms

Devices in the NICU with alarms include cardiorespiratory monitors, ventilators, pulse oximeters, incubators, and infusion pumps. Checklist items for the assessment of alarms in an NICU include audibility, probability matching behavior, silencing, and suspension behavior and controls.[17–20]

Labels and Displays

Printed labels are frequently used in the NICU for medications, laboratory specimens, and breast milk; visual displays and signs are used to convey important messages about the patient (eg, the patient's name and gender, isolation precautions, developmental care measures to be followed), medical equipment (eg, signs that indicate the size and insertion depth of an endotracheal tube), or the environment. Thus, labels and displays often carry safety-critical information. Ideally, labels and displays should use text that is sufficiently large, with adequate contrast between the text and the background, using unambiguous terms that cannot be confused with other terms. Specific checklist topics include visual characteristics, legibility, readability, redundancy, emphasis, and salience.[21–24] The complete checklist for labels and displays is provided in Appendix 1, as an example of the checklist series.

Procedures and Task Guidance

Procedural controls are an important error prevention measure in the NICU, and often the most feasible safety intervention. With human error in general,[25,26] and specifically with NICU incidents, omission of procedural steps has been identified as a common error type. The checklist for procedures and task guidance facilitates the review of omission affordances for specific errors and the use of reminders and checklists.[27–28]

Device Usability

The provision of care in the NICU involves the use of numerous medical devices that perform various functions critical to patient safety. Each unit has its own mix of devices, which makes the context of use and review of equipment unique to each environment. The checklist for device usability uses a heuristic approach to guide usability review, or testing, for devices that are in service, or as a guide to support evaluation and safety considerations related to the procurement of new equipment.[14,29]

Alertness

The effects of fatigue on performance have been well established and the NICU is a 24/7 operation with some staff categories known to work 24-hour shifts. This checklist directs attention to the deployment of preventive countermeasures such as shift design and rotation, and operational countermeasures such as napping and light exposure.[30,31]

Information Systems

The introduction of automation into health care through tools such as the electronic medical record, computerized provider order entry, and information management systems, to improve safety and quality, has the illusion of removing the role of the human and their concomitant failings from the system of care. A recent review[32] cautions about the folly of such an illusion, however, and suggests that such development increases the need for human factors and especially training, interface design, and interaction design. Particular attention should be paid to understanding the workflow patterns of clinical work before introducing automated systems. An in-depth understanding of such workflow patterns and how they might be altered with the perturbation caused by the introduction of the new information system can enable the smooth introduction of such systems.

Physical Environment

The physical environment (eg, lighting, noise, distraction, reach, position) influences the ability of a health professional to perform his or her task successfully, accurately, and efficiently. Physical dimensions of NICU work are affected by the position of equipment and patients. The performance of tasks inside an incubator affects visual acuity and posture. Physical ergonomics has been shown to adversely affect quality and product defects during manufacturing.[33] With many NICUs now building new patient-care areas and with the increasing trend to build single-room NICUs, the design of the physical environment becomes especially important. The construction of these new NICUs offers unique opportunities to design the physical layout optimally from a human factors perspective. Although providing patient care in individual patient rooms may provide significant advantages, it can also have undesirable effects on monitoring of patients and on team interactions.

In recent years there has been increasing interest in the application of methods of lean production (best known as the method responsible for the success of the Toyota Production System) to health care.[34,35] An important principle of lean methods is that a clean, well-ordered workplace facilitates optimal work and the improvement of work. A methodology used in lean production is the 5-S system, which consists of sort, set-in-order, shine, standardize, and sustain. Sort means that all items in the work environment should be classified as being essential or nonessential, and unnecessary material causing clutter in the workplace should be removed. Set-in-order means that the remaining necessary materials and equipment should be organized, labeled, and laid out, preferably using visual cues (the visual workplace) in a way that facilitates work and minimizes wasted motion and effort. Shine indicates that the workplace should be clean and well maintained through regular inspections. Standardize refers to the use of standard layouts in the work environment and standard processes of accomplishing work. Sustain refers to the need for 5-S methods to become an integral and deep-rooted part of the organization, not a transient fad. This result can be achieved through promotional and communication campaigns in the organization, and through 5-S training of all employees.

Device Design

The opportunity for the application of human factors science begins with the concept and design of devices. Usability of devices often seems to be an afterthought. For example, 1 in-depth analysis of an early design of a patient-controlled analgesia device indicated a complex and confusing control process that likely contributed to many errors.[36] Device design can be evaluated to assess the following basic concepts: is the display visible and legible, and are the controls logically positioned? The use of usability heuristics such as those evaluated by Zhang and colleagues,[29] and originally developed by Nielsen and Mack[14] for use in computer software, can improve the likelihood that a novice review will identify usability shortcomings in device design. However, it is likely that a more informed and expert review is necessary to perform a thorough evaluation to counteract political and administrative priorities involved in large capital acquisitions.[37]

Product Selection and System Design

There are requirements for human factors review in the design of medical devices.[11] However, even with this requirement, studies have shown a potential for a wide range of usability and design-related errors to occur with contemporary infusion pumps.[29,37] One recent analysis of incidents in the NICU[38] also indicated that human factors usability problems played a role in errors involving ventilators. Most administrative and clinical personnel who are charged with purchasing decisions are not sufficiently skilled in understanding human factors principles to be able to evaluate scientifically the different equipment choices under consideration. Therefore, they should seek the advice of human factors experts, given the widespread and long-lasting effect of such purchase decisions.[37] If there is a significant cost differential among reviewed products, a decision may need to include an estimate of cost/benefit for the life of the device, to convince decision-makers to overlook these financial disparities. An evidence-based review, however, may also provide the rigor needed for an informed decision. Evaluations should consider user requirements and be based on a comprehensive understanding of how a product will be used and obtained with methods such as HTA.[10,39–43]

Introducing Change

Often the introduction of a change in a QI project involves only the education of providers. However, a QI project informed by human factors science would include other interventions, based on the relevant situation, equipment, processes, and environment. For instance, a frequent quality deficiency involves the omission of steps or practice requirements. To simply provide education may miss the opportunity to introduce other changes to equipment, materials, environment, or procedural (cognitive) aids that follow from an analysis of omission affordances.[27]

SUMMARY

HFE presents a formidable contribution to QI in the NICU. The science behind the fundamental principles concerning the design of work systems that match the needs of the people who work in them is sound and is applied widely in other safety-critical situations. Early application of HFE in NICUs has shown the usefulness of these methods for frontline teams working to improve quality, reliability, and safety. The inclusion of human factors considerations in the design of structure and process has the potential to improve outcomes for patients and families and to improve the comfort and usability of work systems for providers who work in them. New technologies and continual change must be informed and designed through the application of HFE methods and principles to realize the full potential of QI.

APPENDIX 1: LABELS AND DISPLAYS

This checklist has been developed to facilitate a unit's assessment of human factors that relate to labels and displays and error potential in the NICU. The intent is to provide you with guidance in your review of materials, processes, equipment, and environment. Feedback on this checklist and label- or display-related errors should be conveyed to the author, Jim Handyside at jim@improvisionhealthcare.com.

See the Human Factors Checklist Series Overview[16] (see **Table 2**) for general information and instructions about these checklists.

Human Factors of Labels and Displays

Labels and displays communicate essential information, from patient identification to physiologic status or drug dosage. The way in which this information is visually presented is important in minimizing the risk of error.[2,7]

Perception is not just the automatic translation of what we see. We often infer or assume certain meaning based on our expectations or the context of the present situation or what has happened in the past.[44] Making the visual presentation as clear as possible is essential to ensure that the correct meaning is understood.

Under ideal conditions most labels or displays seem adequate. There are times when conditions are not ideal: lighting is low, labels are partially obscured, or glare disrupts the image. The demographics of most organizations suggest that aging further heightens the need for a cautious approach to how information is presented, with a decline in visual acuity with age.[21,45,46]

Several label-related errors are reported in the medical errors system at www.NICQ.org. The following illustrates some of the reported issues:

- Frozen breast milk received from a referring hospital in a different container than is normally used. A nurse obtained a similar nonstandard container of breast milk from the freezer and fed the baby before noting that the label indicated the milk belonged to another patient.
- Wrong breast milk labeled with similar patient's name and sent to NICU.
- Giving breast milk to wrong patient (similar last names on label).
- Near miss: laboratory labels were placed at the wrong patient's bedside.
- Breast milk was thawed, warmed, and gavaged in the wrong infant. The label was wet and faint; the names were similar.
- Breast milk container did not have the required patient identification label. The handwritten label was covered by a "Thaw" sticker.
- Patient's bedside drawer had a carton of Enfamil with iron 24 cal/oz in it and a half-empty bottle on top of the bedside table. Patient was ordered Enfamil with iron 20 cal/oz. Both kinds of bottles have yellow labels.
- A near miss occurred in which a vial of phenylephrine was placed on an anesthesiology cart in the bin in which atropine is to be stored. The stocking technician made the mistake, which was identified by the anesthesiologist. The 2 vials are almost identical in appearance, but in 2 different classes, and confusion could have resulted in a death.
- A gavage tube feeding by a pump was given via the respiratory lavage port of a Ballard in-line suction catheter, despite all lines and ports being appropriately labeled. The Ballard lavage port allows any size syringe or extension tubing to be connected.

Attention to human factors of labels and displays reduces the likelihood of error. Other aspects of labels and displays are also important, such as the process for ensuring that correct labels are applied, education on the content of device displays and how to interpret them, and the use of bar code labeling systems. This checklist addresses human factors related to how information appears on the label or display. It is also important to recognize, as the tube feeding incident described earlier illustrates, that labeling alone is not always adequate and other control measures should be used whenever possible.

Examples of labels include medication labels, breast milk, specimens, embossing cards, patient identification, equipment labels, tubes, and containers.

Examples of displays include screens, liquid crystal display (LCD) panels, and monitors associated with syringe pumps, ventilators, pulse oximeter, cardiorespiratory monitors, isolettes, and other devices.

Labels and Displays: Human Factors Principles

The visual presentation of information requires a consideration of the physical characteristics (how information is presented) to ensure that it is communicated with the least possibility for error. The following principles apply to all forms of visual communication, including labels and device displays. These principles will serve as a guideline as you work through the checklist. Although many may be intuitively obvious, they are based on research reported in the literature on human factors and applied psychology.[2,5–12] These principles should be consulted for guidance as you work through the checklist, as an aid to conducting other safety analysis (eg, RCA) or when considering new labels and displays.

The principles are listed under these categories[24,47–51]:

- Design of message: physical features of the label or display (eg, typeface, size)
- Message transmission: environmental factors (eg, viewing angle, lighting)
- Message receipt: personal factors (eg, visual ability, situation knowledge).

Design of message

Legibility of the message on a label or screen display affects the user's ability to discriminate among or recognize letters, numbers, and other characters. It is influenced by shape, size, contrast, color, and the quality of printing, reproduction, or projection on the screen.

- Use simple and familiar fonts. Sans-serif fonts (eg, Arial) are more legible than serif fonts (eg, Times New Roman)

Viewing distance (in/ft) (m)	Character height (mm)
28 in (0.7)	2–5
3 ft (0.9)	3–7
6 ft (1.8)	7–13
20 ft (6.1)	22–43

- Avoid fonts that have characters that are similar (eg, letter "O" and zero "0")
- Use of all upper case letters reduces legibility and should be avoided unless the text is brief.
- Limit the use of bold or italic type.
- See table for character height and viewing distance.

Color combinations:

Best

Black letters on a white background

Black on yellow

Good

Dark blue on white

Green on white

Yellow on black

White on black

Avoid using black on dark red, green, and blue.

Avoid the use of color in low-light conditions. Do not rely on color as the only distinguishing characteristic; provide redundancy to ensure meaning is clear.

Readability refers to the ease of reading words or numbers when the individual characters are legible.

- Avoid the use of italics or bold for long strings of text.
- Vertical space between lines should be greater than 25% of the overall font height.
- Use ink that will not smear under conditions of use
- Labels should be printed on nonglossy paper. If labels are protected by plastic it should have a matte finish to reduce glare.
- Ensure that the placement of labels on curved surfaces does not distort text to adversely affect legibility.
- Place labels in a position that minimizes damage to the message.
- Highlighter, borders, or underlining can be used for emphasis but should not distort the message text or be the only distinguishing characteristic.
- Icons can be an effective supplement to printed text when they are clear and understood. Icons should not be used alone; always provide a text description to reduce confusion.
- Bar code labels must also include readable text.

Message transmission

- Labels and displays should be viewed at 90° to the line of sight.
- Labels and displays should be oriented horizontally or easily moved to that position.
- If displays are viewed in low light, the device should have an illuminated display screen or have supplemental lighting.
- Task lighting should be available for reading labels when ambient lighting is maintained at low levels.

Message receipt

Comprehensibility is a measure of how reliably someone interprets a message. It depends on prior knowledge, language skills, expectation, habit, routine, location, and the context in which the message is viewed.

- Keep messages on labels brief and concise
- Avoid ambiguous words and abbreviations.
- Provide redundancy in the message (eg, name and identification number; supplement color-coding and symbols with text).
- Have someone test-read labels to verify clarity of meaning.
- For items that look similar, add unique markings and store in separate places.

Using the Label and Displays Checklist

Preparation

Before you begin a walk-through it will be helpful to:

- Identify and obtain all relevant policies, procedures, guidelines, and protocols directing the use of labels and devices with displays.
- Compile an inventory of important safety-critical labels and displays in the unit.
- Identify any recently recorded incidents or near misses involving labels or device displays.

Assessment Team

- This checklist can be conducted in 2 separate walk-through assessments: 1 with attention focused on labels and the other for device displays. Responsibility and job titles may vary in your unit; use discretion in forming the assessment team but include people in the know and those who have the authority to make changes.

- The core team for the labels assessment should include those people in your unit who are involved in the creation and use of labels: nurse, clerical support, pharmacist, other support personnel.
- The core team for the displays assessment should include those people who set up and use device displays: nurse, respiratory technician, biomedical engineer.
- Ad hoc members: physician, nurse educator, administrative leader, purchasing representative.

Responses

Grade your assessment under each question using this scale. Your responses will not be evaluated but rather used by you to help plan and direct necessary changes to improve patient safety. Each question has subpoints to guide your assessment.

A. This characteristic is adequate at this time.
B. This characteristic is being modified or changed.
C. This characteristic requires further investigation.
D. This characteristic is not adequate.

For each of the questions note if there have been any incidents or near misses in your unit related to the question topic.

Record notes while on the walk-through.

HUMAN FACTORS CHECKLIST: LABELS AND DISPLAYS

Point-of-care ergonomics

Are processes established to ensure correct labels are applied?

- Prepared labels are accessible and well marked.
- Label printing equipment and materials are organized and marked to minimize confusion.

Grade:
Notes:

Are labels legible and readable?

- Labels follow principles for legibility and readability.
- Verify this by finding and examining labels in use.
- The conditions of use do not damage labels or otherwise interfere with readability.
- Bar code labels include readable words corresponding to the code information.

Grade:
Notes:

Are product labels unique and clearly marked?

- Labels with similar color schemes are supplemented with clear and unique markings and stored separately.

Grade:
Notes:

Are display screens on devices legible and readable?

- Devices are positioned horizontally and at right angles to the line of sight.
- The whole display screen is visible with no obstruction.
- Test the readability from angles and distances that would be encountered while providing care.
- Adjustments to display content and characteristics are consistent with human factors principles.

Grade:
Notes:

Point-of-care environment

Is there adequate ambient or task lighting available to read labels?

- Overhead room lighting is adequate when on and supplemented with task lighting if required.

Grade:

Notes:

Are device displays illuminated with minimal glare?

- LCD panels have back lighting, or supplemental lighting is available if needed.
- Screens are set with adequate brightness and contrast; color choice matches human factors principles when possible.
- Ambient or task lighting does not produce distracting glare on screens.

Grade:

Notes:

Individual human factors

Are staff familiar with human factors principles for message design, transmission, and receipt?

Handmade or nonstandard labels are consistent with human factors principles.

Grade:

Notes:

Are staff aware of their personal vision characteristics and do they make adjustments to accommodate?

- Staff know how to adjust lighting or displays if required.
- Staff know when to adjust displays to meet their visual capacity and when displays should remain standard.

Grade:

Notes:

Team and group factors

Is there a process for communicating changes in labels or displays?

- Staff alert each other about changes they make in labeling or individual adjustments they make to displays.
- Display screen content and layout are standardized whenever possible.

Grade:

Notes:

Are people using standard abbreviations, symbols, and color codes?

- Use of abbreviations is avoided (preferred) or standardized.
- Symbols and color are used only to supplement a message that is also provided in words.

Grade:

Notes:

Organizational and management factors

How are labels, labeling systems, and devices with displays selected and implemented?

- Human factors principles are used as criteria in the selection process.
- Trials of labels and devices include evaluation of legibility, readability, and other human factors in consideration of error potential.

Grade:
Notes:

Is compliance with established procedures for labels and displays periodically reviewed?

Grade:
Notes:

REFERENCES

1. Donabedian A. Evaluating the quality of medical care. The Milbank Memorial Fund Quarterly 1966;44:166–206.
2. Meister D. The history of human factors and ergonomics. Mahwah (NJ) USA: Lawrence Erlbaum Associates; 1999.
3. Salvendy G. Handbook of human factors and ergonomics. 3rd edition. Hoboken (NJ): John Wiley; 2006. p. 5–24.
4. Cooper JB, Newbower RS, Long CD, et al. Preventable anesthesia mishaps: a study of human factors. Anesthesiology 1978;49:399–406.
5. Cooper JB, Newbower RS, Long CD, et al. Preventable anesthesia mishaps: a study of human factors. 1978. Qual Saf Health Care 2002;11:277–82.
6. Carayon P. Handbook of human factors and ergonomics in health care and patient safety. Mahwah (NJ): Lawrence Erlbaum Associates; 2007.
7. Scanlon MC, Karsh BT, Densmore EM. Human factors engineering and patient safety. Pediatr Clin North Am 2006;53:1105–19.
8. Johnson CW. Why did that happen? Exploring the proliferation of barely usable software in healthcare systems. Qual Saf Health Care 2006;15(Suppl 1):i76–81.
9. Karsh BT, Holden RJ, Alper SJ, et al. A human factors engineering paradigm for patient safety: designing to support the performance of the healthcare professional. Qual Saf Health Care 2006;15(Suppl 1):i59–65.
10. Lane R, Stanton NA, Harrison D. Applying hierarchical task analysis to medication administration errors. Appl Ergon 2006;37:669–79.
11. ANSI/AAMI. Human factors design process for medical devices. 2001;HE:74.
12. Preece J, Rogers Y, Sharp H. Interaction design: beyond human-computer interaction. New York: J. Wiley & Sons; 2002.
13. Rosson MB, Carroll JM. Usability engineering: scenario-based development of human-computer interaction. 1st edition. San Francisco (CA): Academic Press; 2002.
14. Nielsen J, Mack RL. Usability inspection methods. New York: Wiley; 1994.
15. Kushniruk A. Evaluation in the design of health information systems: application of approaches emerging from usability engineering. Comput Biol Med 2002;32: 141–9.
16. Handyside J. Systematic application of human factors and ergonomics in the neonatal ICU. Proceedings of Healthcare Systems Ergonomics and Patient Safety Conference. Strasbourg (France), June 25–27, 2008.
17. Woods DD. The alarm problem and directed attention in dynamic fault management. Ergonomics 1995;38:2371–93.
18. Bliss JP, Gilson RD, Deaton JE. Human probability matching behaviour in response to alarms of varying reliability. Ergonomics 1995;38:2300–12.
19. Edworthy J, Stanton N. A user-centred approach to the design and evaluation of auditory warning signals: 1. Methodology. Ergonomics 1995;38:2262–80.

20. Edworthy J, Hellier E. Fewer but better auditory alarms will improve patient safety. Qual Saf Health Care 2005;14:212–5.
21. Phillips RJ. Why is lower case better. Appl Ergon 1979;10:211–4.
22. Kodak E. In: Rodgers SH, editor. Ergonomic design for people at work, vol. 1. Belmont (CA): Lifetime Learning Publications; 1983.
23. Sanders MS, McCormick EJ. Human factors in engineering and design. New York: McGraw-Hill; 1993.
24. Wilkins AJ, Nimmo-Smith MI. The clarity and comfort of printed text. Ergonomics 1987;30:1705–20.
25. Reason J. Human error. Cambridge (UK): Cambridge University Press; 1990. p. 184–7.
26. de Brito G. Towards a model for the study of written procedure following in dynamic environments. Reliab Eng Syst Saf 2002;75:233–44.
27. Reason J. Combating omission errors through task analysis and good reminders. Qual Saf Health Care 2002;11:40–4.
28. Piotrowski MM, Hinshaw DB. The safety checklist program: creating a culture of safety in intensive care units. Jt Comm J Qual Improv 2002;28:306.
29. Zhang J, Johnson TR, Patel VL, et al. Using usability heuristics to evaluate patient safety of medical devices. J Biomed Inform 2003;36:23–30.
30. Dawson D, Campbell SS. Timed exposure to bright light improves sleep and alertness during simulated night shifts. Sleep 1991;14:511.
31. Bonnefond A, Muzet A, Winter-Dill AS, et al. Innovative working schedule: introducing one short nap during the night shift. Ergonomics 2001;44:937–45.
32. Lee JD. Review of a pivotal human factors article: "humans and automation: use, misuse, disuse, abuse". Hum Factors 2008;50:404.
33. Eklund JAE. Relationships between ergonomics and quality in assembly work. Appl Ergon 1995;26:15–20.
34. Graban M. Lean hospitals: improving quality, patient safety, and employee satisfaction. Boca Raton (FL): CRC Press; 2009.
35. Printezis A, Gopalakrishnan M. Current pulse: can a production system reduce medical errors in health care? Qual Manag Health Care 2007;16:226–38.
36. Lin L, Isla R, Doniz K, et al. Applying human factors to the design of medical equipment: patient-controlled analgesia. J Clin Monit Comput 1998;14:253–63.
37. Nemeth C, Nunnally M, Bitan Y, et al. Between choice and chance: the role of human factors in acute care equipment decisions. J Patient Saf 2009;5:114–21.
38. Snijders C, van Lingen RA, Klip H, et al. Specialty-based, voluntary incident reporting in neonatal intensive care: description of 4846 incident reports. Arch Dis Child Fetal Neonatal Ed 2009;94:F210–5.
39. Zhang J, Johnson TR, Patel VL, et al. Safety for medical devices with integral information technology. Advances in patient safety: from research to implementation, vol. 2. Rockville (MD): AHRQ, Publication No. 05-0021-2. Agency for Healthcare Research and Quality; 2005.
40. Phipps D, Meakin GH, Beatty PC, et al. Human factors in anaesthetic practice: insights from a task analysis. Br J Anaesth 2008;100:333–43.
41. Callan JR. Gwynee JW. Human factors principles for medical device labeling. Food and Drug Administration (FDA Contract No. 223-89-6022). 1993. Available at: http://www.fda.gov/CDRH/dsma/227.html. Accessed January 8, 2010.
42. Degani A. On the typography of flight-deck documentation. (NASA contract report 177605). Moffett Field (CA): NASA Ames Research Center; 1992.

43. Degani A, Wiener EL. The human factors of flight-deck checklist the normal checklist. (NASA contract report 177549). Moffett Field (CA): NASA Ames Research Center; 1990.
44. Wickens CD, Hollands J. Engineering psychology and human performance. Upper Saddle River (NJ): Prentice Hall; 2000.
45. Haigh R. The aging process: a challenge for design. Appl Ergon 1993;24(1): 9–14.
46. Rayner K, Kaiser JS. Reading mutilated text. J Educ Psychol 1975;67:301–6.
47. Rodgers SH, editor. Ergonomic design for people at work, vol. 1. Belmont (CA): Lifetime Learning Publications; 1983.
48. Sanders MS, McCormick EJ. Human factors in engineering and design. 6th edition. New York: McGraw-Hill; 1987.
49. Smith SL. Letter size and legibility. Hum Factors 1979;21(6):661–70.
50. Woodson WE, Conover DW. Human engineering guide for equipment designers. 2nd edition. Berkeley (CA): University of California Press; 1964.
51. Wiedenbeck S. The use of icons and labels in an end user application program: an empirical study of learning and retention. Behav Inf Technol 1999;18(2): 68–82.

Random Safety Auditing, Root Cause Analysis, Failure Mode and Effects Analysis

Robert Ursprung, MD, MMSc[a,*], James Gray, MD, MS[b,c]

KEYWORDS

- Failure mode and effects analysis • Root cause analysis
- Random safety auditing

Improving quality and safety in health care is a major concern for health care providers, the general public, and policy makers.[1–4] Errors and quality issues are leading causes of morbidity and mortality across the health care industry.[5–9] In adult intensive care units, nearly half of all patients suffer at least 1 adverse drug event; 1 in 5 of these patients suffer death or disability from the event.[10]

Gaps in the quality and safety of health care, however, are not limited to the care provided to adults. There is strong published evidence that patients in the neonatal intensive care unit (NICU) are at high risk for serious medical errors.[11–14] Kaushal and colleagues[11] showed that adverse drug events in the NICU occur at a rate that is 8 times those published for hospitalized adults. Anonymous reports of voluntary error from 54 NICUs reveal errors in virtually all domains of care.[15]

Although these published reports provide a valuable overview of safety issues in health care, the research methods typically do not lend themselves to use by frontline providers. To facilitate compliance with safe practices, many institutions have established quality-assurance monitoring procedures including voluntary incident reporting, chart auditing, and automated data mining of laboratory, pharmacy, and case mix data.[16–22] Although these methods may improve error detection, they can be time-consuming, costly, and do little to involve frontline providers. To address these concerns, some quality and patient safety programs use safety methods borrowed from other industries that may improve the quality and safety of patient care more efficiently and more effectively.[23–29]

[a] Pediatrix Medical Group, Cook Children's Medical Center, Department of Neonatology, 801 Seventh Avenue, Fort Worth, TX 76104, USA
[b] Division of Newborn Medicine, Harvard Medical School, USA
[c] Division of Clinical Informatics, Department of Neonatology, Beth Israel Deaconess Medical Center, Boston, MA, USA
* Corresponding author.
E-mail address: robert_ursprung@pediatrix.com

Clin Perinatol 37 (2010) 141–165
doi:10.1016/j.clp.2010.01.008 perinatology.theclinics.com
0095-5108/10/$ – see front matter

Three techniques that have been found useful in the health care setting are failure mode and effects analysis (FMEA), root cause analysis (RCA), and random safety auditing (RSA). When used together, these techniques are effective tools for system analysis and redesign focused on providing safe delivery of care in the complex NICU system (**Table 1**).

RANDOM SAFETY AUDITING

RSA, also known as random auditing, or random process auditing, is an intuitive method that can be applied by frontline clinical staff to enhance quality and safety in a busy work environment. Rather than attempt to monitor all procedures, processes, or process elements in clinical care, this methodology focuses on monitoring a subset of error-prone points in the system. From this subset, items are selected at random for measurement. Immediate feedback can be provided to frontline clinical staff, and subsequent aggregate analysis permits robust coverage of complex systems over time.

Characteristics of RSA that make it attractive to health care include its low cost to implement, minimal requirements for training of staff, the ability to detect errors (many of which are not easily detectable by other means), and perhaps most importantly, the flexibility of the methods. Audit questions can be created, eliminated, or revised as safety/quality priorities change. The auditing methods can be adapted to the culture and workflow of a given work setting.

The Center for Patient Safety in Neonatal Intensive Care (the Center) adapted RSA methodology to the health care setting as a novel approach to improve quality and patient safety.[12,30–33] More than just a tool to detect errors, RSA has the potential to reduce future errors through the identification of system failures that contribute to gaps in quality and safety. Further, RSA incorporates features of evidence-based behavior change agents, including audit and feedback, self-efficacy, social norms, and reinforcement.[23,34,35]

Table 1
Effective tools for system analysis and redesign for safe delivery of care in the complex NICU system

	FMEA	RCA	RSA
Approach	**Proactive**	**Reactive**	**Maintenance**
Key concept	What could go wrong	What went wrong	Are critical system components working?
Technique	Failure modes: What could go wrong? Failure causes: Why would it go wrong? Failure effects: What are the consequences?	Team analysis of event: Why did event occur – proximate and root causes? (5 "Whys") Design correction	Continuous monitoring of high-priority system elements (may have been previously identified by RCA or FMEA)
Comment	Risk prioritization: failure modes and effects are given scores to determine the magnitude of risk Analysis of cause: Enables system redesign of high-priority processes	Analysis of past system failure is focused on system redesign to prevent future errors	Focused on identifying and correcting system breakdowns before patient harm can occur

Initial Use in the Health Care Setting

The usefulness of RSA in the health care setting was first shown in an NICU in a tertiary care children's hospital.[12] The 5-week single-unit study detected more than 300 errors, representing such diverse aspects of care as alarm settings, patient identification, hand hygiene, labeling of tubes, syringes, and medications. In addition to identifying and counting errors, the audit tool stimulated productive discussions among clinicians, because the audits identified major remediable gaps in performance. These bedside discussions, in conjunction with feedback of summarized audit data to staff and management, led to rapid changes in policy and practice.

For example, the audits revealed that only 9% of NICU patients wore their patient identification (ID) band as stipulated by unit policy. This finding is especially concerning in light of data showing NICU patients are at high risk for misidentification.[13] An RCA (see next section), prompted by the audit data, identified several barriers to use of the identification system. These barriers included such circumstances as the frequent removal by bedside clinicians of the hard plastic ID band to avoid abrasions and lacerations of fragile infant skin. In addition, even when these bands were not causing skin breakdown, they were often removed to facilitate intravenous (IV) access. Bands were often not replaced because the process to procure a new one was labor intensive for the bedside nurse (**Fig. 1**). Prompt process changes, including purchase of an ID band that addressed nursing concerns, resulted in sustainable compliance rates greater than 90%.[12]

Although this initial study of RSA was conducted in a research paradigm with a dedicated research nurse, a subsequent follow-up study showed that RSA conducted by frontline providers detected errors at the same rate as a research team auditing concurrently. The authors' experience has shown that RSAs may reduce future errors in 4 important ways: (1) identifying system failures, (2) increasing provider awareness of issues relevant to quality and safety, (3) involving more staff in improvement efforts, and (4) exploiting advantages of the audit and feedback loop.

A

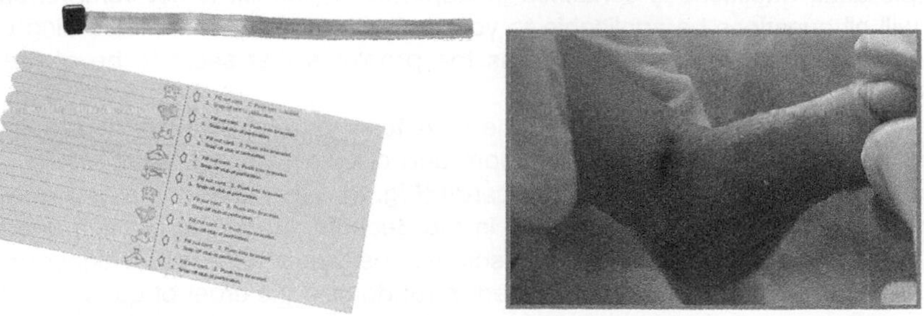

B

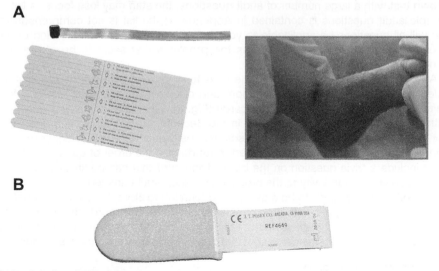

Fig. 1. (*A*) The plastic ID bands were felt to damage preterm infant's skin and when moved to facilitate IV access, the process for procuring a new band was labor intensive for the bedside nurse. (*B*) A softer ID band that could be moved was substituted, resulting in a sustainable 10-fold increase in compliance with unit policy regarding ID band location.

The ease of adoption of RSA was shown by the Vermont Oxford NIC/Q 2002 Quality Improvement Collaborative. A survey of NICUs participating in this collaborative found 26 of 44 NICUs implemented RSA within 6 months of receiving an RSA toolkit and educational presentation.[36] NICUs documented improvement in diverse aspects of care, including hand hygiene, patient identification, breast milk administration, pain management, appropriate labeling of IV tubing, and preprocedure time-outs. When these units were asked to identify the most valuable aspects of RSA implementation in their unit, the responses included "error detection," "error detection and subsequent educational opportunity," "education and feedback to the staff," "education and reinforcement of practice expectations," "multidisciplinary collaboration," "involving more staff in patient safety (increased team spirit)," "showing change over time, both in areas needing improvement and areas performing well."

Three of the 26 participating NICUs reported an adverse experience. These units reported that some staff felt they were being watched. This barrier can be overcome by improving multidisciplinary participation in auditing and development of a culture of safety, a blame-free environment concerning auditing, and feedback of audit results.

Implementing RSA in Your Unit

"One time" preparation work before implementation of RSA

Successful implementation of RSA requires customization of the audit questions and methods to fit the policies, culture, and workflow of your unit (**Fig. 2**). Implementation begins with the selection of a multidisciplinary audit team. This team needs a leader and should include participants from any discipline the audit questions will assess (eg, nursing, nurse practitioner, respiratory therapist, pharmacist, attending physician, trainees).

The initial task for the RSA team is to identify the unit's quality and safety priorities. The team then creates a list of relevant audit questions. The authors suggest starting with 5 to 15 items. Although it may be tempting to focus on a larger number of items, this is not recommended for initial implementation. The authors' experience has shown that with a large number of audit questions, the staff may lose focus. A list of sample audit questions is contained in Appendix 1; the list is not comprehensive, nor will all questions be applicable to your unit. In addition, some rewording of the questions may be required to address the problems that seem to be of greatest concern in an individual NICU.

After refining a list of audit items, the RSA team must determine the process for selecting 1 question each day at random and documenting the audit results. Most units choose to print a deck of audit cards (**Fig. 3**). Each card contains 1 question, with multiple copies of each question in the deck (ie, 10 copies of each question). For items of special high priority, the deck may be "weighted," with a higher proportion of those cards. The deck is shuffled to randomize the order of questions. Many units include a trivia question on the back of the card that can be shared with staff during auditing to add levity to the process and keep staff engaged.

In addition, there needs to be a designated location to store the audit cards before and after their use. Many units have chosen to create an audit card storage box. The more attractive the box, the less likely it will be accidentally thrown away or misplaced. The box can serve as a reminder to staff that quality and safety are priorities in your unit.

Daily Implementation of RSA

The specific methods are flexible and should be tailored to fit the dynamics of workflow in the NICU. In general, one card should be chosen daily to audit and every relevant piece of equipment or patient should be assessed for that question. Depending

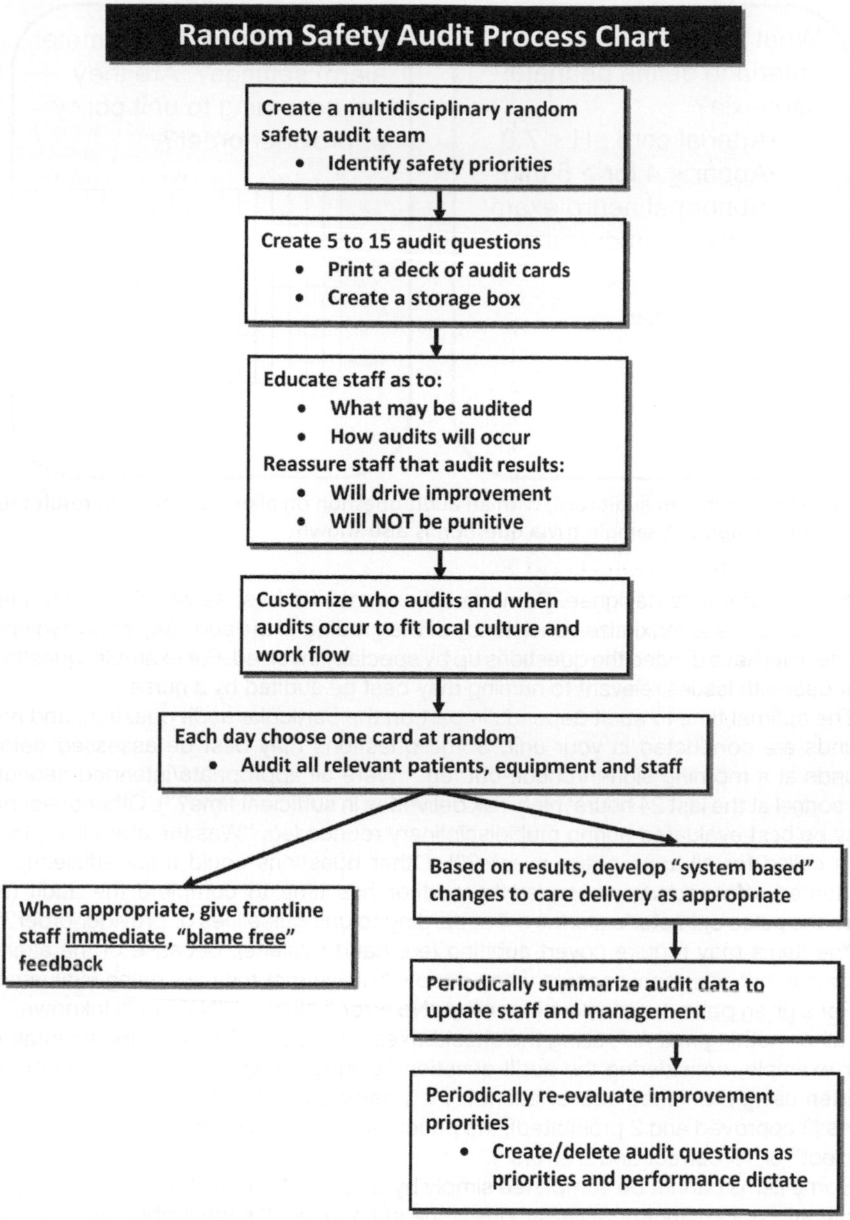
Random Safety Audit Process Chart
Create a multidisciplinary random safety audit team
• Identify safety priorities
Create 5 to 15 audit questions
• Print a deck of audit cards
• Create a storage box
Educate staff as to:
• What may be audited
• How audits will occur
Reassure staff that audit results:
• Will drive improvement
• Will NOT be punitive
Customize who audits and when audits occur to fit local culture and work flow
Each day choose one card at random
• Audit all relevant patients, equipment and staff
When appropriate, give frontline staff immediate, "blame free" feedback
Based on results, develop "system based" changes to care delivery as appropriate
Periodically summarize audit data to update staff and management
Periodically re-evaluate improvement priorities
• Create/delete audit questions as priorities and performance dictate

Fig. 2. Random safety audit process chart.

on the priorities and the areas of concern, you may choose to audit only a certain group of patients. One example of a relevant patient subgroup might be level III patients. If your unit has more than 1 rounding team, these teams may audit different items. Auditing weekend and night shifts should be considered, as differing issues might arise during these compared with day shifts.

Depending on the specific question, the auditor (the person completing the audit card) might be a charge or staff nurse, attending physician, trainee, respiratory therapist, or

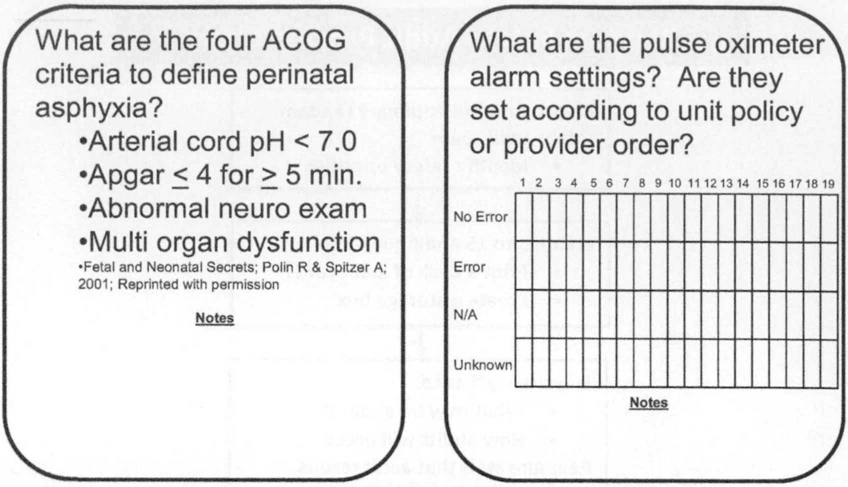
What are the four ACOG criteria to define perinatal asphyxia?
•Arterial cord pH < 7.0
•Apgar ≤ 4 for ≥ 5 min.
•Abnormal neuro exam
•Multi organ dysfunction
•Fetal and Neonatal Secrets; Polin R & Spitzer A; 2001; Reprinted with permission
Notes
What are the pulse oximeter alarm settings? Are they set according to unit policy or provider order?
1 2 3 4 5 6 7 8 9 10 11 12 13 14 15 16 17 18 19
No Error
Error
N/A
Unknown
Notes

Fig. 3. Sample random audit card, with an audit question on alarm settings and result table to record the audit. A sample trivia question is also shown.

another appropriate designee. Some questions may be best served by having a few trained auditors to maximize consistency of the grading of the audit (eg, hand hygiene). Some units have divided the questions up by specialty involved. For example, questions that deal with issues relevant to nursing may best be audited by a nurse.

The optimal time to audit depends in part on the particular audit question, and how rounds are conducted in your unit. Some questions may best be assessed before rounds at a morning sign-in/check-out (eg, "Were all appropriate/intended neonatal personnel at the last 24 hours' high-risk deliveries in sufficient time?"). Other questions may be best evaluated during multidisciplinary rounds (eg, "Was the attending physician called for all appropriate events?"). Other questions could most efficiently be evaluated after rounds whenever the auditor has time to complete the audit (eg, "Are the pulse oximeter's alarms set according to unit guidelines or provider order?"). Some items may require covert auditing (eg, hand hygiene), because of the altered behavior that commonly occurs when people believe that they are being evaluated.

For a given patient, each item is scored "No error," "Error," "N/A" or "Unknown," in an all-or-nothing manner, using the checkboxes on the card for rapid documentation. For example, considering the audit question "During the last 48 hours, were orders written using prohibited abbreviations?", if a particular set of orders has 5 abbreviations (3 approved and 2 prohibited), the patient should be scored "Error" (not "Mostly correct" or "3 correct and 2 errors").

Some items cannot be completed simply by a yes/no from the team and will require verification by an auditor reviewing the issue at hand (eg, "Is the Ambu bag and mask appropriately set up at the bedside?"). The space under "Notes" is intended to allow brief descriptions of errors detected to assist in differentiating trivial from more significant errors when summarizing data. Neither patient nor provider names should appear on the audit card. For auditing to detect errors effectively, the staff must believe the goal is to improve patient care, not to punish providers. On completion of the audit, the card should be stored in a secure location. Used cards can then be collected every 2 to 4 weeks for analysis, allowing summarized feedback of the audit results to frontline staff and management. The audit card deck can be refreshed with new cards as needed.

Monitoring/Feedback of RSA Data to Your Unit Staff

Many audit questions lend themselves to providing immediate feedback to frontline providers. Timely feedback completes the loop of audit and feedback behavior change, a key strength of RSA.[34] Timely feedback is more likely to modify provider behavior than no feedback, or feedback that is delayed (which is common for incident reports).

The local champion should summarize the audit results periodically (eg, every other week or monthly) to allow summarized data to be presented to unit staff and management. Audit results can be presented as graphs over time, optimally with a run chart or statistical process control chart. The optimal method to communicate feedback varies from unit to unit, but could include announcements at staff meetings, e-mails, and posters in break rooms.

Some audit items are subjective (eg, "Was the attending physician called for all 'appropriate' events?"). The compliance percentage in such situations may be of limited value, yet the results may still have some importance in the way that overall care is managed in the NICU. These questions can prompt multidisciplinary discussions that can expose weak systems or processes, and reinforce expectations among unit staff.

The list of items audited is not intended to be comprehensive or static. When problems have been addressed and repeat audits show compliance, it may be appropriate to audit these items less frequently or eliminate them from audit altogether. Conversely, as new concerns arise, new audit questions can be added.

RSA facilitates monitoring of a broad range of complex systems for errors and quality deficiencies without the need for significant infrastructure or resource allocation. RSA involves frontline staff in quality and safety efforts, becoming more than just a tool to detect errors. Auditing has the potential to reduce future errors and provide a method for correction of system failures before they become ingrained in daily practice.

ROOT CAUSE ANALYSIS

RCA (perhaps more appropriately termed root causes analysis) is a methodology for identifying the basic or causal factors that underlie variation in performance.[37] RCA has been used to investigate industrial accidents for decades and has been common in the health care setting since the 1990s.[38] The Joint Commission (JC), the principle health care accrediting organization in the United States, now requires organizations under its jurisdiction to perform an RCA in response to every sentinel event. The JC views RCAs and the resultant actions plans as confidential.

The JC defines a sentinel event as, *an unexpected occurrence involving death or serious physical or psychological injury, or the risk thereof.*[39] Some organizations also choose to perform RCA on near-miss events.

Although it is a retrospective approach to error analysis, the goal of RCA is to prevent future adverse events, through correction of the root causes underlying system vulnerabilities that facilitate errors. The sine qua non of RCA is an intense focus on human factors and system vulnerability characteristics that contribute to errors, and away from personal blame. The RCA can be broken down into 5 key steps (**Box 1**).

(1) Identification of sentinel or other important events that require an RCA

The initial phase for the development of an RCA program includes defining criteria for which events require review with RCA. Once these criteria are defined, a mechanism to identify these events and alert relevant staff is needed.

Box 1
Key steps in RCA

1. Identify sentinel or other important events that require an RCA
2. Assemble a team
3. Diagram the process: What happened?
4. Why did the event happen? Moving from proximate to root causes
5. Development and implementation of an action plan

(2) Assemble an RCA team

It is essential to have the RCA team led by a person with training and experience in RCA. Although the composition of the RCA team varies with each event, it should always be multidisciplinary, including frontline staff with intimate knowledge of the event, and personnel with knowledge of the systems and processes that might have played a role in the event. Furthermore, the team should include senior leadership of the organization, who can facilitate implementation and monitoring of the RCA action plan.

For example, the RCA team evaluating a sentinel event in which an enteral medication was given intravenously should include at least a physician, a nurse, a pharmacist, and a senior hospital manager. At least 1 team member should be experienced in leading an RCA. Depending on the circumstances of the error and workflow at the institution, the team might also include a pharmacy technician, a patient care technician, information systems staff, a unit manager, a nurse practitioner, and physician trainees. Not all team members necessarily participate in every aspect of the RCA.

(3) Diagram the event, reconstruct the process: What happened?

A structured framework should be followed during RCA (see Appendix 1 for a sample framework created by the JC[39]). The initial step is to describe what happened in detail through medical record review and interviews with relevant personnel, patients, and family. To facilitate accuracy, this review should occur as quickly as possible after the event. The description of the episode should include who was affected, what area or services were involved, and when the event occurred. As the details of what happened are identified, the steps in the process, as designed, should also be determined.

(4) Why did the event happen? Moving from proximate to root causes

After the initial reconstruction and description of what happened, the focus of the team shifts to understanding why the event occurred. To be thorough and credible, the analysis should progress from the immediately visible (proximate) causes in the clinical processes to the deeper root causes in the systems supporting care. Each proximate cause typically has underlying root causes. To expose root causes, the team should start with a proximate cause and ask "Why did this happen?" The team repeats this question until the underlying root causes are identified (**Box 2**, **Fig. 4**). Typically 5 iterations of asking why should be sufficient ("5 Whys"). This process is repeated for each proximate cause.[40] Many find a flow diagram or Ishikawa diagram to be helpful in working through and documenting this discovery process (**Fig. 5**).

For example, consider an event in which a child receives a 10-fold medication overdose. One potential series of events follows.

A physician ordered 10.0 mg of gentamicin. A dose of 100 mg is mistakenly read by the pharmacist because of the presence of a trailing zero and the use of a fax machine to transmit this order to the pharmacy. The pharmacist filled the order without reviewing the patient's weight, perhaps because it was not readily available in the pharmacy. The nurse did not double-check the medication dose before administration possibly because appropriate dosing references were not available at the bedside.

(5) Development and implementation of an action plan

Once the sequence of events and the underlying root causes are determined, the RCA team should focus on reengineering the systems or processes that facilitated the error. Not all systems or processes are modifiable. The potentially modifiable root causes can be prioritized for systems reengineering.

Proposed changes may need to be tested before or after large-scale implementation. The action plan should document who is responsible for implementation, the time frame for implementation of change, and how the effectiveness of the interventions in reducing risk will be assessed.

Barriers to Effective RCA

Some RCAs do not produce improvement because they are performed incorrectly.[41,42] Having an experienced and effective leader is therefore essential. Flawed RCAs can also result when the team places undue emphasis on finding the single most important root cause, ignoring lesser possible causes. Uncovering all root causes is important to allow the most effective and efficient systems-based interventions to be implemented. Additional barriers to effective RCA and action plan implementation can include lack of resources, uncooperative colleagues, and unsupportive management. Thus, having support from institutional or units leadership and a team leader with experience or knowledge of the RCA process and potential pitfalls is essential.

Box 2
Framework for an RCA and action plan in response to a sentinel event

1. What human factors were relevant to the outcome?
   a. Were the staff trained and competent?
   b. Was staffing ideal?
   c. Was communication among participants adequate?
   d. Was the environment appropriate for the task?
   e. Was the culture conducive to risk identification and risk reduction?
2. How did the performance of equipment affect the outcome?
3. What controllable environmental factors contributed to the outcome?
4. What uncontrollable factors contributed to the outcome?
5. Information systems: was all appropriate information
   a. Available?
   b. Accurate?
   c. Complete?
   d. Unambiguous?
6. Other contributing factors

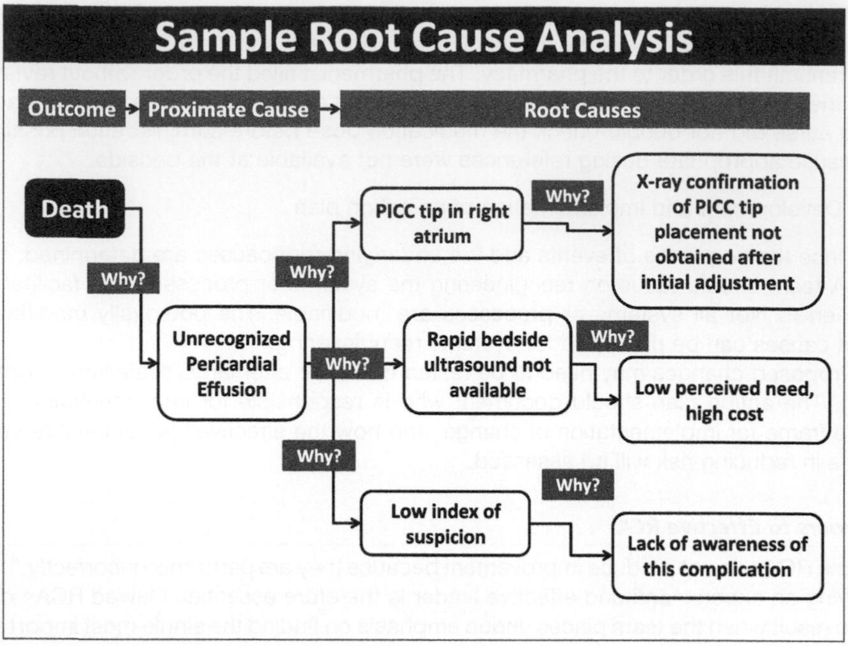

Fig. 4. Sample RCA of a death related to an unrecognized pericardial effusion (proximate cause). RCA showed multiple root causes that contributed to the death. PICC, peripherally inserted central catheter.

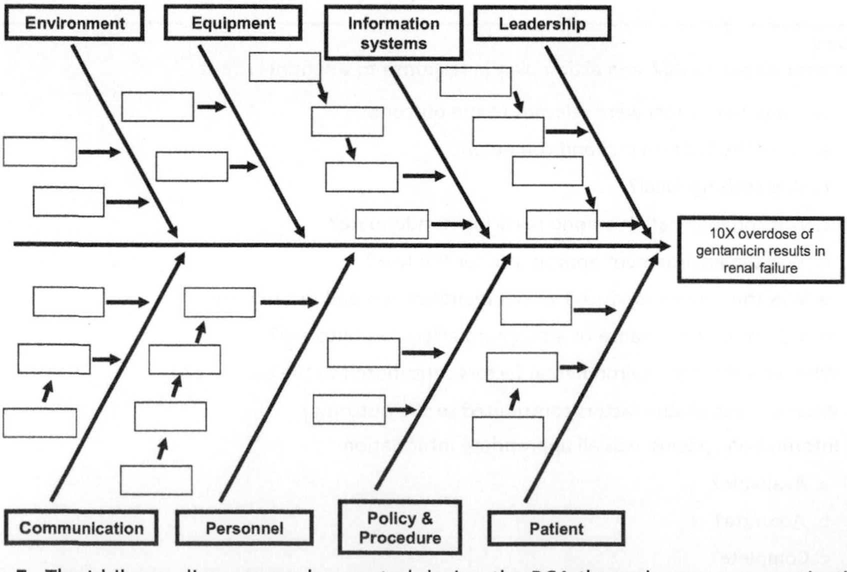

Fig. 5. The Ishikawa diagram can be created during the RCA through open communication among RCA team members. The category headings are flexible and should be adapted to the individual event. The RCA team should identify as many contributory factors as possible, moving from superficial (proximate) causes to deeper root causes.

Adapted from industry, RCA methodology is now well accepted and commonplace in the health care setting. RCA is an important qualitative tool facilitating learning from errors. A multidisciplinary team including an experienced leader and senior leadership from the organization is essential for RCA to lead to a functional action plan that can mitigate future hazards.

FAILURE MODE AND EFFECTS ANALYSIS

FMEA (also known as failure mode, effect, and criticality analysis) is a valuable tool for improving patient safety. Unlike RCA, FMEA is a proactive risk reduction technique that attempts to identify the possibility of future system failures that could affect patient care processes and, ultimately, the patient. Properly implemented, inclusion of an FMEA-based approach to risk reduction addresses JC requirements that ensure that "an ongoing, proactive program for identifying risks to patient safety and reducing medical/health care errors is defined and implemented." Often compared with hazard analysis and critical control points, a method used extensively in food safety programs, FMEA has a long history of successful use in the engineering and software industries. As a nonstatistical method, FMEA can easily be taught to multiple members of the health care team.

Although various approaches to perform FMEA exist, all FMEA implementations share a common conceptual framework.

Failures: Failures are undesirable or unintended deviations, or errors that affect a process or system.
Modes: Modes are the way in which the process or system can fail.
Effects: Effects are the consequences that result from a process or system failure.
Analysis: Analysis is an examination of the way that individual processes or process failures might interact to determine the ultimate outcome seen from the process. In addition, the analysis phase identifies methods to decrease the frequency of or mitigate the consequences of process failure.

Box 3 lists the steps suggested in the generic FMEA process described by the JC.[43,44] Other approaches including that outlined in the Veterans Administrations Health Care Failure Mode and Effect Analysis (HFMEA) can be found elsewhere.[29]

Identifying a High-risk Process

High-risk processes may have a high frequency of failure or may have low failure rates but each failure is likely to lead to significant adverse consequences. High-risk processes that are candidates for FMEA include clinical processes, such as accurately identifying patients during encounters, procedural processes, such as identifying the physician responsible for a patient's care out of hours, or administrative processes, such as ensuring a suitable supply of equipment within the NICU. The presence of new equipment or systems within a unit, such as smart pumps or computerized provider order entry (CPOE), may introduce new care processes that can be prone to error because of their novelty. Potential topics within an NICU include, but are not limited to, patient identification, medication administration, stabilization before, during, or following transport, blood product use, and timely and complete sharing of information with families.

Assembling a Team

Teams involved in FMEA should include members from all disciplines involved in the identified process, but generally should be limited to 10 members or less. Team

Box 3
JC generic FMEA

1. Select a high-risk process and assemble a team
2. Diagram the process
3. Brainstorm the potential failure modes and determine the effects
4. Prioritize failure modes
5. Identify root causes of failure modes
6. Redesign the process
7. Analyze and test the new process
8. Implement and monitor the redesigned process

Data from Joint Commission Resources Inc. Failure mode and effects analysis in healthcare: proactive risk reduction. 2nd edition. Oakbrook Terrace (IL): Joint Commission Resources; 2005.

members might include non-NICU staff such as radiology or ultrasound technicians, consulting services, parents, or even staff from affiliated hospitals (eg, if the process spans institutions). Inclusion of an individual not familiar with the process may also lend a fresh perspective. A successful team includes not only those individuals who can characterize the process, identify failure modes, and understand their effect but also individuals who are needed for the design and implementation of new processes. Consideration should be given to the use of an external facilitator to lead the group through subsequent steps. It is not necessary that the facilitator has domain knowledge of the process, but rather this individual should stimulate the participation of all team members and keep the group moving forward in the FMEA process.

Diagram the Process

All the steps that are required in the process should be sequentially identified and placed into a flowchartlike presentation. Use of a large whiteboard with erasable markers or a blank wall covered with sticky notes can facilitate the iterative nature of this endeavor. Planning for more than a single session can provide participants with an opportunity to identify and focus on hidden steps within a complex process. Once complete, or at interim stages, a digital camera can be used to make copies of the process. Two representations may be needed: the way that the process is intended to occur and the way that it actually occurs. Once completed, various preexisting formats exist for final documentation of the process.

Identify Failure Modes

Brainstorming is used to identify the potential ways in which failures could occur during each step of the process. Brainstorming need not proceed in the sequential manner outlined in the flowchart, but rather should be a stream-of-consciousness exercise for the participants. Examples of potential failure modes during the use of a CPOE system may be the selection (either by human or computerized action) of an incorrect medication or medication dosage for a patient. While conducting this portion of the exercise, no attempt should be made to narrow the list of potential failure modes.

Prioritize Failure Modes

Here the potential critical degree of each failure mode is estimated. Criticality is a complex construct that attempts to measure the relative importance of a failure mode through consideration of its likelihood, potential for detection, and seriousness (as measured by severity of potential effects). The JC does not require that any particular rating scale be used. Individual institutions often create new or adapt existing scales to suit their own particular circumstances. A review of various approaches is available elsewhere.[38,43]

An example of 1 approach is seen in the Veterans Administration HFMEA 4-category schema (**Fig. 6**, HFMEA matrix), which includes frequent (likely to occur several times per year), occasional (probably will occur several times in a 1- to 2-year period), uncommon (possibly may happen in a 5-year period), and remote events (may happen once in a 6- to 30-year period). Similarly, within this framework categorization of seriousness occurs along another 4-point axis that includes catastrophic (ie, could lead to death), major (ie, could lead to permanent loss of body function), moderate (ie, could lead to increased length of stay for 1 or 2 patients), and minor (ie, effect is unlikely to be noticed). For each FMEA, a risk level for immediate action should be determined.

After categorizing the frequency and seriousness of a failure mode, the ability to detect it should be considered. Failures at 1 stage of a process can be mitigated if the failure is readily observed. Even a serious failure that occurs frequently may have little effect on patients if it is noted at once and downstream steps are able to respond to the previous failure. In comparison, tightly coupled processes in which there is little ability to buffer the effects of previous failure are more likely to lead to a cascade of events that result in patient harm.

Identify Root Causes of Failure Modes

The RCA techniques described earlier can be applied to enable system redesign of the identified high-priority processes. Emphasis must be placed on identification of root causes, not just proximate causes of the failure modes.

Redesign the Process

The team should then focus on ways in which to redesign the process by considering the most critical failure modes identified. In general, there are 3 approaches to redesign: the prevention of failure modes; improved detection of failures; and implementation of recovery processes that mitigate the effects of failure (ie, prevent failures that do occur from reaching the patient).

Analyze and Test the New Process

Before implementation of the newly designed process, team members should consider performing another FMEA on the newly created process. Although it is

		SEVERITY			
		Catastrophic	Major	Moderate	Minor
PROBABILITY	Frequent	16	12	8	4
	Occasional	12	9	6	3
	Uncommon	8	6	4	2
	Remote	4	3	2	1

Fig. 6. HFMEA matrix. Each failure mode is assigned a criticality index based on the cross product of its probability and severity.

tempting to examine only the modified steps, this approach can miss important interactions between new and existing steps that may lead to errors.

Implement and Monitor the Redesigned Process

As mentioned earlier, the implementation of newly designed processes can dramatically alter the function of existing clinical care in unforeseen ways. As part of any system reengineering, an active plan for ongoing monitoring of the new process should be created and implemented.

FMEA Summary

FMEA through its systematic, proactive approach to safety can identify error-prone systems and prevent the effects of medical error from reaching the patient. Complete and successful review of a clinical process using FMEA requires the commitment of significant resources, but is likely to result in a valuable return on investment. If viewed solely as a mandate that must be completed to ensure compliance with regulations, FMEA is likely to be performed in a manner that will not achieve its full potential value.

REFERENCES

1. Kohn LT, Corrigan J, Donaldson MS. To err is human: building a safer health system. Washington, DC: National Academy Press; 2000.
2. Institute of Medicine (US). Committee on Quality of Health Care in America. Crossing the quality chasm: a new health system for the 21st century. Washington, DC: National Academy Press; 2001.
3. Page A Institute of Medicine (US). Committee on the Work Environment for Nurses and Patient Safety. Keeping patients safe: transforming the work environment of nurses. Washington, DC: National Academies Press; 2004.
4. Institute of Medicine (US). Committee on Redesigning Health Insurance Performance Measures Payment and Performance Improvement Programs. Performance measurement: accelerating improvement. Washington, DC: National Academies Press; 2006.
5. Brennan TA, Leape LL, Laird NM, et al. Incidence of adverse events and negligence in hospitalized patients. Results of the Harvard Medical practice study I. N Engl J Med 1991;324(6):370–6.
6. Leape LL, Brennan TA, Laird N, et al. The nature of adverse events in hospitalized patients. Results of the Harvard Medical practice study II. N Engl J Med 1991; 324(6):377–84.
7. Wilson RM, Runciman WB, Gibberd RW, et al. Quality in Australian health care study. Med J Aust 1996;164(12):754.
8. Vincent C, Neale G, Woloshynowych M. Adverse events in British hospitals: preliminary retrospective record review. BMJ 2001;322(7285):517–9.
9. Baker GR, Norton PG, Flintoft V, et al. The Canadian adverse events study: the incidence of adverse events among hospital patients in Canada. CMAJ 2004;170(11):1678–86.
10. Andrews LB, Stocking C, Krizek T, et al. An alternative strategy for studying adverse events in medical care. Lancet 1997;349(9048):309–13.
11. Kaushal R, Bates DW, Landrigan C, et al. Medication errors and adverse drug events in pediatric inpatients. JAMA 2001;285(16):2114–20.
12. Ursprung R, Gray JE, Edwards WH, et al. Real time patient safety audits: improving safety every day. Qual Saf Health Care 2005;14(4):284–9.

13. Gray JE, Suresh G, Ursprung R, et al. Patient misidentification in the neonatal intensive care unit: quantification of risk. Pediatrics 2006;117(1):e43–7.
14. Simpson JH, Lynch R, Grant J, et al. Reducing medication errors in the neonatal intensive care unit. Arch Dis Child Fetal Neonatal Ed 2004;89(6):F480–2.
15. Suresh G, Horbar JD, Plsek P, et al. Voluntary anonymous reporting of medical errors for neonatal intensive care. Pediatrics 2004;113(6):1609–18.
16. Cullen DJ, Bates DW, Small SD, et al. The incident reporting system does not detect adverse drug events: a problem for quality improvement. Jt Comm J Qual Improv 1995;21(10):541–8.
17. Jha AK, Kuperman GJ, Teich JM, et al. Identifying adverse drug events: development of a computer-based monitor and comparison with chart review and stimulated voluntary report. J Am Med Inform Assoc 1998;5(3):305–14.
18. Classen DC, Pestotnik SL, Evans RS, et al. Computerized surveillance of adverse drug events in hospital patients. JAMA 1991;266(20):2847–51.
19. Rozich JD, Haraden CR, Resar RK. Adverse drug event trigger tool: a practical methodology for measuring medication related harm. Qual Saf Health Care 2003;12(3):194–200.
20. Miller MR, Elixhauser A, Zhan C. Patient safety events during pediatric hospitalizations. Pediatrics 2003;111(6 Pt 1):1358–66.
21. Miller MR, Zhan C. Pediatric patient safety in hospitals: a national picture in 2000. Pediatrics 2004;113(6):1741–6.
22. Sharek PJ, Horbar JD, Mason W, et al. Adverse events in the neonatal intensive care unit: development, testing, and findings of an NICU-focused trigger tool to identify harm in North American NICUs. Pediatrics 2006;118(4):1332–40.
23. United States. Agency for Healthcare Research and Quality, University of California San Francisco-Stanford Evidence-Based Practice Center. Making health care safer: a critical analysis of patient safety practices. Rockville (MD): Agency for Healthcare Research and Quality, U.S. Dept. of Health and Human Services; 2001.
24. Piotrowski MM, Hinshaw DB. The safety checklist program: creating a culture of safety in intensive care units. Jt Comm J Qual Improv 2002;28(6):306–15.
25. Kendell J, Barthram C. Revised checklist for anaesthetic machines. Anaesthesia 1998;53(9):887–90.
26. Agency for Health Care Policy and Research. AaAM, 2006. Continuous quality improvement tool released by AHCPR. Available at: http://www.ahrq.gov/news/press/qitoolpr.htm. 1998. Accessed December 10, 2009.
27. Benneyan JC, Lloyd RC, Plsek PE. Statistical process control as a tool for research and healthcare improvement. Qual Saf Health Care 2003;12(6):458–64.
28. Reason JT. Human error. Cambridge (UK): Cambridge University Press; 1990.
29. DeRosier J, Stalhandske E, Bagian JP, et al. Using health care failure mode and effect analysis: the VA National Center for patient safety's prospective risk analysis system. Jt Comm J Qual Improv 2002;28(5):248–67, 209.
30. Juran JM, Godfrey AB. Juran's quality handbook. 5th edition. New York: McGraw Hill; 1999.
31. Russell JP, ASQ Quality Audit Division. The quality audit handbook: principles, implementation, and use. 3rd edition. Milwaukee (WI): ASQ Quality Press; 2005.
32. Mills CA, American Society for Quality Control, Quality Audit Technical Committee. The quality audit: a management evaluation tool. New York: McGraw-Hill. Milwaukee (WI): ASQC Quality Press; 1989.
33. Tunner JR. A quality technology primer for managers. Milwaukee (WI): ASQC Quality Press; 1990.

34. Grol R, Grimshaw J. From best evidence to best practice: effective implementation of change in patients' care. Lancet 2003;362(9391):1225–30.
35. Leape LL, Berwick DM, Bates DW. What practices will most improve safety? Evidence-based medicine meets patient safety. JAMA 2002;288(4):501–7.
36. Ursprung R, Edwards WH, Horbar JD, et al. Random patient safety audits: introduction of a novel safety tool to a large NICU collaborative, Poster Presentation, Pediatric Academic Society Annual Meeting, Washington, DC, May 16, 2005.
37. Wilson PF, Dell LD, Anderson GF. Root cause analysis: a tool for total quality management. Milwaukee (WI): ASQC Quality Press; 1993.
38. Root cause analysis in health care: tools and techniques. 4th edition. Oakbrook Terrace (IL): Joint Commission Resources; 2009.
39. Sentinel events policy and procedures. 2007. Available at: http://www.Jointcommission.org/SentinelEvents/PolicyandProcedures/. Accessed April, 2009.
40. Commission TJ. Sentinel event forms and tools. 2009. http://www.jointcommission.org/SentinelEvents/Forms/. Updated April 1, 2009. Accessed December 14, 2009.
41. Wu AW, Lipshutz AK, Pronovost PJ. Effectiveness and efficiency of root cause analysis in medicine. JAMA 2008;299(6):685–7.
42. Berry K, Krizek B. Root cause analysis in response to a "near miss". J Healthc Qual 2000;22(2):16–8.
43. Joint Commission Resources Inc. Failure mode and effects analysis in health care: proactive risk reduction. 2nd edition. Oakbrook Terrace (IL): Joint Commission Resources; 2005.
44. Gray JE, Goldmann DA. Medication errors in the neonatal intensive care unit: special patients, unique issues. Arch Dis Child Fetal Neonatal Ed 2004;89(6):F472–3.
45. Bischoff WE, Reynolds TM, Sessler CN, et al. Handwashing Compliance by Health Care Workers: The Impact of Introducing an Accessible, Alcohol-Based hand Antiseptic. Arch Intern Med 2000;160:1017.
46. Available at: http://www.cdc.gov/handhygiene/. Accessed March 9, 2010.
47. Schelonka RL, Chai MK, Yoder BA, et al. Volume of blood required to detect common neonatal pathogens. J Pediatr 1996;129(2):275–8.
48. Kilbride HW, Wirtschafter DD, Powers RJ, et al. Implementation of evidence-based potentially better practices to decrease nosocomial infections. Pediatrics 2003;111(4):e519–33.
49. O'Grady NP, Alexander M, Dellinger EP, et al. Guidelines for the prevention of Intravascular Catheter-Related Infections. Pediatrics 2002;110:e51.
50. Raad II, Hohn DC, Gilbreath BJ, et al. Prevention of central venous catheter-related infections by using maximal sterile barrier precautions during insertion. Infect Control Hosp Epidemiol 1994;15:231–8.
51. Available at: http://www.cdc.gov/mmwr/pdf/rr/rr5111.pdf. Accessed March 9, 2010.
52. Farr BM. Understaffing: a risk factor for infection in the era of downsizing? Infect Control Hosp Epidemiol 1996;17(3):147–9.
53. Suresh G, Horbar JD, Plsek P, et al. Voluntary anonymous reporting of medical errors for neonatal intensive care. Pediatrics 2004;113:1609–18.
54. The Joint Commission, 2010 National Patient Safety Goals. Available at: http://www.JointCommission.org/PatientSafety/NationalPatientSafetyGoals/. Accessed March 9, 2010.
55. Nowlen TT, et al. Pericardial effusion and tamponade in infants with central catheters. Pediatrics 2002;110:137–42.
56. Kaushal R, Bates DW, Landrigan C, et al. Medication errors and adverse drug events in pediatric inpatients. JAMA 2001;285(16):2114–20.

APPENDIX 1: POTENTIAL RANDOM AUDIT QUESTIONS

Questions focusing on infection control

1. Does this patient's bedside have an alcohol hand rub dispenser easily accessible, which delivers product properly? Score each bedside independently.
   - Compliance with hand hygiene is directly tied to convenience of use, thus the dispenser should be in close proximity to the bed, without obstacles to reaching the dispenser. Further, the dispenser should not be empty or clogged, such that 1 "pump" or "squirt" delivers sufficient product for hand hygiene.[45,46]
2. Is this antimicrobial soap dispenser delivering product properly (ie, it is not empty or clogged, such that 1 pump or squirt delivers sufficient product for hand hygiene)? Score each dispenser independently.
   - Compliance with hand hygiene is directly tied to convenience of use.[45,46]
3. Are there gloves of various sizes (ie, small, medium, and large) easily accessible from this patient's bedside? Score each bedside independently.
4. Is lotion (provided by the hospital free of charge) easily accessible to this patient's bedside and is it functioning properly (ie, not empty or clogged)? Score each dispenser independently.
   - Skin irritation is a major deterrent to compliance with hand hygiene; the US Centers for Disease Control and Prevention (CDC) recommend lotions be available free of charge.[46]
5. Is this sink working properly, with water temperature that is not too hot?
   - Hot water leads to greater skin irritation; skin irritation leads to lower hand hygiene compliance.[46]
6. Is this paper towel dispenser functioning properly (ie, not empty or malfunctioning)? Score each dispenser independently.
   - Compliance with hand hygiene is directly tied to convenience of use.[45,46]
7. Are there hand hygiene reminders (ie, posters, flyers, stickers) visible in the NICU?
   - Education is essential for any successful hand hygiene improvement effort.[46]
8. Was there feedback of the unit's most recent hand hygiene compliance rates to NICU staff (ie, a poster displayed in a break room, an e-mail, discussion at staff meetings, other)?
   - Education is essential for any successful hand hygiene improvement effort. Feedback to staff of the current hand hygiene compliance rate is recommended.[46]
9. Does this staff member know the most recent hand hygiene compliance rate specific to their role (ie, nursing, respiratory therapist, neonatal nurse practitioner [NNP], physician) in the NICU? Audit as many staff members as time allows.
   - Education is essential for any successful hand hygiene improvement effort. Feedback to staff of the current hand hygiene compliance rate is recommended.[46]
10. Are any NICU clinical staff wearing artificial nails? Score each caregiver independently.
    - Those wearing artificial nails are more likely to harbor gram-negative pathogens on their fingertips than those with natural nails before and after hand-washing.[46]
11. For any patients who had a blood culture obtained in the last 48 hours, is there documentation of site and amount of blood sent for culture and does it meet your local guidelines concerning the volume of blood collected?
    - Follow your laboratory's recommendations. Most experts recommend 1 mL as the minimum volume of blood for a neonatal blood culture; sensitivity of the

culture increases with increasing blood volume.[47] Some recommend use of 2 blood cultures per evaluation.[48]

12. Are any patients in the unit on vancomycin or aminoglycosides (eg, gentamicin, tobramycin)? If so, were indicated drug-monitoring levels performed at the appropriate times?
13. If any patients are being treated for infections in which there is a positive culture and known antimicrobial sensitivities, has the antibiotic coverage been narrowed appropriately? Examples:
    - Changing from vancomycin and gentamicin to vancomycin alone when treating *Staphylococcus epidermidis* (also known as coag-negative staph).
    - Changing from vancomycin to oxacillin when treating methicillin sensitive *Staph aureus*.
14. If this infant was on antibiotics for a rule-out sepsis evaluation that was initiated 48 to 96 hours ago (2–4 days), were the antibiotics discontinued at less than or equal to 48 hours from the time of the evaluation, or is there justification for the continuation of antibiotics?
    - The goal of this question is to evaluate if nonindicated doses of antibiotics are being administered.
15. If this patient has a central line (eg, umbilical artery catheter, umbilical venous catheter, Broviac catheter, peripherally inserted central catheter [PICC]) were maximal barrier precautions used during its insertion?
    - Maximal barrier precautions (cap, mask, sterile gloves, sterile gown, and large sterile field) have been shown to reduce catheter-related bloodstream infections when compared with use of minimal barrier precautions (sterile gloves and a smaller sterile field) during central line insertion.
    - As an alternative, you could audit this question during the insertion of a central line.[46,49,50]
16. If the history and physical (H&P) examination or accompanying documentation gives the results of the mother's hepatitis B surface antigen (HbsAg) status as anything but negative, was the infant treated per the *American Academy of Pediatrics (AAP) Red Book* Guidelines?
    - Obtain the result of mother's HBsAg during the infant's initial 12 hours of life.
    - If mother's HBsAg is positive or if the result cannot be obtained during the infant's initial 12 hours of life, the *AAP Red Book* advocates the following treatment:
    - Term infants: hepatitis B vaccine during the initial 12 hours of life, if mother's HBsAg is positive, also give HB immune globulin (HBIG) during the initial 7 days of life.
    - Preterm infants more than 2 kg: hepatitis B vaccine and HBIG during the initial 12 hours of life.
17. Concerning infants delivered in the last 24 hours. Was this infant screened for group B streptococcal (GBS) infection risk and if appropriate treated according to the CDC's guideline (or your hospital's guideline)?
    - Use of the CDC's guideline has drastically reduced the incidence of early onset GBS infections.[51]
18. Does the H&P document mother's GBS status, whether or not the mother received intrapartum antibiotic prophylaxis and for what duration, and any sepsis risk factors (including preterm labor, maternal fever, symptoms of chorioamnionitis)?
19. Is the IV tubing labeled according to unit policy and has not expired?

20. Is the NICU understaffed from a nursing standpoint today? Define understaffed per your local standard.
    - Understaffing is a predictor of poor adherence to hand hygiene and is an independent risk factor for blood stream infection.[46,52]

Hand hygiene (HH) monitoring form.

HH monitoring instructions:

1. Be positioned to observe as many bed spaces as possible simultaneously, while still being able to track and record activities correctly. Generally, this is 2 to 4 bed spaces.
2. HH monitoring should be done as part of routine quality monitoring. Other tasks (eg, checking alarm settings, chart review) should be mixed in so that HH is not perceived as the main focus.
3. Make a tick mark for each HH opportunity observed in the "No. of opportunities" row; record the total number of ticks in the total column.
4. Make a tick mark for each HH opportunity performed correctly ("No. performed correctly" row); record the total number of ticks in the total column.

This section is placed on the back of the HH monitoring form.

These random audit questions were originally developed by the Center for Patient Safety in Neonatal Intensive Care in conjunction with the Vermont Oxford Network's iNICQ collaborative.

Questions focusing on safety

1. If anyone at the bedside participated in a surgical or invasive procedure at this patient's bedside during the last 7 days (ie, chest tube, lumbar puncture [LP], PICC/umbilical line placement or adjustment), was there a final verification process, such as a time-out, to confirm the correct:
    - Patient and
    - Procedure and
    - Site (when applicable; ie, right or left)
      using active (not passive) communication techniques?
    - Patient misidentification is a common source of error in the NICU.[53,54]
2. If a verbal medication order was given/received during the last 24 hours (by someone currently at the bedside), did verification read-back occur in each instance?[54]
3. Is there a procedure note written for all procedures done within the last 48 hours?
    - Including:
    - Intubation
    - Umbilical line
    - Peripheral arterial line
    - PICC or other central line
    - LP
    - Chest tube insertion
    - Paracentesis/thoracentesis
4. Were indicated drug-monitoring levels performed during the last 48 hours?
    - Aminoglycoside antibiotics
    - Vancomycin
    - Phenobarbitol/phenytoin
    - Prothrombin time and partial thromboplastin time tests: If on anticoagulation dosing with heparin

Hand Hygiene (HH) Monitoring Form

Date: _________ Total time observed: ______ minutes Total # of patients observed: ______ patients

Observer: ____________________ Total # of patients on precautions: ______ patients

Staff Member		Precautions Followed [1]	Total	HH prior to initial patient contact [2]	Total	Gloves donned as per standard precautions [3]	Total	HH after glove removal [4]	Total	HH before inserting / manipulating invasive devices [5]	Total	HH when leaving the bedside after contact [6]	Total	Comments
Nurse	#opportunities													
	#performed correctly													
NNP	#opportunities													
	#performed correctly													
Respiratory Therapist	#opportunities													
	#performed correctly													
Clinical Assistant	#opportunities													
	#performed correctly													
Neo-natologist	#opportunities													
	#performed correctly													
Surgeon	#opportunities													
	#performed correctly													
Consultant	#opportunities													
	#performed correctly													
Other	#opportunities													
	#performed correctly													

[a] Precautions followed: Applies only to patients on isolation precautions (eg, contact, droplet). Give credit only if all components of the specific type of precautions are followed.

[b] HH Before initial patient contact: Give credit only if the caregiver practices HH immediately before patient contact, or has practiced HH on leaving an immediately adjacent bed space (on their way to the current patient's bed space). If the caregiver has practiced HH at some other intensive care unit location, HH must be repeated, if only to breed good habits and reassure family members.

[c] Gloves donned: Per CDC standard precautions policy, gloves are required before contact with: mucous membranes, nonintact skin or wounds, body fluids, excretions/secretions.

[d] HH after glove removal: always required (hands are easily contaminated when removing gloves).

[e] HH before inserting/manipulating invasive devices: HH is required (even if gloves are donned). Invasive devices include any intravascular catheter (including the catheter sites, dressings, and administration set), bladder catheters, chest tubes, endotracheal tubes (including suctioning, manipulating of ventilator tubing connections), any other devices inserted into sterile body sites.

[f] HH when leaving the bedside after contact:.Contact refers to: for patients not on precaution, contact with the patient or their bed (incubator/warmer/crib); for patients on precautions, the above plus the patient's general environment (eg, supporting equipment, dedicated computer keypad).

- Anti-factor Xa: If anticoagulated with enoxaprin (low molecular weight heparin)

5. Have the positions of the current central venous lines (CVLs) and surgical drains/tubes been verified by radiograph and repositioned if necessary?
   - Inappropriate location of a central catheter tip is associated with significant complications[55]
6. Was a diagnostic test (ie, laboratory test, radiograph, other) ordered and not obtained during the last 48 hours (not including test scheduled for the future)?
7. Was a diagnostic test (ie, laboratory test, radiograph, other) repeated because of a technical or procedural problem during the last 48 hours?
   - For example, blood specimen clotted or patient not positioned properly for radiograph
8. Was there a delay in informing parents of a significant clinical event/change in clinical status during the prior 48 hours?
9. In the last 2 days, did suboptimal communication within or to the team adversely affect clinical management?
   - For example:
     - Important information not communicated during rounds or during checkout
     - Delay in reporting of a consult
     - Delay in reporting of a diagnostic test (laboratory test/radiology/echo)[54]
10. Did an endotracheal tube, surgical drain/tube, or CVL migrate out of its appropriate location during the last 48 hours?
11. Are there medications or syringes at the patient's bedside in violation of or not labeled according to unit policy?
    - Medication errors are exceptionally common in the NICU.[56]
12. Was the attending physician called for all appropriate events?
13. Is the patient ID band appropriately located (according to unit policy), and was it verified at the beginning of the shift?[54]
14. If this patient received breast milk for his/her most recent feed, were the breast milk and patient identified according to unit policy and was this documented appropriately?
    - Patient misidentification and administration of breast milk to the wrong infant is common.[53,54]
15. Are the nurse's safety checks appropriately documented for this shift?
16. Are the respiratory therapist's safety checks appropriately documented for this shift?
17. Is the inspection sticker from biomedical engineering current for all pumps, isolettes, and ventilators at the patient's bedside?
18. Is this patient's bedside area devoid of any charts, order forms, or medications belonging to another patient?
19. Is the bedside suction set up according to unit guidelines or provider order (for nonintubated and intubated patients and repogle, chest tube, surgical drain)?
20. Were all orders written during the previous shift reviewed by the incoming and outgoing nurse at shift change?
21. For nil-by-mouth patients only, do the intravenous fluid/medication drips as currently administered equal the total daily fluids order/goal (within 10 mL/kg/d)?
22. Is the patient's weight recorded on the most recent medication order sheet?
23. During the last 48 hours, were orders written using abbreviations prohibited by your hospital?[54]
24. What are the cardiac apnea monitor alarm limits? Are they set according to unit guidelines or provider order?
25. What are the pulse oximeter alarm limits? Are they set according to unit guidelines or provider order?

26. Are the Ambu bag and mask set up according to unit guidelines?
27. Does the H&P contain the:
    a. prenatal screens?
    b. estimated gestational age or estimated date of confinement (including method of assessment)?
    c. medications mother received during pregnancy and labor?
    d. sepsis risk factors?
    e. reason for maternal presentation?
    f. method of delivery, including reasons for:
        i. spontaneous vaginal delivery?
        ii. induced vaginal delivery (why induced)?
        iii. cesarean section (why cesarean performed)?
28. Were all appropriate neonatal personnel notified of a high-risk delivery in sufficient time to respond appropriately?
29. Were all appropriate/intended neonatal personnel at the high-risk delivery on time?
30. Is the delivery room (DR) appropriately set up for a delivery, and are all appropriate supplies needed for delivery available? If you keep relevant supplies in the DR (audit each DR) or in a box/bag you bring with your team (audit each box/bag). Include in your assessment items such as:
    a. Functioning laryngoscope with 00, 0, and 1 sized blades
    b. Endotracheal tubes: 2.5, 3.0, 3.5
    c. Stylet
    d. Tape
    e. Appropriate sized masks for various sized infants
    f. Appropriate suctioning equipment: bulb suction, suction tubing, meconium aspirator, DeLee suction, other
    g. Other
31. If appropriate, was an antenatal consult done by the neonatology team before delivery? If not, please document why.
32. If this patient had an antenatal consult done by the NICU team, was the information available to the team at the time of delivery after delivery?
33. Did a registered nurse sign off on an order that used prohibited abbreviations?
34. Did the pharmacy sign off on an order that used prohibited abbreviations?
35. Are all consents appropriately filled out and signed by the parent and appropriate hospital personnel?
36. Was the patient's pain evaluated during the last 12 hours and documented in the medical record?
37. Was pain control used according to unit guidelines?
38. Were all medications/fluids requiring a double check by unit policy done so including appropriate documentation?
39. Have the eye examinations been done at the appropriate postconceptual age?
40. Are the arterial line monitor alarms on and set according to unit guidelines or a provider order?
41. Is all the breast milk in the refrigerator/freezer labeled and stored according to unit policy?

These random audit questions were originally developed by the Center for Patient Safety in Neonatal Intensive Care in conjunction with the Vermont Oxford Network's iNICQ collaborative.

Appendix 2: A framework for RCA and an action plan

Level of Analysis		Questions	Findings	Root Cause	Ask "Why?"	Take Action
What happened?	Sentinel event	What are the details of the event? (Brief description)				
		When did the event occur? (Date, day of week, time)				
		What area/service was affected?				
Why did it happen?	The process or activity in which the event occurred	What are the steps in the process, as designed? (A flow diagram may be helpful here)				
What were the most proximate factors?		What steps were involved in (contributed to) the event?				
(Typically special cause variation)	Human factors	What human factors were relevant to the outcome?				
	Equipment factors	How did the equipment performance affect the outcome?				
	Controllable environmental factors	What factors directly affected the outcome?				
	Uncontrollable external factors	Are they truly beyond the organization's control?				
	Other	Are there any other factors that have directly influenced this outcome?				
		What other areas or services are affected?				

This template is provided as an aid in organizing the steps in an RCA. Not all possibilities and questions will apply in every case, and there may be others that will emerge in the course of the analysis. However, all possibilities and questions should be fully considered in your quest for root cause and risk reduction. As an aid to avoiding loose ends, the 3 columns on the right are provided to be checked off for later reference:

- "Root cause?" should be answered "Yes" or "No" for each finding. A root cause is typically a finding related to a process or system that has a potential for redesign to reduce risk. If a particular finding that is relevant to the event is not a root cause, be sure that it is addressed later in the analysis with a "Why?" question. Each finding that is identified as a root cause should be considered for an action and addressed in the action plan.
- "Ask 'Why?'" should be checked off whenever it is reasonable to ask why the particular finding occurred (or did not occur when it should have), to drill down further. Each item checked in this column should be addressed later in the analysis with a "Why?" question. It is expected that any significant findings that are not identified as root causes themselves have roots.
- "Take action?" should be checked for any finding that can reasonably be considered for a risk reduction strategy. Each item checked in this column should be addressed later in the action plan. It will be helpful to write the number of the associated action item on page 3 in the "Take action?" column for each of the findings that requires an action.

(*continued on next page*)

Appendix 2 (*continued*)

Level of Analysis		Questions	Findings	Root Cause	Ask "Why?"	Take Action
Why did that happen? What systems and processes underlie those proximate factors?	Human resources issues	To what degree are staff properly qualified and currently competent for their responsibilities?				
(Common cause variation here may lead to special cause variation in dependent processes)		How did actual staffing compare with ideal levels?				
		What are the plans for dealing with contingencies that would tend to reduce effective staffing levels?				
		To what degree is staff performance in the operant process(es) addressed?				
		How can orientation and in-service training be improved?				
	Information management issues	To what degree is all necessary information available when needed? Accurate? Complete? Unambiguous?				
		To what degree is communication among participants adequate?				
	Environmental management issues	To what degree was the physical environment appropriate for the processes being performed?				
		What systems are in place to identify environmental risks?				
		What emergency and failure mode responses have been planned and tested?				
	Leadership issues: – Corporate culture	To what degree is the culture conducive to risk identification and reduction?				
	– Encouragement of communication	What are the barriers to communication of potential risk factors?				
	– Clear communication of priorities	To what degree is the prevention of adverse outcomes communicated as a high priority? How?				
	Uncontrollable factors	What can be done to protect against the effects of these uncontrollable factors?				

Action plan	Risk reduction strategies	Measures of effectivevness
For each of the findings identified in the analysis as needing an action, indicate the planned action expected, implementation date and associated measure of effectiveness…OR…	Action item 1:	
If after consideration of such a finding, a decision is made not to implement an associated risk reduction strategy, indicate the rationale for not taking action at this time	Action item 2:	
Check to be sure that the selected measure will provide data that will permit assessment of the effectiveness of the action	Action item 3:	
Consider whether pilot testing of a planned improvement should be conducted	Action item 4:	
Improvements to reduce risk should ultimately be implemented in all areas where applicable, not just where the event occurred. Identify where the improvements will be implemented	Action item 5:	
	Action item 6:	
	Action item 7:	
	Action item 8:	
Cite any books or journal articles that were considered in developing this analysis and action plan:		

Pay for Performance in Neonatal-Perinatal Medicine—Will the Quality of Health Care Improve in the Neonatal Intensive Care Unit? A Business Model for Improving Outcomes in the Neonatal Intensive Care Unit

Alan R. Spitzer, MD

KEYWORDS

- Health care costs in the United States
- Neonatal intensive care
- Pay for performance
- Measurements of quality in health care

The seemingly endless upward spiral of health care cost has provoked intense debate throughout the United States about how best to approach this problem. In 2008, total national health expenditures were expected to increase by 6.9%, or twice the overall inflation rate. Total spending in 2007 was $2.4 trillion, or $7900 per person.[1] Total health care spending currently represents 17% of the gross domestic product. If it continues unchecked, United States health care spending is anticipated to rise at similar rates for the next decade, reaching approximately $4.3 trillion in 2017, or 20% of the gross domestic product.[1] In neonatal medicine alone, the cost of infant care has risen steeply, with approximately $20 billion spent in 2008 to cover the cost of premature births alone in this country.[2] These numbers do not include the

The Center for Research, Education, and Quality, Pediatrix Medical Group, 1301 Concord Terrace, Sunrise, FL, USA
E-mail address: Alan_Spitzer@pediatrix.com

Clin Perinatol 37 (2010) 167–177
doi:10.1016/j.clp.2010.01.010
perinatology.theclinics.com

additional dollars spent on follow-up care for these infants, which is often expensive and life-long, especially if the child is encumbered by common complications of neonatal intensive care, such as cerebral palsy, developmental delay, short bowel syndrome, chronic lung disease, or retinopathy of prematurity.

Although the figures are real, the total impact of these expenditures is incalculable in terms of the effect that it has on the primary contributors to health care—American businesses, the federal government, and the family. As the cost of care rises, the ability of businesses, especially smaller businesses, to sustain health insurance for their employees becomes increasingly limited. Faced with alarming increases in policy rates, many firms are being forced to drop health care benefits or have employees shoulder more of the insurance burden. In challenging economic times, with mortgages defaulting at an unprecedented rate[3] and unemployment rising higher than it has been in many decades,[4] families are hard pressed to maintain their coverage for care. Lastly, the largest national insurer, the federal government, is challenged by an increasing deficit and the depletion of Medicare and Medicaid dollars. As a result of this financial turmoil, it is evident that overall health care delivery in this country may become severely impaired without some form of intervention. No wonder the question increasingly being asked is: How do we get the greatest value for every dollar spent in the delivery of health care?

To date, no clear solutions have been forthcoming. In the White House and in Congress, the resolve to create a new template for health care is obvious, but the path forward is unclear.[5] The devil, as always, is in the details of determining how to proceed and in deciding the form for health care in the twenty-first century.

Because neonatal medicine is so expensive—a small population of infants produces very high health care costs—there has been a fair amount of attention given to this group of patients. An idea that has received increasing attention in this discussion is pay for performance (P4P). This article discusses the concept of P4P, examines what potential benefits and risks exist in this model, and investigates how it might achieve the desired goals if implemented in a thoughtful way.

PAY FOR PERFORMANCE

P4P programs are not an entirely new, but have been around as a concept for the past decade.[6] During the past 5 years, P4P initiatives have been proliferating at a significant rate, with various sides debating both the potential benefits of P4P, as well as the difficulties with this approach. The basic concept underlying P4P is simple: Instead of reimbursing physicians on a fee-for-service basis, which tends to encourage additional testing, surgery, and procedures, P4P provides incentives to physicians based upon the quality of their outcomes. By providing reimbursement based upon results of care and not on the number of procedures, the process aligns the goals of the insurer, which wants to pay for the best possible result; with those of the provider, who is reimbursed for the quality of care that is delivered; and, most importantly, with those of the patient, who receives the primary benefit of this effort. Theoretically, as providers strive to further improve outcomes and enhance the quality of care, the overall cost of care should decline, patients should need less medical care (especially intensive hospital care if preventive measures are embraced), and providers should continue to thrive as they are rewarded for reducing the needs of patients.

Defining Quality

While the concept of P4P appears to be sound overall, a number of issues can potentially interfere with the success of this initiative. Perhaps the most fundamental difficulty is simply defining what *quality* means in health care. This elusive term connotes many things to different people. The meaning often seems to depend upon the perspective in which one approaches health care. From the patient's point of view, quality care may simply mean an empathetic physician who has sufficient time to sit and listen to the patient's concerns while offering sound advice on how best to manage the issues at hand. Measurement of "quality" in such a scenario will be elusive at best, yet these actions by a physician may elevate the patient's sense of well-being and improve the patient's symptoms.

In contrast, from the insurer's perspective "quality" may mean shorter lengths of stay in the hospital for a particular provider's group of patients. For example, in neonatal intensive care, some physician groups appear to be far more adept than others at coordinating hospital care, so that they consistently demonstrate a shorter length of stay. Commonly, a less efficient group may explain away the results by claiming that patients in the other practice are less ill or that they comprise an entirely different patient population. However, good data suggest that the application of evidence-based quality-improvement efforts can dramatically alter outcomes, such as length of stay.[7,8]

The real question, however, is whether length-of-stay improvement is truly indicative of "quality" of health care. Many would argue that reduced length of stay has little to no bearing upon quality of care whatsoever. Parents of neonatal intensive care unit (NICU) patients in particular, when confronted with a request to take a former 24-week gestation baby home at 1700 to 1800 g—a baby who has been out of an isolette for less than 24 hours—may perceive this suggestion as marginal quality of care at best. Even when it is explained to them that the baby is feeding orally, does not need any oxygen or other respiratory support, and can maintain body temperature, their readiness to accept the responsibility for the infant, who was very recently critically ill, may simply not be reasonable at that time. The parents might then view the doctor's incentives as being too directly aligned with those of the payer in simply trying to save dollars at the parents' personal expense and at the expense of the baby's well-being. For many families, this process would appear to be financially motivated and *quality* would not be a term that they would find particularly applicable in this situation.

If shorter length of stay is not quality, then what is quality? Is it fewer cases of retinopathy of prematurity or of necrotizing enterocolitis in the NICU? What if your NICU has a very low rate of retinopathy of prematurity, but a relatively high rate of necrotizing enterocolitis? Do these outcomes represent a quality NICU or not? The elusive nature of quality is thus readily apparent when one attempts to define a high-performing NICU versus one with poorer outcomes. Providers themselves tend to be highly selective when attempting to define the quality of care in their NICU. If they have had great success in reducing rates of retinopathy of prematurity or bronchopulmonary dysplasia, they may tout these results as evidence of "quality," even though they may be aware that their rate of late-onset infection is strikingly high. Also, one of the commonly seen, highly disappointing facts about many quality improvement initiatives is that, by focusing on a particular problem, a nonspecific improvement may be readily detected (the Hawthorne effect). Once the desired improvement goal is reached and the team moves to a new project, the previous improvement in outcome may subsequently be lost.

Thus, defining *quality* in outcomes is far from simple and quite elusive in many instances. Therefore, one of the great challenges in P4P is to formulate a definition of *quality* that aligns the interests of patients, providers, and payers. Somehow, the process must be viewed as scientifically valid, fair to all parties, and of true, inherent value to the patient.

The Need for Data

No P4P effort can be considered without data that has been carefully collected and validated for accuracy. One of the commonly voiced ideas in the current health care environment is that the introduction of electronic health records and computerized physician order entries will immediately improve care and alter health outcomes. Most simply put: They will not achieve these effects without thoughtful attentiveness to data entry, initiatives to enhance and codify chart documentation, precise extraction of data from a compiled database, and well-designed "toolkits" or "clinical pathways" designed to improve clinical outcomes.

The widespread use of the computer has produced the common expression "garbage in equals garbage out." Before one can evaluate the value of any information extracted from a database, one has a number of issues to confront: How are the data entered into the electronic health record? Are most data entered via data fields or drop-down so that consistency can be assured across charts and especially across institutions? Are definitions for clinical events precise enough so that the findings, assessments, or diagnoses of one physician can be compared with those of another? Do the data flow smoothly from the point of chart entry into the database without being corrupted by some technical process? If the database is deidentified for research purposes, does the HIPAA (Health Insurance Portability and Accountability Act of 1996) deidentification process itself somehow alter the data collection within the system?

The extensive process of meticulous validation of such systems is often given little consideration in the planning phases, only to find out later that the extracted data are of little value, since there were far too many inconsistencies in the processes or the definitions of events. As an example, early in the development of the Pediatrix Medical Group BabySteps Clinical Data Warehouse, we had to decide if we could extract information from text fields as well as from drop-down menus or numerical entry fields. As described in more detail elsewhere in this issue, we examined the number of ways in which intraventricular hemorrhage could be described in text fields. Intraventricular hemorrhage is a relatively straightforward event: There is bleeding into or around the ventricular system of the brain, usually in a preterm infant. Surprisingly, more than 1000 different phrases were found for this single clinical problem. To program for all these variations was clearly impossible and, even if one could do it, the drag imposed upon computer speed would have bogged down the system. As a result, we decided that information had to be primarily extracted from only specific drop-down menus or data boxes. Without understanding this process and standardizing the subsequent requirements for data entry, any evaluation of data would have been meaningless. If data are meaningless, then comparisons of data outcomes have even less value.

Similarly, physicians often use certain terminology to mean different things. For example, when a physician speaks of "renal insufficiency" in the neonatal period, what exactly is meant? Is it a concept that depends upon the blood urea nitrogen or creatinine level? Does it always mean renal failure, or does it perhaps refer to something less serious than renal failure, such as a transient decrease in urine output? When we recently examined the use of the term *renal insufficiency* among our neonatologists, it was very apparent that it meant *renal failure* to some, but only *altered renal laboratory values* or *diminished urine output* to others. The creation of a general set of working definitions therefore is paramount to success at data comparisons. While one NICU might have a high rate of "renal insufficiency," which indicates reduced urine output from their style of fluid management, another unit's "renal insufficiency" may, in fact, indicate that their patients are developing transient or permanent renal failure, which requires far more intensive and costly management.

Risk adjustment of data sets is another issue that is somewhat controversial, yet is an important consideration when attempting to make meaningful data comparisons. Risk adjustment accounts for the fact that clinical situations in different care settings are rarely, if ever, identical. Comparisons of rates of necrotizing enterocolitis in an NICU will be vastly different in a tertiary center that cares for many babies with birth weights below 1000 g compared with rates at a community hospital that transfers such infants elsewhere. Late-onset catheter-related blood-stream infections and other similar complications of severe prematurity will also differ among nurseries with different populations of patients. Inner-city hospitals with limited prenatal maternal care will have different outcomes compared with an NICU that serves a more affluent population in which access to prenatal care is a given. Thus, some ability to make valid comparisons between populations is sometimes necessary, and risk adjusting for the many confounding variables that alter outcomes is sometimes mandatory.[9]

Having acknowledged this issue, however, the other side of the coin is that risk adjustment is far too often used as an excuse to justify sub-optimal outcomes. "My babies are different" is a phrase that one often hears when a practice first confronts its outcome data with a sense of disbelief in the way the information looks. In general, however, some acknowledgment that outcome data have been adjusted to account for the common underlying variations is essential to get physicians to effectively and critically evaluate their practice approaches.

MEANINGFUL PAY FOR PERFORMANCE—IDENTIFYING THE PROBLEM

Once outcome data have been settled upon and the potential confounders have been reduced, if not eliminated, from the system, P4P goals can be established. Many of the initial P4P programs, however, have focused more upon improving process rather than affecting actual outcomes. Since P4P has been applied so sparingly in neonatal-perinatal medicine to date, there are few examples of how quality improvement will be approached with the widespread adoption of electronic health records. To gain some insight into this issue, it is helpful to examine some of the objectives outlined, for example, by the federal government's Health IT Policy Committee working to establish objective measures for "meaningful use" of electronic health records. Among its initial goals for 2011 at the time of this writing are to ensure that the records of practitioners indicate, for example:

The percentage of diabetics with A_{1C} determinations
The percentage of hypertensive patients with blood pressure under control
The percentage of smokers who have been offered smoking cessation programs
The percentage of patients over 50 with colorectal screening.[10]

Substantial evidence shows that these public health initiatives enhance care. However, with the focus of these efforts on improved chart documentation, actual improvements in meaningful outcomes as a result of these initiatives may actually be modest. Bringing the blood pressure of hypertensive patients "under control" (at present undefined) does not necessarily reduce the rates of stroke, myocardial infarction, renal failure, or mortality in this population. Although the literature would suggest that rates of morbidity and mortality would fall, it is impossible to be sure unless such outcomes are actually measured.[11] Ideally, one would like to have a database with sufficient data to indicate whether the management of the patient with hypertension in that practice truly did result in better outcomes.

In the Pediatrix Medical Group, the size of the organization provides an ideal clinical setting in which to evaluate real outcome improvement. For a variety of reasons, the company has carefully avoided any form of "corporate practice of medicine," and we never dictate to our physicians or advanced practitioners how they should care for their patients. The objective has instead been to provide a high level of current, evidence-based knowledge and training, both in live meetings and in online educational programs, to enhance our physicians' ability to care for their patients. In some instances, problem-oriented toolkits are created with a very broad educational base for physicians, nurses, and parents, so that they can more effectively care for the infant. In addition, practices are given immediate access through real-time outcomes through our BabySteps Data Warehouse so that physicians can constantly monitor each infant's progress and decide upon the implementation of additional measures.

Simultaneously, at the corporate level, the management teams can gain access to outcome data from the practices in their region, and they can evaluate practice performance in a number of ways. For P4P initiatives, one of the necessary steps is to directly look at the practice variation in a series on hospitals. **Fig. 1** shows the striking range of outcome variation in late-onset sepsis in the neonate in a varied group of

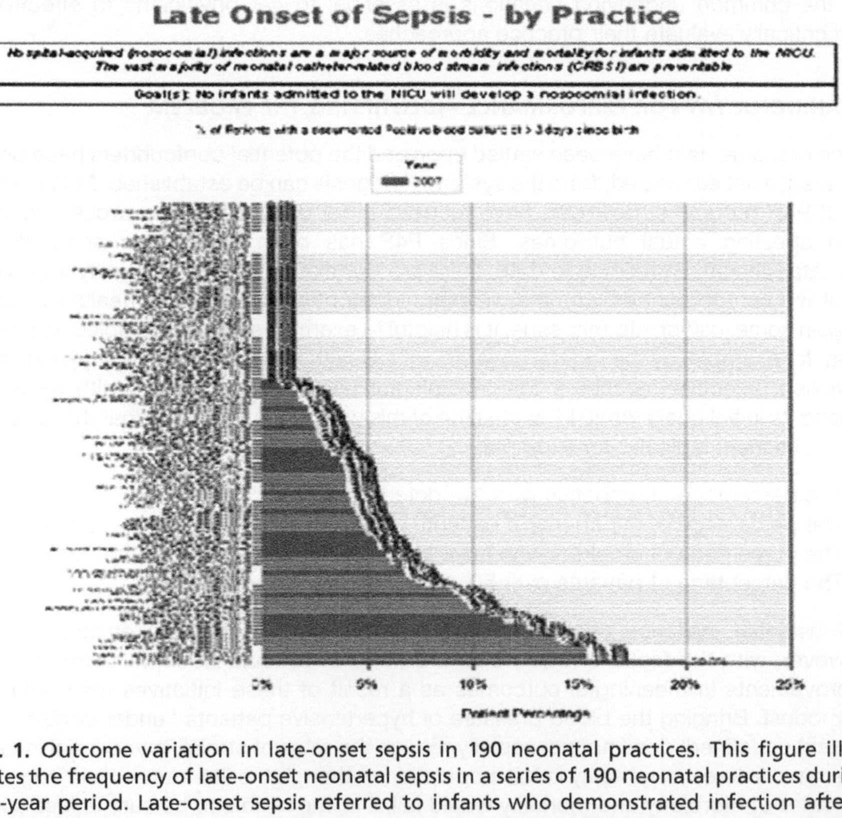

Fig. 1. Outcome variation in late-onset sepsis in 190 neonatal practices. This figure illustrates the frequency of late-onset neonatal sepsis in a series of 190 neonatal practices during a 1-year period. Late-onset sepsis referred to infants who demonstrated infection after 1 week of life. The incidence of infection ranges from 2% to 18% in nurseries that manage patients beyond this age.

practices. The incidence of late-onset septicemia ranges from about 2% to approximately 18% in some NICUs (some smaller NICUs have a rate of 0%, but they rarely keep infants for a sufficient duration to encounter this problem). While some of the variation can be explained away by risk adjustment and comparison of like-sized institutions, one is still left with a striking amount of variation among hospitals in one of the most critical neonatal outcomes. Once Pediatrix Medical Group has identified a problem that appears to result in a significant variation in outcomes among practices, that problem becomes a potential project for P4P. Without this level of variation, it becomes far more difficult to initiate meaningful change, since there is really no "benchmark" standard that one can attempt to reach. Also, outcome levels that are nearly the same would suggest that most practices are probably performing near an optimal level, else one or more of those practices would have initiated a process of improvement. However, it is always possible that many, if not all, practices are going to demonstrate a certain level of outcome until a novel approach or technology arrives on the scene. There may then be an opportunity to reestablish a benchmark and have other practices strive to reach the new level.

PAY FOR PERFORMANCE: THE SEQUENCE AND APPROPRIATE MOTIVATION

In attempting to create a mechanism through which improvement in NICU outcomes can be obtained through P4P, one needs to develop a series of questions that carefully outlines the thinking sequence that defines the process of rewarding improvement. This sequence might be considered as follows:

1. What is the problem that appears to need attention?
2. How serious is the problem? How much of an impact does it have on patients or society?
3. How readily and accurately can the outcome be measured?
4. Is there sufficient variation in the outcome to be meaningful from one NICU to the next?
5. What is the desired benchmark outcome?
6. How is this outcome achieved in the benchmark NICU?
7. What evidence can be applied to foster improvement in the outcome in other NICUs?
8. What is the intervention strategy for improvement based upon the evidence?
9. When should the evaluation and reevaluation of the outcome occur?
10. What level of outcome should be incentivized?
11. How much of an incentive is necessary to achieve the desired goal?
12. How should the incentive be distributed among the NICU caregivers?
13. Is it possible to sustain this level of achievement?
14. Does the achievement level result in improved parental satisfaction?

In working through these questions, it is evident that countless hours of discussion might ensue among any group of clinicians who attempted to agree upon a series of common answers. It is not always simple to answer such questions as: What constitutes a "serious" problem? How do we determine a benchmark practice? Is the evidence sufficiently clear that a certain practice is desirable? and How much of an incentive is needed to produce an agreed upon level of performance? In general, however, it is not difficult to identify a specific issue in the NICU that often provokes heated debate. Such issues are often highly amenable to a P4P approach. For example, some NICUs appear to discharge many of their graduates on breastfeeding, while others have a low rate of success in this area. The value of breast milk over formula has long been evident, yet there is great variation in NICU performance in this area. Furthermore, failure to continue breast feeding is a concern that is commonly shared by physicians, nurses, and parents alike. One could, therefore, determine a goal that at least two thirds of premature NICU graduates should be discharged on breast-milk feeding, as an initial standard to work toward. The team then needs to determine the appropriate reward and how it should be distributed among the various caregivers, since the nursing staff, in addition to the medical team, plays a very large role in such a process.

One of the primary questions that arises at this point, especially if the reward is financial, is: Where do those dollars come from and what amount would be appropriate? To date, many of the initiatives that have emerged have focused incentives more on rewarding better charting documentation rather than affecting real outcome change. As an example, a clinician who documents that a neonate leaving the NICU has received mandated state metabolic screening and hearing testing might receive a modest additional final-day allocation from the third-party payer for noting these aspects in the chart. As previously noted, however, indicating that these screens were performed does not ensure an outcome change unless infants with abnormal screens are followed-up with appropriate care. Furthermore, there are two inherent risks in such situations: (1) that the reimbursement is so trivial that it fails to move the caregivers to perform the necessary documentation and (2) that the third-party payer may actually reduce reimbursement if such documentation is inadvertently omitted. This latter approach, perhaps best entitled "punish for nonperformance," represents a potential risk that can emerge in the P4P system. A variation on this theme would be to only promise that reimbursement for care would not be reduced if the goals were met. But whether one is rewarded or punished for improved charting, does this truly represent a better "quality" of care? Better charting as a primary goal of "quality care," while desirable, is only part of the answer, since little evidence in the neonatal literature actually indicates that improved charting leads to meaningful enhancements in outcomes. As noted earlier, the entire concept of "quality" in health care truly remains elusive.

If one can agree upon a quality measure, however, what then constitutes an adequate incentive to achieve the goal level? To date, the projects that have been studied have rarely resulted in dramatic gains, most likely because the dangled carrot was not sufficiently enticing. Furthermore, in a situation in which health care reform is likely to lead to decreased reimbursement at several levels—to payer and provider alike—will there be adequate resources to fund such initiatives and where will these dollars come from? The clinician engaged in a P4P program will, of necessity, have to balance the enhanced compensation against the added work involved to determine whether the effort is worth it. Some have suggested a 2% added reimbursement for certain P4P initiatives. If this is the reward for checking off a box that indicates that retinopathy of prematurity screening has been performed at the appropriate time, it may be performed, even though the actual compensation may be little more than a few dollars. On the other hand, if 2% is the reward for demonstrating that one's practice has resulted in a one-third reduction in annual rates of retinopathy of prematurity in an extremely low birth weight population, then it is not likely to achieve the desired effect. The extensive effort to deliver such an important, but very broad, outcome would need to have a far greater incentive attached to underwrite the huge additional effort on the part of many NICU personnel.

Lastly, in the discussion of incentive, one cannot overlook current compensation levels for neonatal services. The average reimbursement from Medicaid nationally for a neonatal resuscitation now averages approximately $84. Reimbursement for the hospital day-of-discharge physician care averages $45. Adding a 2% incentive to either of these billing codes, especially if substantial effort and documentation work were involved, would hardly constitute a serious incentive for meaningful enhancement in patient outcome. A clearly defined evaluation of appropriate coding would be a necessity before P4P could ever become a strong methodology for encouraging better patient outcomes.

PAY-FOR-PERFORMANCE RESULTS TO DATE

There is little question that the basic concept of P4P—to reward physician behavior to achieve better outcomes—is intrinsically beneficial. Fee for service, the current approach, rewards volumes of care, but not outcomes, which commonly fail to even enter into the equation. But does P4P actually work in practice? To date, the results are somewhat limited and mixed in the adult and pediatric literature, and virtually nonexistent in the NICU.

Efforts in such areas as diabetes management look encouraging, though longer-term participation and follow-up are still being evaluated. In one study, which involved charting of diabetic management, significant improvement was noted in procedural documentation and outcomes over time.[12] Over a series of twice yearly cycles between 2003 and 2007, physician participation, even with modest reimbursement of $0.60 to $0.70 per member per month, increased and the desired diabetic documentation/outcome goals (eg, blood pressure $<130/80$ mm Hg, low-density lipoprotein <100 mg/dL, hemoglobin $A_{1C}<7\%$) were increasingly met. The investigators attributed this success to physician engagement, office-based education, written action plans, and alignment with internal disease management.

In contrast, however, Rosenthal and colleagues[13] reported in a comparison between a California P4P intervention group and a Pacific Northwest non-P4P group that only marginal gains were realized in the P4P group (primarily for cervical cancer screening). The investigators warned that a "fixed performance target may produce little gain in quality for the money spent and will largely reward those with higher performance at baseline." Similarly, in a large study between 2003 and 2006 by Lindenauer and colleagues,[14] sponsored by the Hospital Quality Alliance and the Hospital Quality Incentive Demonstration, P4P hospitals reported greater improvement in composite measures examined compared with control hospitals. Hospitals reporting in the top 10% received a 2% bonus payment beyond usual Medicare reimbursement, while hospitals in the second 10% were eligible for a 1% bonus payment. All hospitals in the study showed progressive improvement in outcomes, though the P4P hospital improvement was greater during the observation period, especially in four key measures: acute myocardial infarction, heart failure, pneumonia, and overall composite measures. The differences, however, were modest, ranging from 2.6% to 4.1% between groups. Epstein,[15] commenting on that study in an editorial, noted that

> *pay for performance is fundamentally a social experiment likely to have only incremental value. Broad demonstrations and evaluation will probably be helpful. Rather than adopt a single new payment system for all of Medicare, a series of regional models could accelerate learning and allow Medicare officials to find out more about the effect of differing levels of incentives and formulas for payment.*

As indicated, this "experiment" is one that has just begun and the variables remain hard to define.

More recently, Rosenthal[16] wrote that

Earlier this decade, pay for performance took center stage as a tactic for realigning payment with value. Payers' experiences during this period, as well as several major studies, clarified the limitations of this approach—characterized by some as putting lipstick on a pig.

Rosenthal goes on to suggest that broader reforms of reimbursement models are necessary, given the lackluster results of P4P. So the basic question emerges as to whether P4P will ever see the light of day in neonatal-perinatal medicine, given the disappointing results in the adult world so far.

Profit and colleagues,[17] however, writing in *Pediatrics* in 2007, retain some degree of optimism for P4P and outline how one could develop a series of meaningful outcome indicators that could be rewarded. They suggest that a phased approach be used while keeping providers involved in decisions about defining and measuring NICU quality of care, which is likely to be an evolving process. In addition, they note that "heightened attention to measuring (and rewarding) NICU quality should provide unprecedented opportunities to develop valid methods for assessing quality of care, which could have both economic and scientific implications."

Another article recently has pointed out an inherent risk in P4P reporting, however. Doran and colleagues[18] examined the results of introducing a P4P contract among family practitioners in the United Kingdom. In the first year, family practices achieved a high level of achievement in this system, which examined a broad variety of adult outcomes. The investigators noted, however, that "a small number of practices appear to have achieved high scores by excluding large numbers of patients by exception reporting." Thus, the methodology of administration of P4P becomes important, as does the question of patient inclusion into outcome measures. The investigators also note that the size of the financial incentive remains a question and whether it truly made a difference or was the favorable outcome due to the rate of exclusion of complex patients with less optimal outcomes. Clearly, exclusionary reporting must be carefully monitored to be certain that outcomes are not unfairly reported and true patient improvement through P4P is actually taking place.

SUMMARY

P4P in the NICU has not been tested to date to any extent. From the adult literature, it remains unclear if this method of health care reimbursement will be able to achieve its goal of realignment of objectives among payers, providers, and patients, though the underlying concept seems sound. Examination and added incentives for quality outcomes, as opposed to fee for service, would seem to be preferable, especially for the patient. Whether P4P has the ability to achieve a better method of reimbursement will probably be answered during the next few years. As noted by Mangione-Smith and colleagues,[19] children's health services are either not performed or delivered inappropriately more than 50% of the time. Whether P4P can assist children in receiving more timely and appropriate care remains to be seen.

REFERENCES

1. Keehan S, Sisko A, Truffer C, et al. Health spending projections through 2017. Health Affairs Web Exclusive W146 February 2008;21. Available at: www.healthaffairs.orgWebExclusives.php. Accessed January 8, 2010.
2. March of dimes. Available at: https://www.marchofdimes.com/files/66423_MOD-Complete.pdf?src=mod.com. Accessed January 8, 2010.

3. Yu H. U.S. commercial mortgage defaults may rise to 17-year high. Available at: http://www.Bloomberg.com. Accessed June 9, 2009.
4. US Bureau of Labor Statistics. Available at: http://www.bls.gov/. Accessed October 15, 2009.
5. Stolberg SG. Available at: http://www.NYTimes.com. Accessed October 20, 2009.
6. Garcia LB, Safriet S, Russell DC. Pay-for-performance compensation: moving beyond capitation. Healthc Financ Manage 1998;52:52–7.
7. Rihal CS, Kamath CC, Holmes DR Jr, et al. Economic and clinical outcomes of a physician-led continuous quality improvement intervention in the delivery of percutaneous coronary intervention. Am J Manag Care 2006;12:445–52.
8. JBigham MT, Amato R, Bondurrant P, et al. Ventilator-associated pneumonia in the pediatric intensive care unit: characterizing the problem and implementing a sustainable solution. J Pediatr 2009;154:582–7, e2.
9. Madan I, Puri I, Jain NJ, et al. Characteristics of obstetric intensive care unit admissions in New Jersey. J Matern Fetal Neonatal Med 2009;22:785–90.
10. Health Policy Information Technology Group. Available at: http://healthit.hhs.gov/portal/server.pt/gateway/PTARGS_0_10741_887553_0_0_18/Proposed_Revisions_to_Meaningful_Use_post_7_16_2009_FINAL_PT1_508.pdf.
11. Amarenco P, Goldstein LB, Messig M, et al. Relative and cumulative effects of lipid and blood pressure control in the Stroke Prevention by Aggressive Reduction in Cholesterol Levels trial. Stroke 2009;40:2486–92.
12. Foels T, Hewner S. Integrating pay for performance with educational strategies to improve diabetes care. Popul Health Manag 2009;12:121–9.
13. Rosenthal MB, Frank RG, Zhonghe LI, et al. Early experience with pay for performance. JAMA 2005;294:1788–93.
14. Lindenauer PK, Remus D, Roman S, et al. Public reporting and pay for performance in hospital quality improvement. N Engl J Med 2007;356:486–96.
15. Epstein AM. Pay for performance at the tipping point. N Engl J Med 2007;356:515–7.
16. Rosenthal MB. Beyond pay for performance—emerging models of provider-payment reform. N Engl J Med 2008;359:1197–8.
17. Profit J, Zupancic JA, Gould JB, et al. Implementing pay-for-performance in the neonatal intensive care unit. Pediatrics 2007;119:975–82.
18. Doran T, Fullwood C, Gravelle H, et al. Pay for performance programs in family practices in the United Kingdom. N Engl J Med 2006;355:375–84.
19. Mangione-Smith R, DeCristofaro AH, Setodji CM, et al. The quality of ambulatory care delivered to children in the United States. N Engl J Med 2007;357:1515–23.

Collaboration Between Obstetricians and Neonatologists: Perinatal Safety Programs and Improved Clinical Outcomes

Dale P. Reisner, MD[a,b,*], Susan Landers, MD[c]

KEYWORDS

• Perinatal safety • Quality • Teamwork

What higher-risk situation exists than caring for a pregnant woman who actually carries two patients within one body? The best care for the mother may result in preterm birth of the baby. Conversely, the best care for the fetus may place the mother at risk. When multiples are involved, sometimes care is driven by the needs of one fetus, placing the other(s) at risk.

Quality improvement in obstetric care affects both mother and baby. Thus, when assessing patient safety and quality of care, it is logical that perinatalogists and neonatologists work together. Historically, however, that generally has not been the case. When obstetricians created perinatal protocols, neonatologists and pediatricians often were not involved, and vice versa for newborn management plans. In recent years, however, the focus on improving quality of care, patient safety, and avoiding harm has fostered a more cohesive team approach.

The Institute for Healthcare Improvement (IHI) created a perinatal innovation community that began working together in February 2005. That same year, the IHI

[a] CQI for Maternal Fetal Medicine, Pediatrix Medical Group/MEDNAX, USA
[b] Division of Perinatal Medicine, Swedish Medical Center/Seattle, 1229 Madison, Suite 750, Seattle, WA 98104, USA
[c] NICU Nutrition and Lactation Services, Seton Family of Hospitals, Pediatrix Medical Group, Seton Medical Center, 1201 West 38th Street, Austin, TX 78705, USA
* Corresponding author. Division of Perinatal Medicine, Swedish Medical Center/Seattle, 1229 Madison, Suite 750, Seattle, WA 98104.
E-mail address: dale_reisner@pediatrix.com.

Clin Perinatol 37 (2010) 179–188
doi:10.1016/j.clp.2010.01.009 perinatology.theclinics.com
0095-5108/10/$ – see front matter

white paper, "Idealized Design of Perinatal Care," was published.[1] This program was based on the fact that perinatal harm is rare, compared with the total number of births. When problems do occur, however, they can have devastating effects not only on the baby and family, but also on the medical care providers involved. The concept of the highly reliable organization, as used in the aviation industry,[2] has been applied to perinatal units by Knox and colleagues.[3] To be successful, this strategy requires improvement in communication, documentation, and reliable processes in labor and delivery.

Over the past decade, national institutes and professional organizations such as the American College of Obstetricians and Gynecologists (ACOG) and the Association of Women's Health, Obstetric, and Neonatal Nurses (AWHONN), have issued practice bulletins, opinions, and clinical position statements related to improving patient safety and avoiding fetal and maternal injury.[4–7] Individual medical centers and large hospital systems have been working with team approaches to improving patient safety and quality of care. The past year has seen several publications from across the country highlighting how effective this collaborative approach can be.[8–11]

The Codman Award from The Joint Commission is presented to health care organizations for improvements in process and outcome measures that result in better quality and safer health care. In 2007, this award was presented to the Seton Family of Hospitals in Austin, Texas, for its perinatal safety initiative.[8] The following is a detailed description of this successful quality improvement work, which combined the efforts of obstetricians, neonatologists, and hospital personnel. The authors offer it as a model for what might be achieved through this type of broad collaborative effort.

THE SETON FAMILY OF HOSPITALS' EXPERIENCE

Background and Setting

The Seton Family of Hospitals is part of Ascension Health, the nation's largest Catholic nonprofit network of hospitals and related health facilities. Ascension Health developed a perinatal safety priority for action as a result of collaboration between clinical and risk management teams. The main objective of the Seton network's local perinatal safety initiative was to eliminate preventable birth trauma and to improve safety for mothers and babies. This was achieved by creating high-reliability obstetric units that implemented evidence-based obstetric practices.[3] Ascension Health's corporate belief was that improvement in safety for mothers and babies would not only improve care, but also reduce potential malpractice claims.

The Seton Family of Hospitals, comprised of eight acute care hospitals in the Austin and central Texas area, used the four hospitals that provided obstetric services. Four hospitals within the network served as the setting for this perinatal safety initiative: Seton Medical Center, a tertiary care high-risk referral perinatal center with a 40-bed neonatal intensive care unit (NICU) and approximately 4500 deliveries each year; University Medical Center at Brackenridge, an inborn city–county tertiary care center with a 25-bed NICU and approximately 2500 deliveries yearly (this hospital also functions as a pediatric and obstetric residency training facility); and Seton Northwest and Seton Southwest Hospitals, both primary and secondary care facilities delivering approximately 1800 and 1000 babies, respectively, each year.

The Seton multicenter network routinely tracked hospital-level patient safety indicators (PSIs) published by the Agency for Healthcare Research and Quality (AHRQ)[12]; among these indicators is neonatal birth trauma (PSI #17). The network sought to create and maintain a "high-reliability perinatal unit" in each of its facilities.[1,13,14] Low-reliability perinatal units are distinguished by their failure to recognize fetal distress or nonreassuring fetal status, failure to implement a timely cesarean section, failure to properly resuscitate a depressed baby, their inappropriate use of oxytocin, and their inappropriate use of vacuum or forceps.[3]

Quality Improvement Methods

In 2003, Seton formed a multidisciplinary work group to assess certain obstetric procedures and implement changes in labor management, The interdisciplinary team consisted of various types of hospital personnel including senior administrators; each site's medical director; staff physicians from obstetrics (from each site), perinatology, and neonatology; labor and delivery nurses and managers from each site; a network risk management attorney; a network pharmacy administrator; a project data coordinator; and other medical staff support members. In conjunction with Ascension Health's corporate patient safety goals, the work group focused on the five areas of highest risk for obstetric harm (failure to recognize fetal distress, failure to implement a timely cesarean section, failure to properly resuscitate a depressed baby, the inappropriate use of oxytocin, and inappropriate use of vacuum or forceps).

The perinatal safety initiative began with the education of key physician members of the work group, specifically site medical directors, obstetricians, perinatologists and neonatologists. Several physicians traveled to St. Louis, for a day-long training session by the IHI in methods used for obstetric quality improvement (QI). Travel expenses were covered by the Seton Healthcare Network. Subsequently, the work group met on a monthly basis to develop and monitor data and best practices that were shared and implemented by each hospital's perinatal council. The project data coordinator position became fulltime within the first year of the initiative.

Task force members created or revised standardized order sets, which were adopted across all four sites and incorporated into the work flow of the physicians and nurses in each labor and delivery unit. Initially, clinical protocols for the use of oxytocin were reviewed. Key task force members presented regular clinical in-service educational sessions about operative vaginal delivery for labor and delivery nursing staff as well as physicians' grand rounds on operative vaginal delivery and birth trauma.

In conjunction with the IHI, best obstetric practices, as defined by ACOG and AWHONN clinical practice guidelines, were incorporated into the creation of bundles of clinical care. As defined by IHI, a bundle is "a group of evidence-based interventions, or bundle elements, related to a disease or care process, that when executed together, result in better outcomes than when implemented individually." Oxytocin bundles for labor augmentation and elective induction of labor had been developed by IHI.[1] In addition, an operative vaginal delivery (OVD) bundle was developed as a potential birth trauma reduction strategy.

Oxytocin augmentation bundle elements developed by IHI included reassuring fetal status, estimated fetal weight, examination of the cervix within 1 hour before or after start of oxytocin, and absence or management of uterine hyperstimulation. Oxytocin elective induction bundle elements included reassuring fetal status, examination of the cervix within 1 hour before or after start of oxytocin, absence or management of uterine hyperstimulation, and documentation of gestational age greater than 39 weeks or estimated fetal weight (EFW). The locally developed OVD bundle elements included: indications for instrumented delivery, EFW relative to the size of the maternal pelvis, and presentation and station of the fetal head.

The work group provided anonymous data review, engaging physicians through peer comparisons and feedback of their own data describing rates of OVD, elective inductions, and rates of neonatal birth injury. At quarterly intervals, individual physicians' data were compared in a blinded fashion with their peers who delivered babies at the same site and with physicians practicing at other sites within the hospital network.

Compliance with care bundles required documentation of all bundle elements in the medical record by physicians and nurses. Using monthly random chart audits, each site's compliance with documentation of clinical bundles was tracked. A perinatal safety newsletter was published and distributed to all sites at least monthly. Data related to bundle compliance and other performance measures were generated on an ongoing basis for OVD, cesarean section rates, maternal injury, and birth trauma rates; these rates were published in the newsletter.

To promote the use of common terminology for electronic fetal monitoring, joint obstetric physician and nursing fetal monitor strip review sessions were conducted periodically, conforming to use of the common language advocated by the National Institute of Child Health and Human Development (NICHD).[15] Labor and delivery room staff were trained in the use of a customized SBAR communication tool. SBAR (Situation, Background, Assessment, and Recommendation) is a standardized form of communication that helps caregivers, both physicians and nurses, speak about patients concisely and completely. At least quarterly, task force members from each site conducted clinical site visits of the other three network sites. This allowed nursing and physician personnel to witness firsthand significant differences in labor and delivery care practices from site to site.

During 2006, the network sent key nursing managers and educators for special education in simulation obstetric training. Thereafter, interdisciplinary crisis simulation training was implemented at all four labor and delivery sites using a high-fidelity birthing mannequin, Noelle (Gaumard Scientific, Miami, FL, USA). Simulation training focused on communication and teamwork by using medical actors and planned scenarios with the mannequin. Simulations for obstetric emergencies, such as shoulder dystocia and postpartum hemorrhage, were conducted quarterly at each site. Regular, structured team debriefings occurred after each simulation. Best practices were shared via team meetings and conference calls at least quarterly.

The perinatal safety initiative primarily was focused on three areas: (1) tracking compliance for oxytocin elective induction and augmentation bundles, (2) improved communication via the NICHD common language for electronic fetal monitoring and the SBAR tool, and (3) labor and delivery crisis simulation training of nurses and physicians. The primary goal of the initiative had been to eliminate preventable birth injuries. Throughout the initiative, rates of OVD, elective inductions less than 39 weeks' gestation, total cesarean sections (both primary and repeat) and all infant morbidity designated as serious birth trauma were examined. For purposes of tracking serious respiratory illness in near-term babies, the work group defined iatrogenic prematurity as a NICU admitting diagnosis of respiratory distress syndrome (RDS) or transient tachypnea of the newborn (TTN) in inborn infants from 37 0/7 to 38 6/7 weeks gestational age. Babies remaining in normal newborn care with milder forms of TTN were excluded. Differences in hospital length of stay and charges associated with neonatal morbidity from serious birth trauma and respiratory distress of inborn neonates before, during, and after implementation of the perinatal safety initiative were examined.

Infants with birth trauma or respiratory distress were identified by tracking primary or secondary International Classification of Disease codes (ICD-IX) diagnoses, noted by ICD IX codes of 767.0 to 767.9 (representing the AHRQ codes specific for PSI #17 or neonatal birth injury), or the ICD-IX code 767.6 for brachial plexus injury. In addition, infants with gestational ages ranging from 37 0/7 weeks to 38 6/7 weeks gestation, who were admitted to NICU for care with ICD-IX codes for neonatal respiratory distress, including 769 to 770.8, or persistent pulmonary hypertension 747.83, were tracked.

Perinatal Safety Initiative Results

From 2000 to 2007, the Seton network facilities altogether delivered on average 9745 babies annually. During the baseline period (2000 to 2003) before the initiative, the network hospitals delivered 31,290 newborns. Among these deliveries, there were 7.5% OVDs, 3.2% elective inductions less than 39 weeks, 22.5% total cesarean sections, and a rate of 0.3% for serious birth trauma. The period from 2003 to 2004 was considered to be a transition. The perinatal safety initiative, or intervention period, lasted from 2004 to 2007. During this period, the network hospital deliveries totaled 28,130, and the network rates fell incrementally to 4.5% for OVD, to 1.6% for elective inductions less than 39 weeks, and to 0.03% for serious birth trauma. This was a remarkable 90% reduction in the rate of serious birth injury (**Figs. 1** and **2**). During this time period, however, the network cesarean section rate rose to 29.3%.

In January 2007, the network hospitals reported a 36% reduction in the use of vacuum and forceps (from a frequency of 7.4% to 4.7%).[8] Data were examined for unintentional harm that may have resulted from changes in practice related to prolonged second stage of labor when instrumented delivery was not performed, but no evidence was found to substantiate adverse injury to neonates as a result of changes in delivery practices. In addition, the relative change in the percentage of births performed by cesarean section was examined. It had been anticipated that the reduction in OVD would produce a rise in the primary cesarean section rate; although an upward trend in primary cesarean sections has been noted over time, the degree of change was slight, from 22% in 2003, and to 24% in 2007. This was consistent with national trends.[16]

The rate of brachial plexus injury remained stable throughout the perinatal safety initiative, averaging 0.1%, or 1 of 1000 live births. The AHRQ dropped this particular diagnosis from among those codes defining PSI #17 (serious birth injury), as most obstetric experts felt that brachial palsy often occurred spontaneously and was largely uninfluenced by obstetric practices.

During the initiative, the average length of stay for infants admitted to the NICU for birth injury declined by 79% (compared with the baseline years), from 15.8 days to 3.4 days. This denoted a dramatic reduction in the clinical severity of the infants' birth injury. Moreover, total hospital billed charges for NICU care for these infants declined

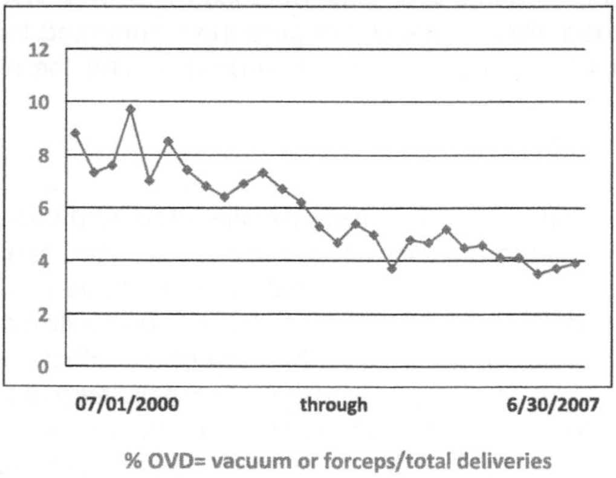

Fig. 1. Operative vaginal delivery (OVD) rate, Seton Family of Hospitals.

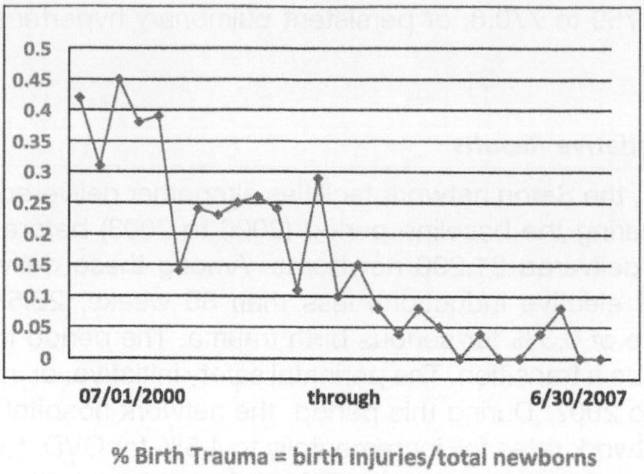

Fig. 2. Birth trauma rate by AHRQ PSIs #17, Seton Family of Hospitals.

by 98% during the intervention, as compared with baseline, from $4,479,898 for the fiscal years 2000 to 2003 to $66,321 for fiscal years 2004 to 2007.[8]

The rate of respiratory morbidity requiring NICU care in near-term babies (iatrogenic prematurity) fell from 0.24% during the baseline period to 0.14% during the initiative. Total length of stay and hospital charges for NICU care for these near-term infants declined from 10 days and $1,825,486, respectively, during the baseline period, to 8 days and $1,010,620 during the intervention period. Although less dramatic, a reduction in the clinical severity of RDS and TTN among near-term babies was noted after the initiative. It appeared that infants admitted to the NICU for both respiratory distress and birth injury were less ill than previously. Comparing baseline with intervention periods, NICU days on oxygen fell from 3.8 to 3.1 days; the number of infants requiring artificial surfactant fell from 12% to 6%, and babies needing nasal continuous positive airway pressure support remained constant at 23% and 20%. The number of infants requiring mechanical ventilation, however, fell from 7% to 3%. Most notably, during the baseline period, 9 of 69 (13%) of these babies with respiratory distress requiring NICU care had been born after elective induction. During the transition period, only one case was delivered after elective induction, and after the initiative began, no cases were associated with elective induction of labor.

Although network hospital charges for neonatal morbidity, especially birth trauma, were reduced drastically as a result of the perinatal safety initiative, it was noteworthy that a similar amount, $4,300,000 in legal defense fees, was saved by the network during the same period. Risk management personnel attributed these savings to the prevention of serious birth trauma cases, thereby obviating the need to defend the care provided to these infants.

Conclusions

Because the initiative was multidisciplinary, multifaceted, and sequential, it is impossible to say just what methods, or quality improvement tools, had the greatest influence on the reductions in birth trauma that were observed. Vital factors in the success of this perinatal safety initiative included the commitment of the network's senior leaders and managers, the public advocacy of the initiative by specific physician and nurse champions at each site, and the interdisciplinary nature of the initiative. Drawing clinicians' attention to OVD and elective inductions may have influenced birth injury rates in and of itself (the Hawthorne effect).[17] Obstetricians appreciated viewing maternal and neonatal morbidity data in a regular and confidential manner, allowing them to compare their morbidity rates with those of their peers. Obstetric nurses greatly appreciated the updates on electronic fetal monitoring nomenclature and training in the use of SBAR tool and high-fidelity mannequins for crisis simulation. More so, they appreciated that their voices in describing current labor and delivery care practices were heard and respected.

This quality improvement initiative was successful because the hospital network allowed a team of personnel to implement small tests of change and allow sequential quality improvement efforts to evolve. With this approach, there was tremendous potential to achieve buy-in and support from some originally skeptical physicians. In addition, giving nurses a voice at the table with physicians and providing physicians with real-time data for self-examination resulted in greater acceptance of the need for change. Clearly, feedback of data to the physicians and nurses actively involved in care is paramount to success in any quality improvement initiative.

OTHER COLLABORATIVE EFFORTS

Recently Published Perinatal Quality Improvement Projects

The Seton Hospitals' work was published in April 2008. In April of 2009, Fisch and colleagues,[9] published their results from Magee Hospital in Pennsylvania in successfully reducing inappropriate inductions, particularly any elective induction under 39 weeks gestation and elective inductions in nulliparas. This paper was a retrospective study that looked at three time frames in 2004, 2005, and, finally, from 2006 to 2007 after a new scheduling process was implemented. Their goal was avoiding unnecessary primary cesarean sections, but they also anticipated that fewer babies would be expected to go to the NICU if no elective inductions occurred until 39 weeks or greater. They began with an educational program but did not see significant improvements until the new scheduling process began to strictly enforce the guidelines. Strong physician and nurse champions were crucial to their success.

Pettker and colleagues,[10] from Yale-New Haven, published their patient safety results in May 2009. They used a collaborative team approach, tracking 10 obstetric-specific outcomes as patient safety interventions were begun over a 2-year period. An adverse outcome index (AOI) of 10 indicators was tracked prospectively over 36 months. Indicators included transfusion, maternal or neonatal death (over 2500 g), fetal birth injury, third or fourth degree perineal lacerations, maternal ICU admission, return to the operating room or labor and delivery unit, uterine rupture, 5-minute neonatal Agar less than 7, and unexpected NICU admission if over 2500 g and for over 24 hours. Their teamwork included nurses, obstetricians, anesthesiologists, neonatologists, administration, and ancillary services. This group's focus was to improve communication and coordination of care. Interventions over 2 years included hiring a patient safety nurse, standardizing protocols and guidelines, team training, electronic fetal monitoring certification, and formation of a patient safety committee. The composite AOI was used, because each individual indicator occurred infrequently. The AOI dropped from 3.25% to 1.75% over 36 months (**Fig. 3**).

In June 2009, Reisner and colleagues[11] published prospective collaborative work on reducing elective inductions at Swedish Medical Center, Seattle. The report included over 29,000 deliveries during a 3.75-year period. A team of all obstetric care providers was formed with a goal of reducing elective inductions, and a particular focus on nulliparous women. Practitioners were educated about risks of induction, and their individual statistics were shared with them. There were existing scheduling parameters that did not allow elective inductions before 39 weeks' gestation, but physicians did have the option for providing evidence of fetal lung maturity by

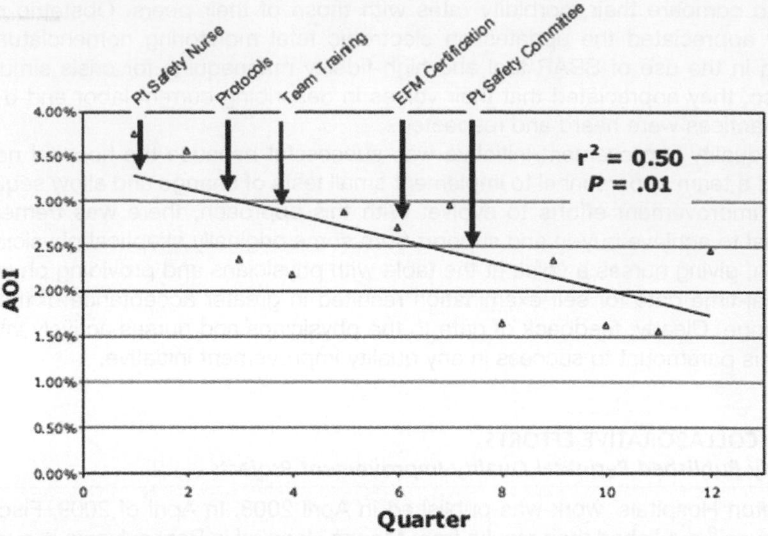

Fig. 3. Adverse outcome index (AOI) trend. Yale-New Haven Hospital, New Haven, Connecticut (YNHH) quarterly obstetric (OB) AOI. Abbreviations: EFM, electronic fetal monitoring; Pt, patient. (*From* Pettker CM, Thung SF, Norwitz ER, et al. Impact of a comprehensive patient safety strategy on obstetric adverse events. Am J Obstet Gynecol 2009;200:492; with permission.)

amniocentesis when gestational age was less than 39 weeks. In the new protocol, elective inductions were limited to 39 weeks or greater, with a favorable cervix (Bishop score of 6 or more). Patients were told they had a standby date when scheduled for any elective induction. Nulliparous elective inductions decreased from 4.3% to 0.8%, a rate which has been sustained now for 5 years (**Fig. 4**). Multiparous elective inductions dropped from 13% to 5%. Hours in labor and delivery were shortened by 4 to 5 hours for spontaneously laboring women, compared with those who were induced. Unplanned primary cesarean sections were significantly lower for both nulliparas and multiparas who were laboring spontaneously, compared with those being induced. The key to success was common, clear goals created by collaboration between the nurses, doctors, midwives, and office and hospital staff members. Sustaining the gains has been a result of continued shared individual and group data support of the guidelines and oversight.

Smaller-Scale Collaborative Projects

Large perinatal safety programs obviously require extensive planning with organizational support for the program itself, data collection/interpretation/reporting, and ongoing monitoring to assure sustainability. Other collaborative projects can be done on a smaller scale with perinatalogists, obstetricians, and family practitioners working with their neonatalogy or pediatric colleagues. Some examples would include collaborative work on a new protocol or guideline for screening and monitoring of potential drug-affected neonates, group B streptococcus management in labor, delivery, and after delivery, or diagnosis and treatment of chorioamnionitis in labor with appropriate newborn monitoring and care.

Another local collaborative project is joint presentations at Morbidity and Mortality or other educational conferences. This year at Swedish Medical Center in Seattle, our neonatologists encouraged a combined grand rounds presentation on the late

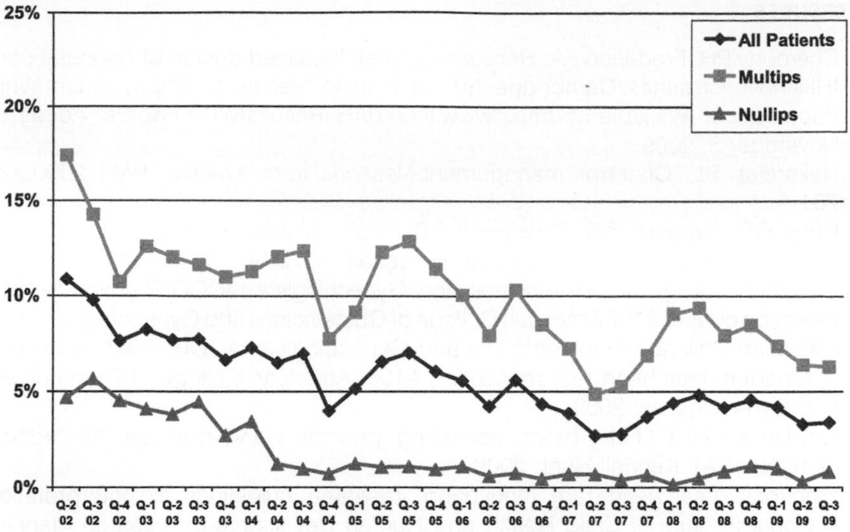

Fig. 4. Elective induction rates by quarter, Swedish Medical Center.

preterm infant titled, "34–37 Week Newborns: More problems than we thought?". The recent outcomes data on 34- to 36-week babies first were presented by a neonatologist who described the higher morbidity and mortality with this group of infants than previously known. A perinatalogist then discussed situations where these babies need delivery for significant maternal or fetal indications, such as preeclampsia, chorioamnionitis, bleeding complications, or other reasons. Part of the perinatal presentation, however, also encouraged obstetricians to reassess current management of a subset of late preterm deliveries, in which delivery at less than 37 or 38 weeks might not be essential.

This type of review challenges the near-term approach of perinatal care in the last decade or more. Recently, Lewis and colleagues[18] published neonatal outcome results in women with mild preeclampsia and amniocentesis evidence of fetal lung maturity delivered between 34 and 37 weeks' gestation. This paper was a retrospective review with its attendant limitations, but it raised some questions regarding management of mild preeclampsia in the late preterm period. The authors emphasized that a risk of immediate morbidity exists for these neonates with planned deliveries, such a NICU admission (31%), RDS (10%), and hyperbilirubinemia (30%), even when lung maturity testing has been performed. Although not a definitive study, it does remind practitioners that one constantly needs to look for new data and reevaluate current practices as one component of perinatal quality improvement.

Benefits of Collaboration

Because pregnancy represents a unique situation with two patients within one, the management of each of the patients necessarily must affect the other. Perinatalogists/obstetricians and neonatologists/pediatricians are often the physician leaders who initiate and help sustain perinatal patient safety and quality care programs. Working collaboratively on these quality improvement projects, protocols, clinical educational efforts, and research is essential to achieve the best outcomes for both mother and baby.

REFERENCES

1. Cherouny PH, Frederico FA, Haraden C, et al. Idealized design of perinatal care: IHI innovation series. Cambridge, MA: Institute for Healthcare Improvement White Paper, 2005. Available at: http://www.ihi.org/IHI/Results/WhitePapers. Accessed November 3, 2009.
2. Helmreich RL. On error management: lessons from aviation. BMJ 2000;320:781–5.
3. Knox GE, Simpson KR, Townsend KE. High reliability perniatal units: further observations and a suggested plan for action. ASHRM J 2003;23:17–21.
4. American College of Obstetricians and Gynecologists. ACOG Practice Bulletin. Induction of labor #107 American College of Obstetricians and Gynecologists; 2009.
5. American College of Obstetricians and Gynecologists. ACOG Practice Bulletin. Intrapartum fetal heart rate monitoring #106. American College of Obstetricians and Gynecologists; 2009.
6. Lyndon A, Ali L. Fetal heart monitoring principles and practice. 4th edition. Dubuque (IA): Kendall-Hunt; 2009.
7. Electronic fetal heart rate monitoring: research guidelines for interpretation. National Institute of Child Health and Human Development Research Planning Workshop (1997). J Obstet Gynecol Neonatal Nurs 1997;177:635–40.
8. Mazza F, Kitchens J, Akin M, et al. The road to zero preventable birth injuries. Jt Comm J Qual Patient Saf 2008;34(4):201–5.
9. Fisch JM, English D, Pedaline S, et al. Labor induction process improvement. Obstet Gynecol 2009;113:797–803.
10. Pettker CM, Thung SF, Norwitz ER, et al. Impact of a comprehensive patient safety strategy on obstetric adverse events. Am J Obstet Gynecol 2009;200:492, e1–e8.
11. Reisner DP, Wallin TK, Zingheim RM, et al. Reduction of elective inductions in a large community hospital. Am J Obstet Gynecol 2009;200:674, e1–e7.
12. Agency for Healthcare Quality and Research. Patient safety indicators. Available at: www.qualityindicators.ahrg.gov/psi_overview.htm. Accessed November 3, 2009.
13. Nolan T, Resar R, Haraden C, et al. Improving the realiability of health care. IHI Innovation Series white paper. Available at: www.IHI.org. Accessed November 3, 2009.
14. Mazza F, Kitchens J, Kerr S, et al. Eliminating birth trauma at Ascension Health. Jt Comm J Qual Patient Saf 2007;33(1):15–24.
15. Macones GA, Hankins GD, Spong CY, et al. The 2008 National Institute of Child Health and Human Development workshop report on electronic fetal monitoring: update on definitions, interpretation, and research guidelines. Obstet Gynecol 2008;112(3):661–6.
16. Ecker J, Frigoletto F. Primary caesarean rate of vaginal birth after previous caesarean delivery (VBAC) in the US, 1989–2004, and total caesarean rate, 1989–2005. N Engl J Med 2007;356:885–8.
17. Leung WC, Chan BC, Ma G, et al. Continued reduction in the incidence of birth trauma and birth asphyxia related to instrumental deliveries after the study period: was this the Hawthorne effect? Eur J Obstet Gynecol Reprod Biol 2007;130:165–8.
18. Lewis DF, McCann J, Wang Y, et al. Hospitalized late preterm mild preeclamptic patients with mature lung testing: what are the risks of delivery? J Perinatol 2009; 29:413–5.

Delivery Room Intervention: Improving the Outcome

Wade D. Rich, RRT, CCRC[a], Tina Leone, MD[a], Neil N. Finer, MD[b,*]

KEYWORDS

• Video review • Neonatal resuscitation • Delivery room

Although most infants pass through the delivery room (DR) with little more than a quick drying and a physical examination, more complex neonatal resuscitation remains a frequently practiced and critically important intervention. Currently it is estimated that more than 400,000 infants in the United States each year require some assistance in the DR, and that intensive resuscitation is required in 1% of all deliveries. A 2001 survey[1] suggested that 10.6% of infants required bag and mask ventilation at birth.

Although there have been several important single-center studies describing physiologic responses to resuscitation, there are still few prospective randomized trials that evaluate these interventions. Establishing good baseline data through unbiased observation, and measuring outcomes based on monitored data, will allow these types of studies to be performed in the future.

MEASUREMENT OF INTERVENTION AND OUTCOMES

Video Recording

We initiated a quality improvement program in 1999 and began to video record neonatal resuscitations in our dedicated resuscitation suite and 1 additional obstetric operating room.[2] Our ongoing quality improvement program involving the video and analog data recording of high-risk deliveries and the subsequent review of such resuscitations,[3] and our prospective database of all neonatal intubations,[4] have allowed us to critically evaluate and modify our own practices, and the resuscitation environment.

Videotaping can be an effective training and quality assurance tool and allows the timely recognition of many systematic and procedural errors. Apart from the presence of a dedicated observer, it is the simplest method currently available for objectively

[a] Division of Neonatology, University of California San Diego, 402 Dickenson Street, Suite 1-140, San Diego, CA 92103-8774, USA

[b] Division of Neonatology, University of California San Diego Medical Center, 200 West Arbor Drive, San Diego, CA 92103-8774, USA

* Corresponding author.

E-mail address: nfiner@ucsd.edu

Clin Perinatol 37 (2010) 189–202

doi:10.1016/j.clp.2010.01.011

perinatology.theclinics.com

evaluating that the correct intervention was chosen, and that the intervention was correctly applied by individuals and teams during resuscitations. The videotape can be reviewed by many observers, avoiding or reducing individual observer bias, can be replayed for clarification, contains accurate timing information, and the verbal communication during the resuscitation is not subject to recall bias. The audio recording has proven invaluable in assessing communication during resuscitation interventions. The audio information is the basis for determining if there has been appropriate communication, with acknowledgment, and whether team members and leaders interacted constructively. If there were delays in instituting appropriate interventions, the available audio information can confirm that the team was aware of the problem and the reason for any delay. These reviews also provide current information on the capability of the personnel responding, and the need for any further educational efforts. The audio recording provides examples of individuals recognizing potential problems during the resuscitation, and the response to this information.

Physiologic Data Recordings

The addition of physiologic measurements to the video recording, including oxygen saturation, pulse rate, Fio_2, tidal volume, or end-tidal carbon dioxide, further improves the usefulness of the DR data collection.[5] Our current practice is to gather oxygen saturation, pulse rate, Fio_2, airway pressure, end-tidal carbon dioxide and audio on all recordings, with an option to collect an electrocardiogram (EKG) using the BioPac data acquisition and Acqknowledge 4.0 software (Biopac Systems Inc, Goleta, CA). This information is collected any time the wired resuscitation bed is used, whether or not a video recording is obtained. All data are collected at 30 Hz, except for EKG, which is collected at 60 Hz. Analysis includes maximum and minimum values for peak inspiratory pressure (PIP) and positive end-expiratory pressure (PEEP), respiratory and heart rates, and an oxygen saturation histogram. We are now able to evaluate significant detail about the actual interventions, and determine whether they were appropriate and were performed correctly (ie, an increase in Fio_2, or an increase in the inspiratory pressure for a bag and mask or intubated breath).

We have frequently found that the medical record documentation of a resuscitation varies considerably from the actual interventions seen on video, including the recording of the number and duration of intubation attempts, the duration of positive pressure breaths, or continuous positive airway pressure (CPAP), and, on occasion, even the failure to mention the use of chest compressions.

Recently, we observed an unintended increase in CPAP/PEEP during a resuscitation (**Fig. 1**). We believed that this occurred through the inadvertent twisting of the CPAP dial on the T-piece. Without these recordings we would have been unaware of this situation. We immediately provided education to all caretakers to monitor the PEEP/CPAP levels during resuscitation and be aware that such changes were possible, with potentially dire consequences.

There are other parameters that should be more continuously monitored in the minutes following birth and these include the infant's temperature, measures of tissue oxygenation, and, perhaps, blood pressure. There is a need to evaluate newer techniques to provide such information to the resuscitation teams during this critical period.

TEAM AND LEADERS

The Team

When evaluating team function, 2 distinct outcomes should be measured. These include evaluating whether the intervention was the correct one, and whether the

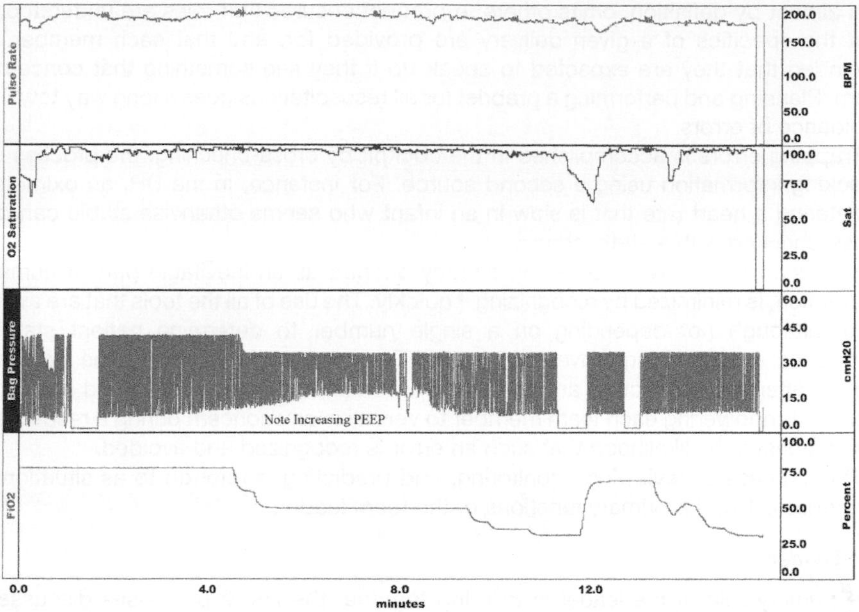

Fig. 1. Data recording of DR intervention. Note inadvertent increase in PEEP as seen on third channel (airway pressure).

intervention was performed correctly. Initial video review of resuscitations at the University of California San Diego Medical Center revealed several problems in the conduct of the resuscitation involving the team, the leader, or both. These problems included more than 1 person doing a single task; other tasks that were not performed at all, such as providing a continuous communication of the infant's heart rate; the lack of the provision of blow-by oxygen or cricoid pressure during intubation; and poorly coordinated or completely uncoordinated compressions and ventilation.

The ideal qualities and functions for the team and its leader were developed using the observations of Cooper and Wakelam.[6] These qualities and functions included adequate preparation, having resuscitation team members who were adaptable, and who coordinated their activities and interventions using acknowledged clear and concise communication, under the direction of a calm and knowledgeable leader.[3] Clear and acknowledged communication is the most basic vital function of a good team, and is the 1 function that fails most frequently. Crew resource management (CRM) is a methodology developed for the training of aircrews during the late 1970s that evolved from a careful evaluation of the role of human error in air crashes.[7] CRM is the basis for much of the team and leader training used in various medical areas. including the operating room, the emergency room, and the DR in our institution. Robert Helmreich, 1 of the original designers of the process, describes the fifth generation of CRM, established in 1997, as an error management tool with 3 fundamental countermeasures.[8] These countermeasures are avoidance, trapping, and mitigation. The use of CRM fundamentals in the DR environment to manage errors and improve outcomes can and should include all of these measures.

Avoiding errors requires some system of pre-event communication, based on an established procedure. Knowing what each team member is supposed to do while in the DR, and providing consistent training to ensure that they know how to perform each of those tasks, eliminates errors such as multiple individuals performing 1 task, and almost by definition, omits others. A prebrief ensures that roles are understood, that the specifics of a given delivery are provided for, and that each member is reminded that they are expected to speak up if they see something that concerns them. Planning and performing a prebrief for all resuscitations goes a long way toward avoidance of errors.

Trapping errors is accomplished in the cockpit by cross-checking, the process of checking information using a second source. For instance, in the DR, an oximeter registering a heart rate that is slow in an infant who seems otherwise stable can be cross-checked with a stethoscope.

Mitigation occurs when an error, already defined as an inevitable part of human interaction, is minimized by recognizing it quickly. The use of all the tools that are available, although not depending on a single number to determine patient status, decreases errors and improves outcomes. Every team member sees the process from a different perspective, and their information should be acknowledged and processed. Empowering each team member to verbalize any concern during a resuscitation increases the likelihood that such an error is recognized and avoided.

This process of reviewing, monitoring, and predicting is referred to as situational awareness, 1 of the primary functions of the team leader.

The Leader

The primary role of the leader is to bring together the first 2 processes discussed earlier, making sure that the correct interventions are chosen and that they are performed correctly. To accomplish these goals, the leader must have what is referred to in CRM as situational awareness, the single most important function of the leader during a DR resuscitation.

If the team has chosen the wrong intervention, or someone is not skilled in a particular task, or they are too busy to carry out a particular intervention, it is up to the leader to recognize this while still maintaining an awareness of the status of the infant. This effort requires a skill called scanning, whereby the leader goes through a mental checklist of critical processes. This list includes checking environmental factors such as bed temperature, technical problems such as not properly assessing heart rate, and communication issues such as not repeating back orders, all while assessing the status of the infant, predicting the future course, and determining the appropriate next step. (We have found that some are uncomfortable with the term orders, as it denotes a military type of rule, but it is simply the best term for a call for a specific action at a specific time.) Scanning should take place every minute to ensure that no errors of omission or commission go unnoticed for a significant period of time.

Communication is the primary framework of CRM and of resuscitation leadership also. A good leader has the ability to provide commands clearly and succinctly, while encouraging and integrating the suggestions of other team members. Our scoring looks for orders that are relayed to a specific person, not the group ("Mary, get me some Epi", not "Get me some Epi"), and that are acknowledged.

Errors that lead to less than optimal outcomes can also occur if everyone at the resuscitation does not believe that they are empowered to stop them. A prebrief should include a specific statement, to be read every time, that encourages everyone that if they see something they are not comfortable with, they should communicate it to the leader. A good team and leader will ensure that once the appropriate interventions are established, they are performed in such a way as to truly decrease errors and improve outcomes.

In a trial incorporated into the advanced life support provider course in the United Kingdom, Cooper and Wakelam[6] showed that a formal leadership program significantly improved leadership performance in the simulated environment of a training scenario. We have taken our previously validated resuscitation scoring tool[9] and added a component to measure leadership skills based on CRM fundamentals. Video review combined with specifically defined errors and acceptable deviations has been shown by Oakley and colleagues[10] to be better than chart review in recognizing management and leadership errors, although less effective in recognizing items like dosing errors that are not easily visualized. This group also noted that the absolute number of management errors was high in their trial because of the nature of video review and its superiority to clinician memory. The most effective way to use a scoring tool during resuscitation is to combine it with a video review.

The leadership skills incorporated into our tool include prebriefing, maintaining situational awareness, reinforcing good communication, empowering team members, and conducting a debrief. The prebrief is simply scored as having occurred or not having occurred. The checklist forces each team member to be prepared and review their own functions during the upcoming resuscitation, and provides a time for questions. For example, a team that has discussed the need for a bag to protect an infant with a gastroschisis is more likely to have one available and use it.

The postbrief is meant to allow for a review, and it is purposefully kept simple, asking 3 questions: "What did we do well?"; "What could we do better?"; and "How could we do it better?"

During the video review, there is another opportunity for a postbrief, and the benefit of this review is that many more individuals can participate and learn from a single team's experience.

Resuscitation Environment

An infant who receives care in a neonatal intensive care unit (NICU) is placed in an environment that provides servo-controlled temperature regulation, continuously monitored vital signs, and oxygen saturation. Supplemental oxygen is provided with a heated, humidified, blended gas source, and positive pressure ventilation is provided by sophisticated devices that provide for consistent, well-monitored ventilation. Historically, however, during the first few critical moments of the same infant's life, the infant may be cared for in a part of a room designed for the delivery and the mother, with less attention to the needs of the resuscitation team and the infant. The heart rate might be determined by palpation or auscultation, and oxygenation was often assessed from the infant's color, a method that has been shown to be ineffective.[11] The bed was most likely an NICU castoff. Ventilation, if required, was provided using a manual device without heat or humidification, which may or may not have adequately controlled the level of PEEP. These differences in environment and management in the crucial first minutes of life seem paradoxic and irrational, and are not based on any controlled outcome data. In addition, in our experience infants with extremely low birth weight (ELBW) stay in the DR following delivery for 22.5 ± 9 minutes, consistent with earlier observations.[12,13] As pointed out by Vento and colleagues[14] high-risk deliveries should be performed in perinatal centers with adequate staffing, in an environmentally appropriate room specifically designed to evaluate and treat newborn infants.

Temperature Support

The accepted standard for preterm infants and nonasphyxiated term infants is an environment that provides for minimal heat loss and optimal metabolic oxygen consumption. These requirements are especially important for infants with ELBW because of their increased surface area to body weight ratio, their immature skin without a well-defined stratum corneum or covering vernix, their lack of subcutaneous tissue, and their poor vasomotor control, all of which can lead to hypothermia following delivery. The International Standard for Infant Warmers (IEC 60601-2-21) requires that a radiant warmer should cut power and sound an alarm if the total output has been higher than 10 mW/cm^2 for more than 15 minutes. As all current warmers are greater than this on 100% power, during prolonged and difficult resuscitations they will reduce heat output to meet this standard. We strongly suggest that servo probes are an essential part of the resuscitation process and can decrease hypothermia and hyperthermia, both of which can be harmful to the neonate. A team member must monitor the heat output if a servo probe is not applied to ensure that the sickest and smallest infants who spend the most time in the DR are protected from hypothermia and hyperthermia.

The use of some type of occlusive wrap has become standard in infants of less than 28 weeks' gestation. The EPICure study found that 36% of infants of 24 and 25 weeks' gestation had NICU admission temperatures less than 35°C.[15] Vohra and colleagues[16] showed that a polyethylene occlusive wrap in preterm infants is associated with a significant increase in mean admission temperature (1.9°C, $P<.001$) and survival ($P = .04$). The improvement in admission temperature has been a consistent finding in multiple studies.[17] Other methods of maintaining temperature (mattress pads[18] and Kangaroo care[19]) also have a positive effect on admission temperature, with skin-to-skin also providing improved bonding between mother and child. The use of hats to maintain temperature has mixed results depending on the material used.[20]

It is probably most sensible to use some combination of these practices in conjunction with skin-temperature probes and servo control of radiant-warmer output to avoid hyperthermia and a drop in the heater output when in full-power manual mode for more than 15 minutes. An increase in the DR temperature also facilitates the maintenance of adequate core temperatures in the infant with ELBW. Admission temperatures that are in the hypothermic range have been associated with increased risk for mortality and late-onset sepsis.[21] Therefore, every effort should be made to keep the preterm infant's temperature within normal limits during resuscitation and transport.

The routine use of servo-controlled infant temperature probes, plastic wrap, and chemical warmers for infants with ELBW, maintenance of an adequate room temperature (we use 85°F), and frequent monitoring of the infant's temperature by the team (every 5 minutes) decrease the incidence of hypothermic and hyperthermic NICU admissions.

Pulse Oximetry

The use of pulse oximetry has been included as a tool in the current textbook of the neonatal resuscitation program, but there is no evidence-based recommendation regarding its use. We instituted the use of pulse oximeters (POs) during resuscitation to provide continuous heart rate and a quantitative determination of oxygenation, 2 of our previously established requirements for a well-controlled resuscitation. In reviewing resuscitations, we found that the current recommendation of intermittent heart rate checks using a stethoscope or cord palpation was inadequate for infants receiving advanced resuscitation and that having a team member assigned to indicate continuous heart rate visually was more helpful in assessing the benefit of any intervention. Oximeters can effectively fulfill this function,[22] although a useful signal is rarely available within 1 minute of birth. Our current observations seem consistent with those of Lundstom,[23] who placed a PO on the right hand of 12 infants in each of their groups of premature infants and noted that useful information was obtained at approximately 3 minutes of age. The use of shorter averaging intervals, maximal sensitivity, and POs with excellent motion artifact rejection should decrease the interval between application and function of the PO in the DR. Continuous palpation/auscultation of heart rate during resuscitation is vital to gauge the effects of resuscitation interventions, and should continue until the PO is operational.

Knowledge of the normative saturation values for infants at the time of delivery is improving. A composite of the increase in Spo_2 in infants following birth is shown in **Fig. 2**,[24] with the red dot approximating the expected fetal Spo_2 of approximately 45% to 55% [25–30] and therefore the Spo_2 immediately after a birth without complications. Targeting an Spo_2 of 70% at 4 minutes and 80% at 7 minutes represents an absolute increase of 5% per minute, and is consistent with previous observations of the increases in Spo_2 following delivery in the preterm nonresuscitated infant.

With minimal experience, it is possible to monitor oxygen saturation in the first few minutes of life. Management by color is inaccurate and inconsistent and is significantly affected by ambient light. Although it is often not functional within the first minute, the early use of the PO in the DR should be the standard for any infant requiring resuscitation.

Supplemental Oxygen

The correct delivery of oxygen requires tools that have become the standard in the NICU environment, but less so in the DR. To use a targeted oxygen strategy, a functioning oximeter as described earlier needs to be available as soon as possible after delivery, with compressed air and an oxygen blender.

There is currently no agreement about the initial or optimal oxygen concentration for resuscitating the infant with ELBW. The current neonatal resuscitation program guidelines indicate that such resuscitation or stabilization may be performed with any oxygen concentration and that a PO should be applied and blenders must be available to facilitate the optimal Spo_2 values during resuscitation. Accumulating evidence in term infants suggests that the initial use of 21% versus 100% oxygen for resuscitation is associated with a significant lowering of mortality.[31,32]

The optimal oxygen saturation values and associated Fio_2 levels for the resuscitation, stabilization, and ongoing care of very preterm infants remain undefined. There have now been multiple small prospective randomized trials comparing the use of lower and higher oxygen concentrations during neonatal resuscitation in preterm infants[33–38] using some range of targeted Spo_2. The outcomes evaluated were

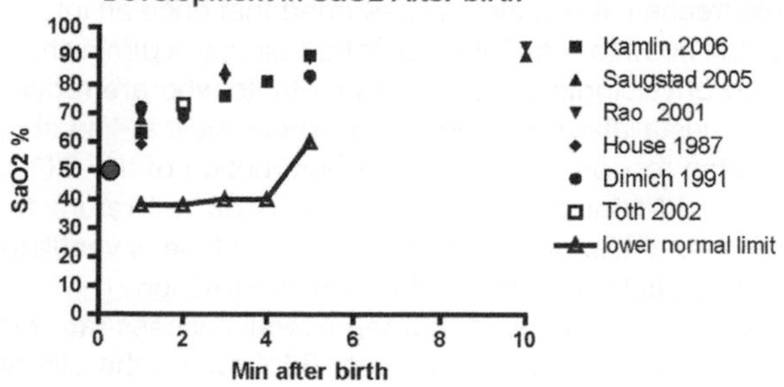

Fig. 2. A composite of the increase in Spo_2 in infants following birth. Red dot represents antenatal oxygen saturation. (*Modified from* Saugstad OD. Oxygen saturations immediately after birth. J Pediatr 2006;148(5):569–70; with permission.)

short-term effects of differing oxygen concentrations on Spo_2 changes immediately after birth. Vento and colleagues[39] reported a decrease in biparietal diameter (BPD) in their low inspired oxygen group, a benefit which has not been reproduced in the other trials. The oxygen level that yields the best long-term outcome in the preterm population has not as yet been determined in a multicenter randomized controlled trial. We use and recommend an initial Fio_2 of between 0.30 and 0.40 for such infants and then attempt to achieve an increase of Spo_2 of approximately 5% per minute to a target of 85% to 90%.[40]

Airway Maintenance

Approximately 85% to 90% of the most immature infants require assisted ventilation as part of their neonatal care. The standard approaches to provision of this support include bag and mask ventilation, followed if necessary by endotracheal intubation. A patent airway is critical during each of these maneuvers. Chest wall movement is the most common method of determining adequacy of ventilation with bag and mask. The visualization of chest rise is often difficult because of operator position, a crowded bed space, infant size, and the use of plastic wrap. The ability to recognize adequate chest rise in the infant with ELBW, a subtle finding that may be confused with abdominal rise, is difficult and requires clinician experience. Tracy and colleagues[41] have shown that hypocarbia and hyperoxia occur frequently in the intubated, ventilated preterm infant during resuscitation when chest rise is used as a marker for determining appropriate ventilatory pressures.

We have introduced the use of a colorimetric, semiquantitative, carbon dioxide detector to assist in the recognition of airway patency during bag and mask ventilation.[42] We found that more than 80% of infants with ELBW receiving bag and mask breaths have evidence of airway obstruction during the initial breaths that may persist for more than 37 breaths and more than 1 minute.[43] These obstructed breaths may often go unrecognized in the absence of a CO_2 detection device and can lead to hypoxia and bradycardia, requiring further, more aggressive, hazardous procedures, such as increased inflating pressures, compressions, or medications, if they are not rapidly recognized and relieved. Such airway obstruction may present an urgent indication for intubation if it cannot be resolved by other means.

The authors and others have shown that the placement of an endotracheal tube (ETT) in a newborn infant is associated with significant adverse physiologic effects, including bradycardia, fluctuations in blood pressure, hypoxia, and increases in intracranial pressure.[44] The most common indications for intubation in the infant with ELBW are (1) absent or inadequate respirations; (2) ineffective or prolonged bag and mask ventilation; and (3) surfactant administration. Because the ETT provides a direct path to the trachea, it is generally assumed that once an infant with no meconium is intubated, the need to monitor for a patent airway is diminished. Our review of video and recorded physiologic parameters in infants who are receiving surfactant, using either a direct-installation method or a purpose-built in-line adaptor, suggests that surfactant is often responsible for partial obstruction of the ETT. As seen in the recording in **Fig. 3**, end-tidal carbon dioxide levels do not return to baseline after administration of surfactant, suggesting a longer transit time of ventilatory gas through a smaller orifice, compatible with a partial airway obstruction.

From our video reviews we showed that the overall success rate for neonatal intubation during resuscitation was approximately 33% within the allotted 20 seconds stated in current guidelines, and 56% successful overall using a 30-second duration.[2] The authors and others have subsequently reported that the failure rate using a 30-second interval is substantially greater for infants of less than 28 weeks' gestation.[45,46]

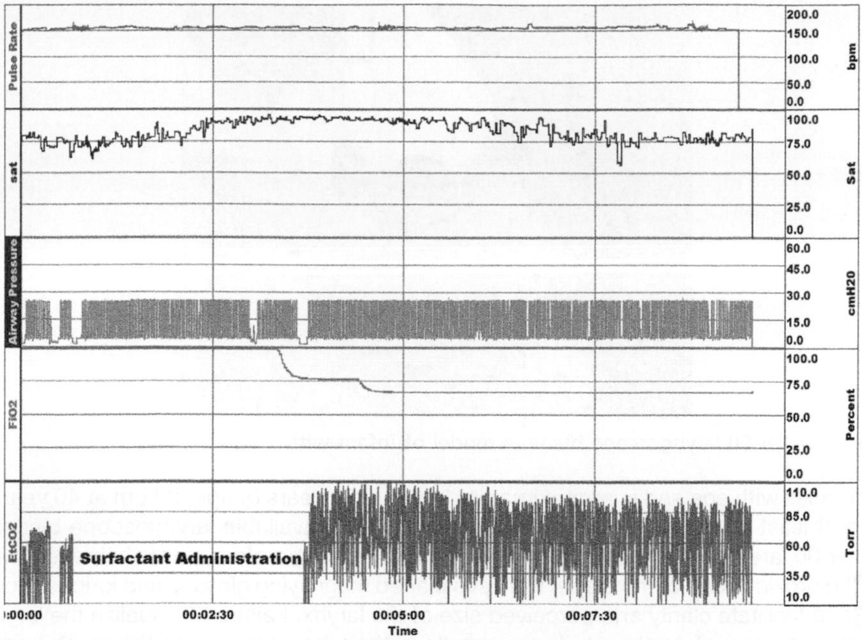

Fig. 3. Data recording during surfactant administration in DR. Note how fourth tracing (end-tidal CO_2) does not return to baseline after administration.

A detailed review of the last 5 years of this database has demonstrated that on average, at least 3 attempts are required for the successful intubation of infants of less than 1000 g birth weight.

Training

Our current practice is to provide individualized resuscitation training for all residents rotating through the NICU. An analysis of this process by Garey and colleagues[47] has shown that repeated training improved resuscitation skills. There does not, however, seem to be a clear relationship between manikin practice and successful clinical intubation skills. Our practice is also to provide feedback by way of video review for all intubations that occur during resuscitation. Although review of video provides significant detail regarding an operator's approach and skill, and increases understanding of what needs to occur, the acquisition of such a skill requires significant real world experience.[48–50] There is no substitute for experience in learning the skill of endotracheal intubation, and adequate resources need to be provided for pediatric residents to allow for mastery of this vital skill.

Current instrumentation is not designed specifically for infants with ELBW and requires manipulation of the infant to achieve adequate visualization of the larynx. The currently available laryngoscope blades, including the Miller 00, do not allow adequate visualization without excessive and often forceful cricoid pressure and change in head position (**Fig. 4**). The size and shape of current blades leave little space in the upper airway in which to insert and pass an appropriately sized ETT through the larynx while maintaining an adequate view of the larynx.

Even with conventional instrumentation, the process of intubation can be improved. The shortest distance that an individual can bring into focus without visual correction

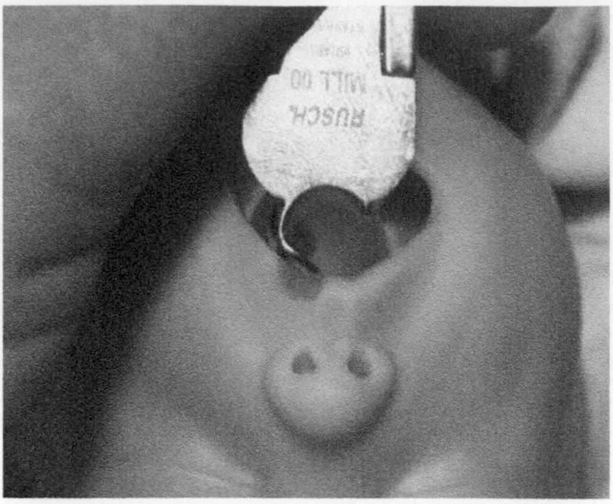

Fig. 4. Miller 00 laryngoscope blade in model of infant with ELBW.

increases with age and is approximately 14 cm at 30 years of age, 22 cm at 40 years, and at least 40 cm by 50 years of age. The smallest available laryngoscope blades, Miller 00, are approximately 6 cm in length and most operators place their eye close to the proximal end of the blade. We have placed magnifying glasses and loupes in our DRs to facilitate clarity and perceived size of the larynx. Failure to visualize the laryngeal inlet adequately almost always results in the tube passing into the much larger and posterior esophagus. Improved tools for intubation of the infant with ELBW will help ensure intubation is accomplished successfully.

T-Piece Resuscitator

The T-piece, a simple pressure-limited manual ventilation device, has gained favor in neonatal resuscitation. We previously studied the ability of our staff (including nurses, respiratory care practitioners, and physicians, including residents, fellows, and neonatologists, and neonatal nurse practitioners) to provide bag and mask ventilation using an anesthesia bag and the Neopuff (Fisher & Paykel, Laguna Hills, CA, USA).[51] The participants were asked to use a specific pressure and rate algorithm. The PIP and PEEP were significantly different between operators using the 2 manual bagging devices, but all operators could generate the target PEEP with the Neopuff ($P<.001$). The PIP was similar for all groups using the Neopuff device.

We also observed that more than 61% of breaths delivered by an anesthesia device failed to stay more than 3 cm of PEEP, whereas 31% failed to reach the prescribed PIP. Oddie and colleagues[52] reported similar results in a preliminary publication comparing 3 devices, 1 of which was a T-piece. They noted that for 15 of 25 studies the operators using a 240-mL bag exceeded the peak target pressure, and that prolonged inflations could be delivered with a T-piece. The use of a device that provides consistent target pressures regardless of the skill level of the operator has the potential to decrease barotrauma and improve pulmonary outcomes. Insuring that the intervention is performed properly requires operator awareness of potential drawbacks like difficulty in increasing pressures and the administration of inadvertently increased CPAP levels.

Outcome Measures

This article focuses on interventions that can improve the outcome of infants resuscitated in the DR. Gestational age and birth weight at delivery are the most important predictors of survival in extremely premature infants. Many additional modifying factors have now been recognized, however, that contribute to the risk of mortality and morbidity for this population, including race, gender, multiple gestation, antenatal steroids, Apgar scores, institutional experience, and illness severity scores.[53,54]

Several outcome measures can be collected early, for example admission blood gases, ideal $Paco_2$, admission temperature, and the need for intubation or surfactant. To power prospective studies using these measures, it is necessary to determine the current baseline data for different populations in the DR. We have reviewed the DR interventions and admission status of 193 infants with ELBW in a single institution between 2001 and 2006.[13] Male sex, prolonged premature rupture of membranes, lack of exposure to prenatal steroids, and an initial blood gas with low pH or high lactate levels were found to be significant independent predictors of early death and severe intraventricular hemorrhage. Mean admission values for temperature, oxygen saturation, and Pco_2 on the first blood gas were 36.4°, 95%, and 66.8 torr, respectively. Larger trials relating DR interventions to short-term outcomes are necessary.

Establishing which DR interventions result in the best outcomes requires planning, teamwork, leadership, and continued analysis by large multicenter randomized trials with adequate power to mitigate the many variables that stand between the initial intervention and the final outcome.

REFERENCES

1. Singhal N, McMillan DD, Yee WH, et al. Evaluation of the effectiveness of the standardized neonatal resuscitation program. J Perinatol 2001;21:388–92.
2. Carbine DN, Finer NN, Knodel E, et al. Video recording as a means of evaluating neonatal resuscitation performance. Pediatrics 2000;106(4):654–8.
3. Finer NN, Rich W. Neonatal resuscitation: toward improved performance. Resuscitation 2002;53(1):47–51.
4. Leone TA, Rich W, Finer NN. Neonatal intubation: success of pediatric trainees. J Pediatr 2005;146(5):638–41.
5. Schmölzer GM, Kamlin OF, Dawson JA, et al. Respiratory monitoring of neonatal resuscitation. Arch Dis Child Fetal Neonatal Ed 2009. [Epub ahead of print].
6. Cooper S, Wakelam A. Leadership of resuscitation teams: 'Lighthouse Leadership'. Resuscitation 1999;42(1):27–45.
7. Cooper GE, White MD, Lauber JK. Resource management on the flightdeck: Proceedings of a NASA/Industry Workshop. (NASA CP-2120). Moffett Field, CA: NASA-Ames Research Center; 1980.
8. Helmreich R, Merritt A, John A. The evolution of Crew Resource Management training in commercial aviation. Int J Aviat Psychol 1999;9(1):19–32.
9. Lockyer J, Singhal N, Fidler H, et al. The development and testing of a performance checklist to assess neonatal resuscitation megacode skill. Pediatrics 2006;118:e1739–44.
10. Oakley E, Stocker S, Staubli G, et al. Using video recording to identify management errors in pediatric trauma resuscitation. Pediatrics 2006;117:658–64.
11. O'Donnell CP, Kamlin CO, Davis PG, et al. Clinical assessment of infant colour at delivery. Arch Dis Child Fetal Neonatal Ed 2007;92(6):F465–7.
12. Du JN, Oliver TK. The baby in the delivery room: a suitable microenvironment. JAMA 1969;207:1502–4.

13. Kimball A, Leone TA, Vaucher Y, et al. Admission status of extremely low birth weight (ELBW) infants over the last five years [abstract]. E-PAS 2007:617932.
14. Vento M, Aguar M, Leone TA, et al. Using intensive care technology in the delivery room: a new concept for the resuscitation of extremely preterm neonates. Pediatrics 2008;122(5):1113–6.
15. Costeloe K, Hennessy E, Gibson AT, et al. The EPICure Study: outcomes to discharge from hospital for infants born at the threshold of viability. Pediatrics 2000;106:659–71.
16. Vohra S, Frent G, Campbell V, et al. Effect of polyethylene occlusive skin wrapping on heat loss in very low birthweight infants at delivery; a randomized trial. J Pediatr 1999;134:547–51.
17. McCall EM, Alderdice FA, Halliday HL, et al. Interventions to prevent hypothermia at birth in preterm and/or low birthweight infants. Cochrane Database Syst Rev 2008;(1):CD004210.
18. Flenady VJ, Woodgate PG. Radiant warmers versus incubators for regulating body temperature in newborn infants Cochrane Database Syst Rev 4 2003;(4):CD000435. DOI:10.1002/14651858.CD000435.
19. Bergman NJ, Linley LL, Fawcus SR. Randomized controlled trial of skin-to-skin contact from birth versus conventional incubator for physiological stabilization in 1200- to 2199-gram newborns. Acta Paediatr 2004;93(6):779–85.
20. Stothers JK. Head insulation and heat loss in the newborn. Arch Dis Child 1981; 56:530–4.
21. Laptook AR, Salhab W, Bhaskar B. Neonatal Research Network. Admission temperature of low birth weight infants: predictors and associated morbidities. Pediatrics 2007;119(3):e643–9 (7):530e4.
22. Kamlin CO, Dawson JA, O'Donnell CP, et al. Accuracy of pulse oximetry measurement of heart rate of newborn infants in the delivery room. J Pediatr 2008;152(6):756–60.
23. Lundstrom KE, Pryds O, Greisen G. Oxygen at birth and prolonged cerebral vasoconstriction in preterm infants. Arch Dis Child Fetal Neonatal Ed 1995; 72(2):F81–6.
24. Saugstad OD. Oxygen saturations immediately after birth. J Pediatr 2006;148(5): 569–70.
25. LeszczynskaGorzelak B, PoniedzialekCzajkowska E, Oleszczuk J. Fetal blood saturation during the 1st and 2nd stage of labor and its relation to the neonatal outcome. Gynecol Obstet Invest 2002;54(3):159–63.
26. Saugstad OD, Ramji S, Rootwelt T, et al. Response to resuscitation of the newborn: early prognostic variables. Acta Paediatr 2005;94(7):890–5.
27. Kamlin COF, ODonnell CPF, Davis PG, et al. Oxygen saturation in healthy infants immediately after birth. J Pediatr 2006;148(5):585–9.
28. Rao J, Yax S, Rao S. The role of oximetry in the first 10 minutes of age after birth [abstract]. E-PAS 2005:3425.
29. House JT, Schultetus RR, Gravenstein N. Continuous neonatal evaluation in the delivery room by pulse oximetry. J Clin Monit 1987;3(2):96–100.
30. Toth B, Becker A, Seelbach-Gobel B. Oxygen saturation in healthy newborn infants immediately after birth measured by pulse oximetry. Arch Gynecol Obstet 2002;266(2):105–7.
31. Saugstad OD, Ramji S, Vento M. Resuscitation of depressed newborn infants with ambient air or pure oxygen: a meta-analysis. Biol Neonate 2005;87(1):27–34.
32. Tan A, Schulze A, O'Donnell CPF, et al. Air versus oxygen for resuscitation of infants at birth Cochrane Database Syst Rev 2005;(2):CD002273.pub3. DOI:10.1002/14651858.CD002273.pub3.

33. Wang CL, Anderson C, Leone TA, et al. Resuscitation of preterm neonates by using room air or 100% oxygen. Pediatrics 2008;121:1083–9.
34. Escrig R, Arruza L, Izquierdo I, et al. Achievement of targeted saturation values in extremely low gestational age neonates resuscitated with low or high oxygen concentrations: a prospective, randomized trial. Pediatrics 2008;121:875–81.
35. Rabi Y, Nettel-Aguirre A, Singhal N. Room air versus oxygen administration during resuscitation of preterm infants (ROAR Study) [abstract]. E-PAS 2008;5127.5
36. Vento M, Moro M, Escrig R, et al. Preterm resuscitation with low oxygen causes less oxidative stress, inflammation, and chronic lung disease. Pediatrics 2009. [Epub ahead of print].
37. Harling AE, Beresford MW, Vince GS, et al. Does use of 50% oxygen at birth in preterm infants reduce lung injury? Arch Dis Child Fetal Neo Ed 2005;90:F401–5.
38. Ezaki S, Suzuki K, Kurishima C, et al. Resuscitation of preterm infants with reduced oxygen results in less oxidative stress than resuscitation with 100% oxygen. J Clin Biochem Nutr 2009;44(1):111–8.
39. Vento M, Moro M, Escrig R, et al. Preterm resuscitation with low oxygen causes less oxidative stress, inflammation, and chronic lung disease. Pediatrics 2009; 124(3):e439–49.
40. Finer N, Leone T. Oxygen saturation monitoring for the preterm infant: the evidence basis for current practice. Pediatr Res 2009;65(4):375–80.
41. Tracy M, Downe L, Holberton J. How safe is intermittent positive pressure ventilation in preterm babies ventilated from delivery to newborn intensive care unit? Arch Dis Child Fetal Neonatal Ed 2004;89(1):F84–7.
42. Leone TA, Lange A, Rich W, et al. Disposable colorimetric carbon dioxide detector use as an indicator of a patent airway during noninvasive mask ventilation. Pediatrics 2006;118(1):e202–4.
43. Finer NN, Rich W, Wang C, et al. Airway obstruction during mask ventilation of very low birth weight infants during neonatal resuscitation. Pediatrics 2009; 123(3):865–9.
44. Kelly MA, Finer NN. Nasotracheal intubation in the neonate: physiologic responses and effects of atropine and pancuronium. J Pediatr 1984;105(2): 303–9.
45. Lane B, Finer N, Rich W. Duration of intubation attempts during neonatal resuscitation. J Pediatr 2004;145(1):67–70.
46. O'Donnell CP, Kamlin CO, Davis PG, et al. Endotracheal intubation attempts during neonatal resuscitation: success rates, duration, and adverse effects. Pediatrics 2006;117(1):e16–21.
47. Garey D, Rich W, Leone T, et al. Supplemental training to improve neonatal resuscitation skills in pediatric residents [abstract]. E-PAS 2009:4322.48.
48. de Oliveira Filho GR. The construction of learning curves for basic skills in anesthetic procedures: an application of the cumulative sum method. Anesth Analg 2002;95:411–6.
49. Mulcaster JT, Mills J, Hung OR, et al. Laryngoscopic intubation: learning and performance. Anesthesiology 2003;98:23–7.
50. Konrad C, Schüpfer G, Wietlisbach M, et al. Learning manual skills in anesthesiology: is there a recommended number of cases for anesthetic procedures? Anesth Analg 1998;86:635–9.
51. Finer N, Rich W, Craft A. Comparison of methods of bag and mask ventilation for neonatal resuscitation. Resuscitation 2001;49(3):299–305.

52. Oddie SJ, Wyllie JP, Matthews J. Lung inflation in neonatal resuscitation; what device should we use? Pediatr Res 2003;53(4):498A.
53. Shankaran S, Fanaroff AA, Wright LL, et al. Risk factors for early death among extremely low-birth-weight infants. Am J Obstet Gynecol 2002;186(4):796–802.
54. Pollack MM, Koch MA, Bartel DA, et al. A comparison of neonatal mortality risk prediction models in very low birth weight infants. Pediatrics 2000;105(5):1051–7.

Comprehensive Oxygen Management for the Prevention of Retinopathy of Prematurity: The Pediatrix Experience

Dan L. Ellsbury, MD*, Robert Ursprung, MD, MMSc

KEYWORDS

- Comprehensive Oxygen Management • Quality improvement
- Retinopathy of prematurity • Very low birth weight infants

In 2003, Chow and coworkers[1] described a striking reduction in retinopathy of prematurity (ROP) after implementation of a structured oxygen management protocol, focused on avoiding hyperoxia and repeated episodes of hypoxia-hyperoxia in very low birth weight infants. This publication generated much interest and discussion in the neonatology community including practices within Pediatrix Medical Group. Some Pediatrix Physician Groups adopted the general approach proposed by Chow and coworkers[1] with similar results,[2–4] as did a number of centers outside of Pediatrix.[5–7] Within Pediatrix Medical Group, discussions continued by intranet discussion forums and presentations at Pediatrix quality improvement conferences. In 2006, the basic principles of avoiding hyperoxia and repeated episodes of hypoxia-hyperoxia were expanded into a Pediatrix quality improvement initiative called "Comprehensive Oxygen Management for the Prevention of Retinopathy of Prematurity" (COMP-ROP).

COMP-ROP was enthusiastically received. Eighty neonatal intensive care units (NICU) formally participated in the initiative, with many more informally participating. The COMP-ROP Collaborative was loosely structured. NICUs were provided with a toolkit containing a basic description of the oxygen management process and multiple tools to facilitate rapid adaptation and implementation of the program within their centers.

Because of the uncertainties and controversies surrounding the definition of "optimal oxygen saturation" in extremely premature infants, rigid oxygen saturation

The Center for Research, Education, and Quality, Pediatrix Medical Group, 1301 Concord Terrace, Sunrise, FL 33323, USA
* Corresponding author.
E-mail address: Dan_Ellsbury@pediatrix.com

Clin Perinatol 37 (2010) 203–215
doi:10.1016/j.clp.2010.01.012 perinatology.theclinics.com
0095-5108/10/$ – see front matter

limits were not mandated.[8,9] Emphasis was placed on NICU staff education, system-based approaches to decreasing hyperoxia, avoidance of large fluctuations in oxygen saturation, ensuring compliance with oximeter alarm use, and using oxygen saturation trending to assist and guide oxygen management efforts.

Between 2003 and 2008, a striking decrease in severe ROP (stage 3, 4, 5, or surgical) was seen in the Pediatrix Network. In infants with birth weights of 400 to 1500 g, severe ROP dropped from 11% in 2003 to 5.8% in 2008 (**Fig. 1**). During this time period, mortality rates remained stable. Necrotizing enterocolitis decreased, then increased during this time period, with 2008 rates very similar to 2003. This pattern was also seen in infants with birth weights greater than 1500 g, who were not included in COMP-ROP. Patent ductus arteriosus and patent ductus arteriosus ligation rates also fluctuated, with 2008 rates remaining similar to 2003. Oxygen use at 28 days of life and at 36 weeks postmenstrual age decreased from 2003 to 2008.

WHY WAS COMP-ROP SUCCESSFUL?

Why did this initiative succeed? Early adopters started the process after Chow and coworkers'[1] publication. The quality improvement infrastructure within Pediatrix Medical Group fostered the spread of this information, eventually formalizing the process as the COMP-ROP program. Berwick[10] describes seven guiding rules for diffusion of innovations, all of which were used in the events leading up to the COMP-ROP initiative and continued in the implementation of the program:

1. Find sound innovations: The structure of the Pediatrix system encourages, by intranet and conferences, continuous discussion and debate of new innovations found in the medical literature.
2. Find and support innovators: The ongoing communication and debate of new innovations includes discussion of the initial successes and difficulties with implementation of new ideas. Successful innovators could be identified despite the size of the network (almost 1000 physicians in 33 states, providing care for approximately 20% of infants receiving neonatal intensive care in the United States).

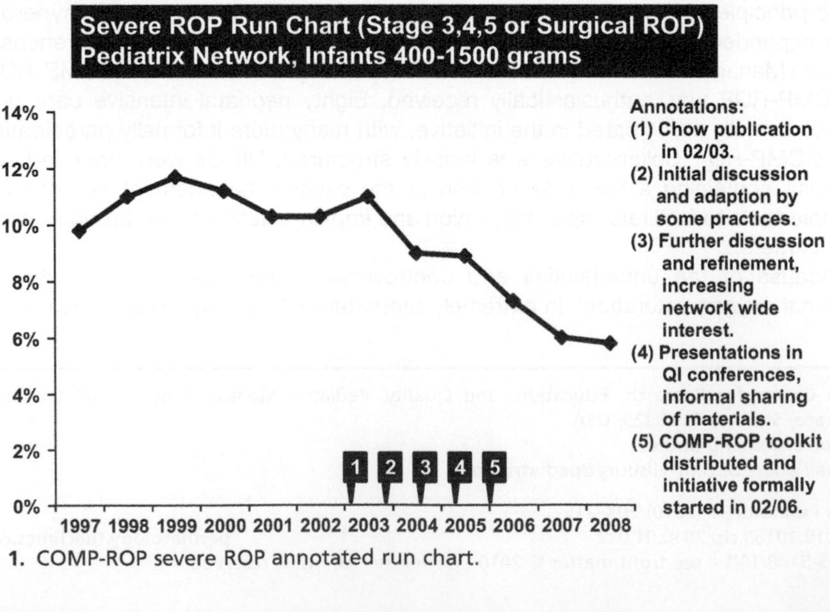

Fig. 1. COMP-ROP severe ROP annotated run chart.

3. Invest in early adopters: The early adopters were identified in these ongoing intranet discussions and quality conferences. Corporate support including mentorship, education materials, conference calls, and so forth was provided to assist these early adopters in effectively implementing the COMP-ROP program.
4. Make early adopter activity observable: The COMP-ROP program was encouraged and promoted by corporate staff in a variety of settings. Although participation was encouraged, it was not mandated.
5. Trust and enable reinvention: As the program was implemented, objections to some components of the program were raised. Elements that were completely acceptable in one center were not accepted in others. All participating centers were encouraged to adapt the program to fit the culture and workflow of their centers.
6. Create slack for change: Center participation was valued at the corporate level and viewed as an important contribution to the practice and the patients. Quality improvement activity was considered a vital part of the practice, not an extracurricular activity.
7. Lead by example: Leaders of the COMP-ROP program were practicing neonatologists who shared their ongoing successes and difficulties with implementation in their own centers.

THE COMP-ROP PROGRAM

This article describes the components of the COMP-ROP toolkit and lessons learned from its dissemination within the Pediatrix network. The toolkit was provided to all Pediatrix practices in electronic format. Educational presentations, sample order sets, bedside signs, surveys to assess knowledge gaps, and other materials were provided. Local adaptation and modification of the materials was encouraged to facilitate acceptance and use in a variety of NICU settings.

Basic Principles

The guiding principles of the COMP-ROP program included the following: (1) the avoidance of hyperoxia and repeated episodes of hypoxia-hyperoxia is associated with reduced incidence of ROP; (2) systems should be redesigned to minimize or eliminate practices that result in periods of hyperoxia; (3) NICU staff should be educated regarding the risks and benefits of supplemental oxygen administration in premature infants, including the limitations of pulse oximetry in detecting hyperoxia; and (4) auditing compliance with oximeter alarm settings, and the percentage of time patients spend below, within, and above the targeted oxygen saturation parameters, should be used to provide short-term feedback on the success of oxygen management practices.

Program Structure

The program was structured to assess baseline ROP outcomes, oxygen management practices, and staff beliefs concerning ROP pathophysiology. Further, the program provided basic instruction in team building, multidisciplinary NICU staff education, and facilitated system-based changes designed to optimize oxygen management. After implementation, periodic review of process, outcome, and balancing measures was followed to assess the impact of COMP-ROP (**Fig. 2**).

The Multidisciplinary COMP-ROP Team

The COMP-ROP toolkit advocated for each unit to create a multidisciplinary ROP team. Ideally, this group would include physicians, nurses, nurse practitioners, and respiratory therapists; inclusion of leadership with the authority to make system-based

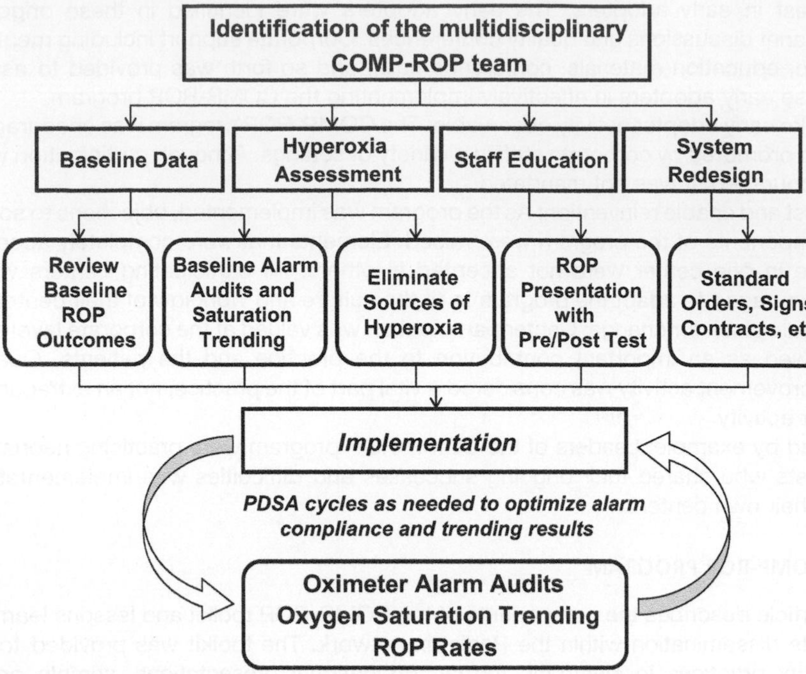

Fig. 2. Structure of the COMP-ROP program.

changes was encouraged. Emphasis was placed on including individuals from different work shifts (days, nights, weekend shifts). Additionally, it was emphasized that COMP-ROP was not a clinical trial or research project, and that the program was meant as a starting point, with adaptation to each center's culture and work flow provided by each project team. Review by an institutional review committee or hospital quality improvement committee was governed by each center's guidelines and regulations for quality improvement activities.

Baseline Data Collection

Certain baseline data were obtained, including ROP outcomes, and several measures of oxygen and oximetry use. These measures were followed throughout the project.

ROP outcomes

ROP data were available through the Pediatrix Clinical Data Warehouse (discussed elsewhere in this issue). The reports provided data on clinical outcomes and certain process measures related to ROP and could be stratified by birth weight, gestational age, NICU patient volume, and inborn-outborn status.

Baseline oximeter alarm audits

A sample oximeter alarm audit tool (**Fig. 3**) was provided to facilitate collection of oximeter alarm settings by bedside audits. The experience was that many centers had poor compliance in setting oximeter alarms in a fashion to minimize exposure to hyperoxic environments. Many centers had no process to consistently order oximeter alarm settings in the population at risk for ROP. Further, many oximeters have a factory

Pulse Oximetry Alarm Audit Tool

Please review the oximeter alarm settings and mark "correct" if they are set appropriately, and "incorrect" if not, according to:

- **the standard oximeter alarm setting orders, OR**
- **a specific order in the chart**

Determine reasons for non-compliance when they occur, and address these as indicated, especially system issues

- **use episodes of non-compliance as educational opportunities**

The overall percent correct should be recorded on a spreadsheet (use the oximeter alarm audit run chart, in excel)

Patient	1	2	3	4	5	6	7	8	9	10
Correct										
Incorrect										

Fig. 3. Sample oximeter alarm compliance audit tool.

default high-saturation alarm setting of 100%. If this default setting is not noticed and altered, infants receiving supplemental oxygen are at risk for excess time in a hyperoxic environment.

Baseline oxygen saturation trend audits

This audit was designed to provide an estimate of the amount of time an infant spent at various oxygen saturations, with emphasis on the proportion of time the oxygen saturation is greater than 95% and the general distribution of saturation values, both high and low. Ongoing measurement of saturation trends was suggested as an important ongoing process measure. Four methods were suggested, discussed next.

Flow-sheet review Nursing or respiratory therapy flow-sheets typically capture oxygen saturations levels. Although flow sheets may provide a general sense of oxygen saturation trends, they are of limited use because of the small number of data points and the potential bias of the documenter; the provider may choose to document the "best" number over the last hour, not the "most representative."

Monitor trend review Many bedside monitors have features that allow trending of vital sign data. Capabilities among monitors vary; however, many machines allow the data of the time spent at various oxygen saturations to be presented graphically, downloaded to a computer, or printed. Rapid feedback of oximetry trends to front-line providers is a powerful behavior change agent.

Peak Po_2 in the first 24 hours As a supplement to the previously mentioned techniques, the Po_2 trend, as determined by arterial blood gases, can be reviewed from the medical record. This observation is limited to babies with arterial catheters, but may be useful for some babies in the first days of life.

Saturation level and oximeter alarm random spot checks This supplementary technique involves simply walking to the bedsides of infants at risk for ROP at a random time and auditing the oxygen saturation, the fraction of inspired oxygen (F_{IO_2}), and the oximeter alarm settings to determine if they are appropriate at that point in time. This "spot check," although not precise, is an additional method to determine general compliance with the desired oxygen management strategies. This technique can be informally used during clinical rounds as part of a random safety audit program.[11]

Hyperoxia Assessment

A hyperoxia assessment survey was provided to enable teams to review the manner in which oxygen is used in their unit. This survey facilitated identification of common sources of hyperoxia, including equipment and practice style issues. Once identified, system reengineering and focused education efforts could address sources of hyperoxic exposure.

Common problem areas include use of unblended (100%) oxygen; use of high oxygen concentrations during routine procedures and handling; overtitration of oxygen in response to alarms; and therapeutic use of hyperoxia, the intentional use of high F_{IO_2} as a treatment.

Delivery room

Determine if blended oxygen is available for infants less than 32 weeks' gestational age, per the 2006 Neonatal Resuscitation Program recommendations.[12] If blended oxygen was not available in the delivery room, a simple mobile cart was suggested that included an air and oxygen tank connected to an oxygen blender.

Transport

Some NICUs historically have used 100% oxygen during both "in-house" and "out-of-house" transports. Neonatal transport incubators are commonly designed to provide blended oxygen. If not, most systems can be adapted to include an air tank and an oxygen blender. Oximetry should be used during transports to enable titration of inspired oxygen.

Nebulizers

100% oxygen is often used as the gas source for nebulizer treatments, creating a significant exposure to hyperoxia for some patients. This issue can be addressed by providing blended oxygen as the nebulizer gas source, or changing to administration by a metered dose inhaler.

Preoxygenation for procedures and cares

Because some infants desaturate when exposed to noxious stimulation (eg, suctioning, heelsticks, diaper changes, and so forth), providers may prophylactically increase the F_{IO_2} to "preoxygenate" the infant. This practice may result in hyperoxia, especially if large increases in oxygen concentration are given. This problem can be addressed by education and modification of nursing protocols focused on minimizing this practice, and using only small incremental increases F_{IO_2} when indicated.

Treatment of apnea

Infants at risk for ROP often desaturate when apneic. Although stimulation of effective breathing typically corrects the transient hypoxia, the initial response of many providers is to increase the patient's F_{IO_2}. Not only is increasing the F_{IO_2} typically ineffective as an initial intervention, it places the infant at risk for an "overdose" of oxygen once respirations are reestablished. This problem can be addressed by education and modification of nursing protocols focused on minimizing this practice, and using only small incremental increases in F_{IO_2} when indicated.

Therapeutic use of hyperoxia

Excess oxygen is given, at times, to intentionally cause hyperoxia for a specific therapeutic purpose. Many of these practices are of little benefit, and may risk significant hyperoxic injury.

Initial transition after delivery Some believe that it is better to give extra oxygen during the first hours after delivery to "enhance transition" or "help the baby recover" from a stressful delivery. There is no evidence that supports this practice. There is evidence that this is detrimental, especially in the preterm infant.[13] This practice should be abandoned.

Pneumothorax A 100% oxygen is sometimes used as a treatment for a nontension pneumothorax ("nitrogen washout"). This practice places a preterm infant at very high risk of significant and severe hyperoxia. Conservative management is often very effective.[14,15] This practice should be abandoned.

Pulmonary hypertension (early) Oxygen is a pulmonary vasodilator and can be beneficial in the management of persistent pulmonary hypertension of the newborn. Maintaining high oxygen saturation levels (>95%) in these infants incurs a significant risk of hyperoxic injury, however, including ROP. This practice should be restricted, and alternative treatment strategies should be used as indicated. Additionally, early pulmonary hypertension should be clearly distinguished from pulmonary hypertension that develops later in the hospital stay in infants with severe bronchopulmonary dysplasia. The infant's retina may be mature in this latter circumstance, or at least past the stage of retinal development where higher oxygen saturations might be detrimental.[16,17]

Staff ROP Education

A major component of COMP-ROP is the educational program. Most health care providers want to provide high-quality clinical care. It was observed that many providers including physicians, nurses, and respiratory therapists had knowledge gaps concerning the pathophysiology of ROP, the physiologic impact of oxygen management practices, and the principles of oximetry. Further, NICU nursing staff and respiratory therapy staff commonly had the foundation of their training in adult medicine, providing a basic knowledge set about the risks and benefits of oxygen that is not fully applicable to premature infants. Oxygen was commonly perceived as a "safe drug" and high oxygen levels were thought to be physiologically beneficial.

The educational program consisted of a premade slide set that discussed the pathophysiology of ROP, risks and benefits of oxygen use in premature infants, and the limitations of pulse oximetry. The educational program also included a discussion of the targeted oxygen management practices described by Chow and coworkers[1] (avoiding hyperoxia and repeated episodes of hypoxia-hyperoxia).

A brief pretest and posttest was provided to determine if adequate knowledge transfer occurred with the educational program, with remedial action if gaps remained. It was suggested to centers that the educational program should be considered mandatory or at least heavily recommended for all NICU staff that manage oxygen, including physicians, nurse practitioners, nurses, and respiratory therapists. The compliance rate with completing the educational program was considered one of the process measures of the project.

System Redesign

As discussed elsewhere in this issue, system reengineering is more likely to achieve sustainable improvement than telling people to "be careful" or to "try harder." The hyperoxia assessment and educational testing typically highlighted systems or processes for reengineering. To effect change in ROP outcomes, development of a structured approach to the use of oxygen and oximetry was emphasized. This process included developing standardized orders for oximeter settings and alarm limits, creating or modifying specific oxygen management nursing protocols, bedside signs, and the use of "oxygen management contracts."

Standardized oximeter alarm orders

Centers were encouraged to develop center-specific oximeter alarm limits to use for all infants at risk for ROP. Two general approaches to use of alarm limits emerged. The alarm limit approach consisted of the alarm limits being placed at the precise borders of the acceptable saturation range (eg, lower alarm at 85%, upper alarm at 93%).[18] Alternatively, other centers preferred to use a targeting approach, which used wide alarm limits, with the staff titrating the inspired oxygen to keep the saturation level within a narrower limit (eg, alarm limits at 80% and 95%, with saturations targeted at 88%–92%). It was believed by some centers that the targeting approach resulted in fewer alarm events and hence fewer opportunities to overadjust the oxygen concentration.

The specific alarm limits and the specific approach (alarm or targeting) was determined by each center. The guiding principles were to use a strategy to minimize hyperoxia by avoidance of saturation levels above 95% when receiving supplemental oxygen and avoiding large fluctuations of the oxygen saturation levels into hyperoxic and hypoxic ranges. Development of standardized orders to reflect the center's chosen approach was recommended.

Further, emphasis was given to ongoing saturation trending as an important process measure to assess the effectiveness of the system redesign and educational interventions. Oxygen management is a complex task. The target saturations and alarm limits are the proverbial tip of the iceberg in oxygen management (**Fig. 4**). As Greenspan and Goldsmith[19] very importantly and astutely observed, "Providers need to understand that cumulative oxygen saturations over time represent a bell-shaped curve, and the role of the health care team is to minimize the tails in both directions."

Default oximeter alarm limits

Many oximeters have a default high saturation alarm setting of 100%. These oximeters typically revert to this 100% default setting each time they are turned off and back on, adversely affecting compliance with the center's agreed on alarm settings. Fortunately, many oximeter default settings can be altered by hospital biomedical engineering personnel to comply with the center's desired alarm settings. This system-based intervention can dramatically increase compliance with desired alarm limits in many centers.

Nursing protocols

Commonly, nursing and respiratory therapy protocols required modifications to be consistent with the desired changes in oxygen management. These modifications commonly included specific details of responding to an oximeter alarm (eg, determine if it is real or motion artifact, observe for spontaneous recovery, assess for a loose probe, and so forth before adjusting the oxygen concentration). Guidelines were often provided on the magnitude of oxygen titration (eg, increase by 2%–5% and observe).

Bedside signs

Bedside signs were frequently used to reinforce desired oximeter alarm limits and the approach to titrating oxygen. Sample signs were provided for customization and

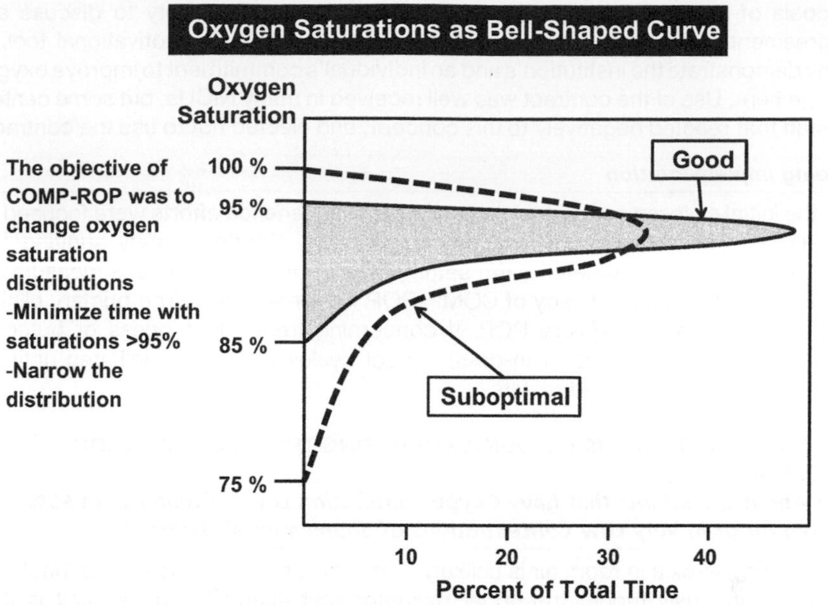

Fig. 4. Oxygen saturation trending curves. While the average oxygen saturation for each curve is similar, the wide distribution seen in the suboptimal curve should be avoided.

personalization at each center. These simple signs were often quite effective, especially in the initial stages of the program, when the oxygen management strategies were still new to the staff (**Fig. 5**).

Oxygen management contract

Chow and coworkers[1] described use of a written oxygen management agreement, or contract, that summarized the approach to oxygen and oximetry use, and was designed to be signed by all NICU staff members. The contract clarifies and reinforces

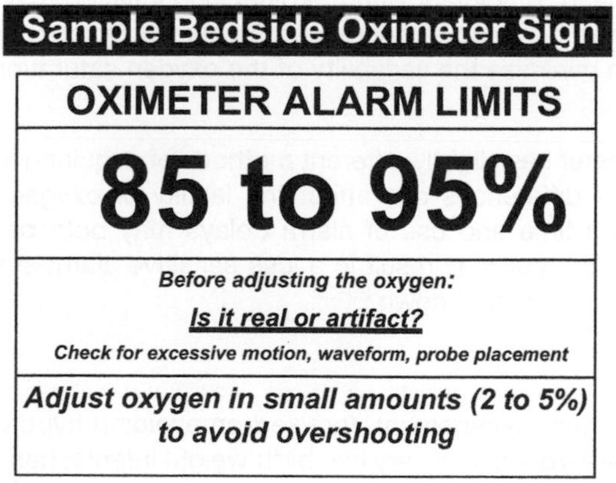

Sample Bedside Oximeter Sign
OXIMETER ALARM LIMITS
85 to 95%
Before adjusting the oxygen:
Is it real or artifact?
Check for excessive motion, waveform, probe placement
Adjust oxygen in small amounts (2 to 5%) to avoid overshooting

Fig. 5. Sample bedside oximeter alarm sign. These were typically modified to reflect the center's preferred oximeter alarm limits. Additional personalization (animals, logos, catchphrases) was often added to draw attention to the sign and reinforce oxygen management principles.

the goals of the program and provides an additional opportunity to discuss any disagreements with the practice changes. It can be used as a motivational tool, to clearly demonstrate the institution's and an individual's commitment to improve oxygen management. Use of the contract was well received in many NICUs, but some centers had staff that reacted negatively to this concept, and elected not to use the contract.

Ongoing Implementation

After the initial assessment and implementation, maintenance efforts were focused on compliance with the oxygen management guideline. Random safety auditing[11] of saturation trends and oximeter alarm settings were suggested process measures to evaluate the short-term efficacy of COMP-ROP implementation. The primary clinical outcome measure was severe ROP. If concerning trends in process or outcome measures were noted, serial plan-do-study-act cycles were to be initiated until the system provided the desired results.

QUESTIONS AND BARRIERS ENCOUNTERED DURING THE IMPLEMENTATION OF COMP-ROP

What About the Infants that have Oxygen Saturation Levels Greater than 95% in Room Air or in Very Low Concentrations of Supplemental Oxygen?

Significant hyperoxia in room air is unlikely. The difficulty in this scenario is that these infants continuously trigger the upper oximeter limit alarm; the alarm limit is then adjusted upward to prevent continuous triggering of the alarm. Unfortunately, many of these infants will require supplemental oxygen again, but the upper alarm limit (now functionally turned off) may not always be reset, creating an opportunity for hyperoxia. There is not a clear system solution to this problem.

What About Infants Whose Oxygen Saturation Level Rapidly Fluctuates and Triggers Alarms Continuously?

Respiratory issues

After ruling out common causes of artifact (eg, soiled or loose probes, motion), one should assess for airway obstruction. Malposition of the endotracheal tube, secretions, and loose taping of the endotracheal tube are common problems. Infants on continuous positive airway pressure may have nasal obstruction or malposition of the prongs or the head. Any infant with marginal lung inflation may show substantial lability in oxygenation because of decreased functional residual capacity. Attention to these issues can minimize the variability of the oxygen saturation levels.

Oximeter issues

Each brand of oximeter has slightly different methods of acquiring and sampling Spo_2 levels. These subtle differences can affect the lability of oxygen saturation levels. Increasing averaging time and use of alarm delays may both be useful in filtering out "nuisance alarms," but may result in a less sensitive alarm system. The optimal use of these techniques is not known.[20–22]

SUMMARY

Comprehensive oxygen management, focused on avoiding hyperoxia and repeated episodes of hypoxia-hyperoxia in very low birth weight infants, has been successfully used for the reduction of ROP. Building on this experience, the COMP-ROP quality improvement initiative was developed to facilitate the spread and refinement of these techniques. The initiative focused on staff education, evaluation and redesign of the processes, and practices involving oxygen use. Monitoring of the effectiveness of the system changes was supported through audits of clinical practice changes, use of oxygen saturation trending data, and the incidence of ROP.

ACKNOWLEDGMENTS

The authors thank the many neonatal nurses, respiratory therapists, and Pediatrix Medical Group clinicians that have participated in COMP-ROP. Their efforts, observations, and refinements have significantly enriched the program and are greatly appreciated.

REFERENCES

1. Chow LC, Wright KW, Sola A, et al. Can changes in clinical practice decrease the incidence of severe retinopathy of prematurity in very low birth weight infants? Pediatrics 2003;111(2):339–45.
2. Ellsbury DL. Quality improvement program for the reduction of retinopathy of prematurity [abstract]. E-PAS 2006;3602.469.
3. Ursprung R, Nedrelow J. Comprehensive oxygen management for the prevention of retinopathy of prematurity [abstract]. E-PAS 2008;634452.8.
4. Sears JE, Pietz J, Sonnie C, et al. A change in oxygen supplementation can decrease the incidence of retinopathy of prematurity. Ophthalmology 2009; 116(3):513–8.
5. Deulofeut R, Critz A, Adams-Chapman I, et al. Avoiding hyperoxia in infants. J Perinatol 2006;26(11):700–5.
6. Vanderveen DK, Mansfield TA, Eichenwald EC. Lower oxygen saturation alarm limits decrease the severity of retinopathy of prematurity. J AAPOS 2006;10(5): 445–8.
7. Wright KW, Sami D, Thompson L, et al. A physiologic reduced oxygen protocol decreases the incidence of threshold retinopathy of prematurity. Trans Am Ophthalmol Soc 2006;104:78–84.
8. Cole CH, Wright KW, Tarnow-Mordi W, et al. Pulse Oximetry Saturation Trial for Prevention of Retinopathy of Prematurity Planning Study Group. Resolving our uncertainty about oxygen therapy. Pediatrics 2003;112(6 Pt 1):1415–9.
9. Tin W, Wariyar U. Giving small babies oxygen: 50 years of uncertainty. Semin Neonatol 2002;7(5):361–7.
10. Berwick DM. Disseminating innovations in health care. JAMA 2003;289(15): 1969–75.
11. Ursprung R, Gray JE, Edwards WH, et al. Real tsime patient safety audits: improving safety every day. Qual Saf Health Care 2005;14(4):284–9.
12. American Heart Association, American Academy of Pediatrics. 2005 American Heart Association (AHA) guidelines for cardiopulmonary resuscitation (CPR) and emergency cardiovascular care (ECC) of pediatric and neonatal patients: neonatal resuscitation guidelines. Pediatrics 2006;117(5):e1029–38.
13. Saugstad OD. Optimal oxygenation at birth and in the neonatal period. Neonatology 2007;91(4):319–22.
14. Carlo WA, Martin RJ, Fanaroff AA. Assisted ventilation and complications of respiratory distress. In: Martin RJ, Fanaroff AA, Walsh MC, editors. Fanaroff and Martin's neonatal-perinatal medicine: diseases of the fetus and infant. 8th edition. St Louis (MO): Mosby Elsevier; 2006. p. 1122–45.
15. Litmanovitz I, Carlo WA. Expectant management of pneumothorax in ventilated neonates. Pediatrics 2008;122(5):e975–9.

16. Supplemental therapeutic oxygen for prethreshold retinopathy of prematurity (STOP-ROP), a randomized, controlled trial. I: primary outcomes. Pediatrics 2000;105(2):295–310.
17. McGregor ML, Bremer DL, Cole C, et al. HOPE-ROP Multicenter Group. High Oxygen Percentage in Retinopathy of Prematurity study. Retinopathy of prematurity outcome in infants with prethreshold retinopathy of prematurity and oxygen saturation >94% in room air: the high oxygen percentage in retinopathy of prematurity study. Pediatrics 2002;110(3):540–4.
18. Castillo A, Sola A, Baquero H, et al. Pulse oxygen saturation levels and arterial oxygen tension values in newborns receiving oxygen therapy in the neonatal intensive care unit: is 85% to 93% an acceptable range? Pediatrics 2008; 121(5):882–9.
19. Greenspan JS, Goldsmith JP. Oxygen therapy in preterm infants: hitting the target. Pediatrics 2006;118(4):1740–1.
20. Rheineck-Leyssius AT, Kalkman CJ. Advanced pulse oximeter signal processing technology compared to simple averaging. I. Effect on frequency of alarms in the operating room. J Clin Anesth 1999;11(3):192–5.
21. Rheineck-Leyssius AT, Kalkman CJ. Advanced pulse oximeter signal processing technology compared to simple averaging. II. Effect on frequency of alarms in the postanesthesia care unit. J Clin Anesth 1999;11(3):196–200.
22. Rheineck-Leyssius AT, Kalkman CJ. Influence of pulse oximeter settings on the frequency of alarms and detection of hypoxemia: theoretical effects of artifact rejection, alarm delay, averaging, median filtering or a lower setting of the alarm limit. J Clin Monit Comput 1998;14(3):151–6.

FURTHER READINGS

Sola A, Rogido MR, Deulofeut R. Oxygen as a neonatal health hazard: call for détente in clinical practice. Acta Paediatr 2007;96(6):801–12.

Saugstad OD. Optimal oxygenation at birth and in the neonatal period. Neonatology 2007;91(4):319–22.

Saugstad OD. Oxygen and retinopathy of prematurity. J Perinatol 2006;26(Suppl 1): S46–50.

Tin W, Gupta S. Optimum oxygen therapy in preterm babies. Arch Dis Child Fetal Neonatal Ed 2007;92(2):F143–7.

Tin W, Milligan DW, Pennefather P, et al. Pulse oximetry, severe retinopathy, and outcome at one year in babies of less than 28 weeks gestation. Arch Dis Child Fetal Neonatal Ed 2001;84(2):F106–10.

Nghiem TH, Hagadorn JI, Terrin N, et al. Nurse opinions and pulse oximeter saturation target limits for preterm infants. Pediatrics 2008;121(5):e1039–46.

Ford SP, Leick-Rude MK, Meinert KA, et al. Overcoming barriers to oxygen saturation targeting. Pediatrics 2006;118(Suppl 2):S177–86.

Goldsmith JP, Greenspan JS. Neonatal intensive care unit oxygen management: a team effort. Pediatrics 2007;119(6):1195–6.

Hagadorn JI, Furey AM, Nghiem TH, et al. AVIOx Study Group. Achieved versus intended pulse oximeter saturation in infants born less than 28 weeks' gestation: the AVIOx study. Pediatrics 2006;118(4):1574–82.

Clucas L, Doyle LW, Dawson J, et al. Compliance with alarm limits for pulse oximetry in very preterm infants. Pediatrics 2007;119(6):1056–60.

Fleck BW, McIntosh N. Pathogenesis of retinopathy of prematurity and possible preventive strategies. Early Hum Dev 2008;84(2):83–8.

Lutty GA, Chan-Ling T, Phelps DL, et al. Proceedings of the third international symposium on retinopathy of prematurity: an update on ROP from the lab to the nursery. Mol Vis 2006;12:532–80.
Gaynon MW. Rethinking STOP-ROP: is it worthwhile trying to modulate excessive VEGF levels in prethreshold ROP eyes by systemic intervention? A review of the role of oxygen, light adaptation state, and anemia in prethreshold ROP. Retina 2006;26(Suppl 7):S18–23.
Askie LM, Henderson-Smart DJ, Irwig L, et al. Oxygen-saturation targets and outcomes in extremely preterm infants. N Engl J Med 2003;349(10):959–67.
Askie LM, Henderson-Smart DJ. Restricted versus liberal oxygen exposure for preventing morbidity and mortality in preterm or low birth weight infants. Cochrane Database Syst Rev 2001;(4):CD001077.
Section on Ophthalmology American Academy of Pediatrics; American Academy of Ophthalmology; American Association for Pediatric Ophthalmology and Strabismus. Screening examination of premature infants for retinopathy of prematurity. Pediatrics 2006;117(2):572–6 [Erratum in: Pediatrics 2006;118(3):1324].
International Committee for the Classification of Retinopathy of Prematurity. The international classification of retinopathy of prematurity revisited. Arch Ophthalmol 2005;123(7):991–9.
Early Treatment For Retinopathy Of Prematurity Cooperative Group. Revised indications for the treatment of retinopathy of prematurity: results of the early treatment for retinopathy of prematurity randomized trial. Arch Ophthalmol 2003;121(12): 1684–94.
O'Donovan DJ, Fernandes CJ. Free radicals and diseases in premature infants. Antioxid Redox Signal 2004;6(1):169–76.
York JR, Landers S, Kirby RS, et al. Arterial oxygen fluctuation and retinopathy of prematurity in very-low-birth-weight infants. J Perinatol 2004;24(2):82–7.
Silverman WA. A cautionary tale about supplemental oxygen: the albatross of neonatal medicine. Pediatrics 2004;113(2):394–6.
Hellström A, Engström E, Hård AL, et al. Postnatal serum insulin-like growth factor I deficiency is associated with retinopathy of prematurity and other complications of premature birth. Pediatrics 2003;112(5):1016–20.
Cunningham S, Fleck BW, Elton RA, et al. Transcutaneous oxygen levels in retinopathy of prematurity. Lancet 1995;346(8988):1464–5.
Poets CF, Wilken M, Seidenberg J, et al. Reliability of a pulse oximeter in the detection of hyperoxemia. J Pediatr 1993;122(1):87–90.
Flynn JT, Bancalari E, Snyder ES, et al. A cohort study of transcutaneous oxygen tension and the incidence and severity of retinopathy of prematurity. N Engl J Med 1992;326(16):1050–4.
Msall ME, Phelps DL, DiGaudio KM, et al. Severity of neonatal retinopathy of prematurity is predictive of neurodevelopmental functional outcome at age 5.5 years. Behalf of the Cryotherapy for Retinopathy of Prematurity Cooperative Group. Pediatrics 2000;106(5):998–1005.
Anderson CG, Benitz WE, Madan A. Retinopathy of prematurity and pulse oximetry: a national survey of recent practices. J Perinatol 2004;24(3):164–8.

Improving the Use of Human Milk During and After the NICU Stay

Paula P. Meier, RN, DNSc[a,b,*],
Janet L. Engstrom, RN, PhD, CNM, WHNP-BC[a], Aloka L. Patel, MD[b],
Briana J. Jegier, PhD[a], Nicholas E. Bruns, BA[c]

KEYWORDS

- Human milk feeding • Newborn intensive care unit
- Milk dose and exposure period • Prematurity-specific morbidity

The feeding of human milk (milk from the infant's own mother; excluding donor milk) during the newborn intensive care unit (NICU) stay reduces the risk of short-and long-term morbidities in premature infants, including enteral feed intolerance, nosocomial infection, necrotizing enterocolitis (NEC), chronic lung disease (CLD), retinopathy of prematurity (ROP), developmental and neurocognitive delay, and rehospitalization after NICU discharge.[1–29] The mechanisms by which human milk provides this protection are varied and synergistic, and appear to change over the course of the NICU stay.[30,31] In brief, these mechanisms include specific human milk components that are not present in the milk of other mammals, such the type and amount of long-chain polyunsaturated fatty acids and digestible proteins, and the extraordinary number of oligosaccharides (approximately 130).[32] Human milk also contains multiple lines of undifferentiated stem cells, with the potential to impact a variety of health outcomes throughout the life span.[33] Other human milk mechanisms change over the course of lactation in a manner that complements the infant's nutritional and protective needs. These mechanisms include immunologic, anti-infective, anti-inflammatory, epigenetic, and mucosal membrane protecting properties.[34–41] Thus, human milk from

Supported by NIH Grant NR010009.
[a] Department of Women, Children and Family Nursing, Rush University Medical Center, 1653 West Congress Parkway, Chicago, IL 60612, USA
[b] Section of Neonatology, Department of Pediatrics, Rush University Medical Center, 1653 West Congress Parkway, Chicago, IL 60612, USA
[c] Rush Medical School, Rush University Medical Center, 1653 West Congress Parkway, Chicago, IL 60612, USA
* Corresponding author. Department of Women, Children and Family Nursing, Rush University Medical Center, 1653 West Congress Parkway, Chicago, IL 60612.
E-mail address: paula_meier@rush.edu

Clin Perinatol 37 (2010) 217–245
doi:10.1016/j.clp.2010.01.013 perinatology.theclinics.com
0095-5108/10/$ – see front matter

the infant's mother cannot be replaced by commercial infant formula or donor human milk, and the feeding of human milk should be a NICU priority.

Recent evidence suggests that the impact of human milk on improving infant health outcomes and reducing the risk of prematurity-specific morbidities is linked to specific critical exposure periods in the post-birth period during which the exclusive use of human milk and the avoidance of formula may be most important.[29–31,42,43] Similarly, there are other periods when high doses, but not necessarily exclusive use of human milk, may be important. This article reviews the concept of "dose and exposure period" for human milk feeding in the NICU to precisely measure and benchmark the amount and timing of human milk use in the NICU. Similarly, the critical exposure periods when exclusive or high doses of human milk appear to have the greatest impact on specific morbidities are reviewed. Finally, the current best practices for the use of human milk during and after the NICU stay for premature infants are summarized.

DOSE AND EXPOSURE PERIOD: PRECISE MEASUREMENT OF HUMAN MILK USE IN THE NICU

Research, practice, and quality improvement initiatives focused on the use of human milk in the NICU have been limited by the lack of a precise, quantitative measure of "human milk feeding" for premature infants.[30] Whereas definitions for "breastfeeding" were standardized for term healthy infants in the early 1990s,[44] these six categorical definitions do not capture the critical components of human milk feeding patterns for NICU infants.[45] In addition, the existing definitions for "human milk feeding" used in studies of premature infants are limited and inconsistent. For example, human milk feeding might vary from receiving "any" human milk to having received a specific volume threshold, such as 50 mL/kg/d.[30] However, the measures usually do not specify *when* the infant received human milk and whether there were periods of exclusive or high doses of human milk feeding. Thus, quality improvement initiatives that focus only on increasing the percentage of NICU infants that are "human milk fed" will be inadequate if specific amounts and time periods of human milk feeding are not specified.

A second category of quality improvement indicators focuses on the use of human milk at the time of NICU discharge. Examples of these indicators include "increasing the percentage of NICU infants that are exclusively breastfeeding or receiving exclusive human milk feedings" at the time of NICU discharge. Although this outcome is precise and easily measured, it fails to capture the infant's human milk feeding history throughout the NICU stay. Similarly, it is dichotomous with respect to the individual infant and mother. For example, a mother who had no desire to breastfeed may have provided her milk for her infant for a significant portion of the NICU stay so that her infant was fed exclusive human milk for a substantial period (eg, 30 or 60 days). However, this mother-infant dyad would be classified as "not breastfeeding" at the time of discharge, even though the mother may have provided human milk throughout the most critical period of the infant's development. Indeed, current evidence suggests there are relatively short, critical exposure periods post birth when exclusive or high amounts of human milk are especially important in optimizing health outcomes for premature infants[30] and reducing the risk of enteral feed intolerance, nosocomial infection, and inflammation-based morbidities such as NEC.[7,27,28,46,47] From a cost outcomes perspective, these morbidities translate directly into higher costs of NICU care[15,48–50] and greater probability of long-term health problems.[10–21] Thus, the infant who receives exclusive human milk feeding in the first month post birth may have a better health outcome than an infant who received low doses of human milk throughout the NICU stay.

Consistent with the emerging clinical and molecular evidence, quality improvement indicators should focus on measuring and benchmarking the "dose and exposure period" for human milk use in the NICU.[31] The *dose* of human milk should be quantitatively measured for each infant, both as a percentage of total enteral feedings and in mL/kg/d for each day of the NICU stay. These simple calculations require only the total amount in milliliters of human milk and nonhuman milk fed to the infant each day. The *exposure period* refers to the specific days during the NICU stay during which the infant received any human milk feeding. For example, 3 quality indicators using dose and exposure period might be: "Increase to 75% the percentage of very low birth weight infants (VLBW; <1500 g) who receive a dose of human milk of at least 80% over the first month post birth"; "Increase to 75% the percentage of extremely low birth weight infants (ELBW; <1000 g) who receive at least 50 mL/kg/d of human milk over the NICU stay"; and "Increase to 75% the percentage of ELBW infants who receive exclusive human milk feeding during the first 14 days post birth." These indicators are evidence-based, precise, objective, measurable, and, as continuous variables, are easily related to health outcomes and cost of care in statistical and economic analyses.

CRITICAL EXPOSURE PERIODS FOR THE USE OF HUMAN MILK

This section reviews the clinical evidence for use of critical exposure periods to conceptualize and measure the dose of human milk feeding for premature infants in the NICU. In addition, the underlying human milk mechanisms and their impact on the development of specific infant organs and systems during these critical exposure periods are detailed. These four critical periods include: colostrum as the transition from intrauterine to extrauterine nutrition; the transition from colostrum to mature milk feedings during the first month post birth; human milk feedings throughout the NICU stay; and human milk feedings after NICU discharge.

Colostrum: The Transition from Intrauterine to Extrauterine Nutrition in Mammals

The first critical exposure period for human milk feeding is the use of colostrum during the introduction and advancement of enteral feedings in the early post-birth period. Colostrum is secreted during the early days post birth when the paracellular pathways in the mammary epithelium are open and permit the transfer of high molecular weight antibodies, anti-inflammatories, growth factors, and other protective components into the milk product.[30,39,51,52] Colostrum, with a profile of growth factors, and anti-inflammatory and anti-infective components similar to amniotic fluid, facilitates the transition from intrauterine to extrauterine nutrition in mammals.[53–60] When colostrum is fed to the infant during the early post-birth period, the high molecular weight protective components of colostrum can pass through the open paracellular pathways in the infant gastrointestinal tract.[56,59] Colostrum feedings are especially important for extremely immature infants because, during the last trimester in utero, the infants would have swallowed approximately 750 mL of amniotic fluid daily.[56,59] An array of growth factors in the swallowed amniotic fluid more than doubles the weight of the intestinal mucosa during this time.[56]

For extremely premature infants, the early administration of colostrum may compensate for the shortened period of in utero amniotic fluid swallowing. Initial colostrum feedings stimulate rapid growth in the intestinal mucosal surface area, facilitate the endocytosis of protein, and induce many digestive enzymes.[53–60] In animal models, the intestinal tract does not mature comparably if colostrum is not the first feeding.[53–60] This observation is true even when initial feedings consist of mature milk from the same mammalian species and are followed by colostrum.[53,55,59] Furthermore, artificial feedings appear to exert a separate detrimental effect when they replace colostrum as initial postnatal nutrition in piglets, including atrophy of the gastrointestinal tract, higher concentrations of inducible nitric oxide synthase in the intestinal tissue, and elevated serum cortisol.[53,55,56,60] These structural and biochemical outcomes have been linked to necrotizing enterocolitis in laboratory animals.[53,60]

Human colostrum is also different from mature milk, with higher concentrations of secretory IgA, growth factors, lactoferrin, anti-inflammatory cytokines, oligosaccharides, soluble CD14, antioxidants, and other protective components.[32,61–64] Recent studies suggest an inverse relationship between the duration of pregnancy and the concentration of these agents in maternal colostrum, meaning that mothers of the least mature infants produce the most protective colostrum.[65] Separate studies suggest that secretion of colostrum may be prolonged by several hours or days following extremely premature birth, and that the additional colostrum-type milk may be a specific protective mechanism for the compromised infant.[36,39] A recent study has also demonstrated the safety and feasibility of oropharyngeally administered colostrum before the introduction of trophic feedings in ELBW infants.[65,66] The mechanisms of protection with oropharyngeally administered colostrum, such as cytokine absorption via the oropharyngeal associated lymphoid tissues (OFALT) with subsequent systemic immunomodulation and the local interference with microbe attachment to the oral mucous membranes, may be additive to trophic feedings and may have a specific role in protection from ventilator-associated pneumonia.[65,66]

The evidence about the importance of colostrum as a first feeding has many implications in the NICU, especially for extremely premature infants who have not been exposed to the growth factors in amniotic fluid during the last trimester. **Box 1** summarizes clinical guidelines for colostrum feeding in the NICU, and **Fig. 1** shows patient information in the form of a handout that summarizes the importance of colostrum feeding for families of NICU infants.

Early Enteral Feedings: Transition from Colostrum to Mature Milk During the First Month Post Birth

A second critical period for high doses of human milk feedings is the first 14 to 28 days post birth, when several studies have demonstrated a dose-response relationship between the amount of human milk received by VLBW and ELBW infants and reduction in the risk for specific clinical morbidities including enteral feed intolerance,[28] nosocomial infection,[7,46] NEC,[24,27] CLD,[47,67] ROP,[47] and the total number of morbidities during the NICU stay.[47] The mechanism by which the feeding of high doses of human milk impacts morbidities during this critical period is linked to structural and functional changes in the gastrointestinal tract that occur as enteral feedings are advanced. Human milk appears to program or stimulate many of these healthy processes, whereas formula appears to exert an independent detrimental effect.[29,68] Unfortunately, no previous study has examined the effect of donor human milk during this transition to full enteral feedings, so the impact of donor milk during this period is unknown.

During the first days of life the gastrointestinal tract, sterile at birth, becomes colonized with an array of commensal and potentially pathogenic bacteria. Many factors surrounding the birth of a premature or NICU infant, such as Cesarean birth, antibiotic use, and delayed enteral feedings, predispose the intestine to a dysbiosis with respect to colonization and maturation.[68–70] However, several independent studies indicate

Box 1
Clinical application for colostrum feeding in the NICU

1. Colostrum should be the first feeding received by the infant.
2. Colostrum may be used for trophic feedings and can also be administered safely via the oropharyngeal route with and/or before trophic feedings.
3. Colostrum should be fed in the order that it is produced, even if it has been previously frozen.
4. After the first 3 to 4 days of exclusive colostrum feedings, colostrum can be alternated with fresh mature milk (to protect infant from microorganisms in the NICU via the enteromammary pathway).
5. Colostrum should be stored in small, sterile, food-grade containers that are easily identifiable in the refrigerator or freezer by the nurse.
6. Colostrum containers should be numbered in the order they were collected, in a manner easily identifiable by the nurse.
7. Small expressed drops of colostrum can be diluted with 1 to 2 mL of sterile water to remove the drops from the pump collection kit and/or to achieve a desired feed volume. Dilution is not necessary for any other reason.
8. Colostrum should not be mixed with fortifier or commercial formula.
9. Removal of colostrum from the breast may be most effective using a combination of a hospital grade electric breast pump and hand expression.
10. Formula should be avoided during the introduction and advancement of colostrum feedings, because formula may exert a separate detrimental effect on gastrointestinal integrity during this critical time.

that human milk, which has both probiotic and prebiotic activity,[32,61,62,71,72] results in a predominantly commensal gut microflora.[73–75] In contrast, even small amounts of formula fed during this time appear to interrupt the protective colonization conferred by human milk.[73–75] Related research indicates that soluble CD14, a pattern recognition molecule that functions as a coreceptor for Toll-like receptors II and IV, is highly concentrated in human milk, at a level up to 20 times higher in milk than in the serum of lactating women.[62,63] In combination, the pre- and probiotics, and soluble CD14 provide the substrates for healthy bacterial-enterocyte crosstalk in the developing intestine.[76]

A second protective mechanism that occurs during the transition from colostrum to mature milk feedings is the closure of paracellular pathways between the enterocytes in the infant's intestine. The closure of the paracellular pathways is positively associated with the volume of human milk feeding.[29] The resulting tight junctions inhibit the translocation of high molecular weight bacteria and their toxins from the lumen of the gut to the bowel wall where they can up-regulate inflammatory processes through activation of the cytokine, interleukin-8.[77–79] With little or no ability to mount a compensatory anti-inflammatory response, the extremely immature infant is susceptible to local inflammatory processes, such as NEC, as well as the spread of inflammation to distal organs such as the lungs, eyes, and brain.[78,80] The specific human milk components that protect from inflammation include pre- and probiotics, oligosaccharides, soluble CD14, transforming growth factor-β, epidermal growth factor, interleukin-10, and lactoferrin, all of which are concentrated most highly in the colostrum.[29,32,34–41,61–63,65,66,71–75,77,78,80] Furthermore, during this critical exposure period, which coincides with the introduction and advancement of enteral feeds,

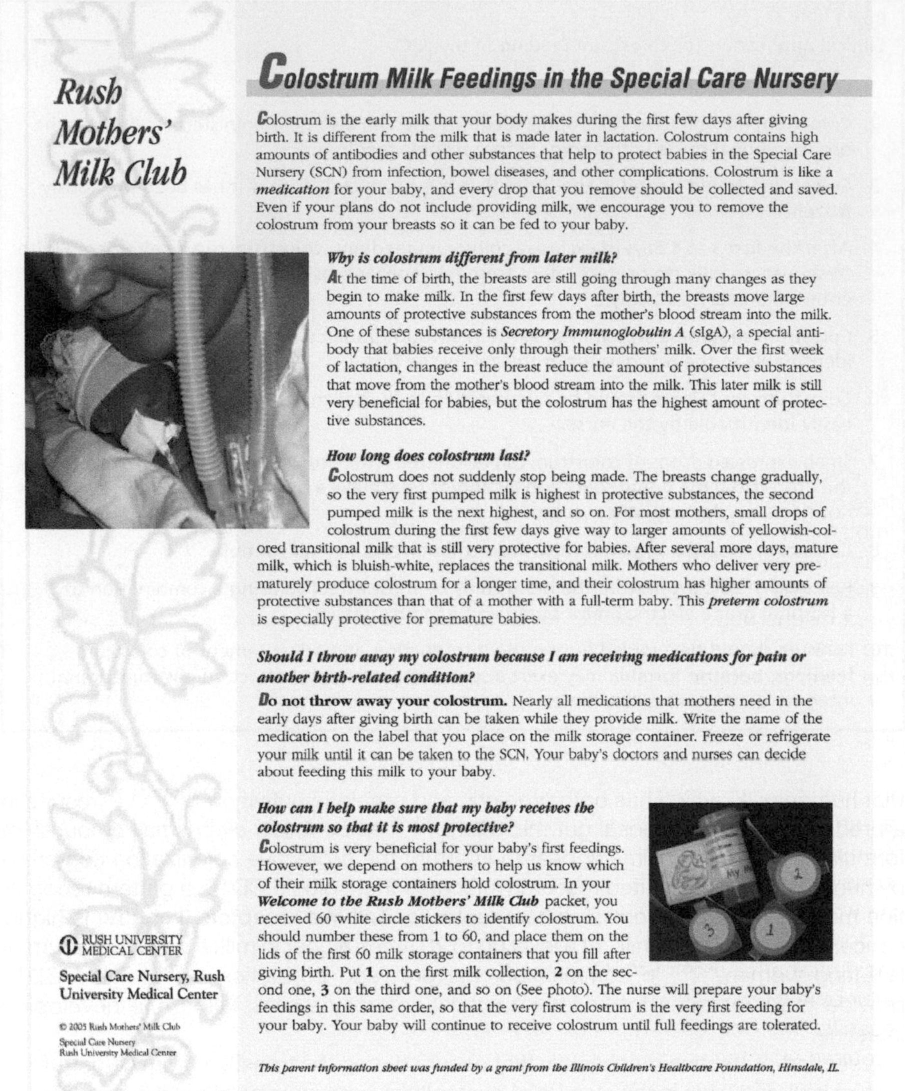

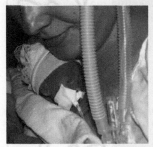
Rush Mothers' Milk Club

Colostrum Milk Feedings in the Special Care Nursery

Colostrum is the early milk that your body makes during the first few days after giving birth. It is different from the milk that is made later in lactation. Colostrum contains high amounts of antibodies and other substances that help to protect babies in the Special Care Nursery (SCN) from infection, bowel diseases, and other complications. Colostrum is like a *medication* for your baby, and every drop that you remove should be collected and saved. Even if your plans do not include providing milk, we encourage you to remove the colostrum from your breasts so it can be fed to your baby.

Why is colostrum different from later milk?

At the time of birth, the breasts are still going through many changes as they begin to make milk. In the first few days after birth, the breasts move large amounts of protective substances from the mother's blood stream into the milk. One of these substances is ***Secretory Immunoglobulin A*** (sIgA), a special antibody that babies receive only through their mothers' milk. Over the first week of lactation, changes in the breast reduce the amount of protective substances that move from the mother's blood stream into the milk. This later milk is still very beneficial for babies, but the colostrum has the highest amount of protective substances.

How long does colostrum last?

Colostrum does not suddenly stop being made. The breasts change gradually, so the very first pumped milk is highest in protective substances, the second pumped milk is the next highest, and so on. For most mothers, small drops of colostrum during the first few days give way to larger amounts of yellowish-colored transitional milk that is still very protective for babies. After several more days, mature milk, which is bluish-white, replaces the transitional milk. Mothers who deliver very prematurely produce colostrum for a longer time, and their colostrum has higher amounts of protective substances than that of a mother with a full-term baby. This ***preterm colostrum*** is especially protective for premature babies.

Should I throw away my colostrum because I am receiving medications for pain or another birth-related condition?

Do not throw away your colostrum. Nearly all medications that mothers need in the early days after giving birth can be taken while they provide milk. Write the name of the medication on the label that you place on the milk storage container. Freeze or refrigerate your milk until it can be taken to the SCN. Your baby's doctors and nurses can decide about feeding this milk to your baby.

How can I help make sure that my baby receives the colostrum so that it is most protective?

Colostrum is very beneficial for your baby's first feedings. However, we depend on mothers to help us know which of their milk storage containers hold colostrum. In your ***Welcome to the Rush Mothers' Milk Club*** packet, you received 60 white circle stickers to identify colostrum. You should number these from 1 to 60, and place them on the lids of the first 60 milk storage containers that you fill after giving birth. Put **1** on the first milk collection, **2** on the second one, **3** on the third one, and so on (See photo). The nurse will prepare your baby's feedings in this same order, so that the very first colostrum is the very first feeding for your baby. Your baby will continue to receive colostrum until full feedings are tolerated.

RUSH UNIVERSITY MEDICAL CENTER

Special Care Nursery, Rush University Medical Center

© 2005 Rush Mothers' Milk Club
Special Care Nursery
Rush University Medical Center

This parent information sheet was funded by a grant from the Illinois Children's Healthcare Foundation, Hinsdale, IL

Fig. 1. Parent information handout about the importance of collecting and feeding colostrum in the NICU. (*Available in* English and Spanish, *Courtesy of* Rush Mother's Milk Club, Rush University Medical Center, Chicago, IL.)

formula appears to exert an independent, proinflammatory effect.[29,32,34–41,61–63,65,66,71–75,77,78,80]

Dose of Human Milk During the NICU Stay

Five well-controlled studies of four cohorts of extremely premature, VLBW, or ELBW infants have linked the dose of human milk feedings (mL/kg/d) received throughout the NICU stay with specific health outcomes during or after the NICU stay.[5,6,25,26,47]

However, only one of these studies examined the effect of specific exposure periods within the NICU stay, and found that high doses of human milk during the first 14 days post birth were most highly associated with the advantageous health outcomes that were noted throughout the NICU stay.[47] In 3 of the 4 cohorts, premature infants who received the highest doses or exclusive feedings of fortified human milk had shorter hospital stays than formula-fed infants, despite the fact that the human milk–fed infants grew either at a similar rate[47] or more slowly[5,6] than the formula-fed infants. Although the remaining studies[25,26] did not find a feeding related trend in hospital-based morbidities or length of the NICU stay, they established a dose-response relationship between the amount of human milk received during the NICU stay and better health outcomes during the first 18 and 30 months of age, corrected for prematurity.

In separate studies, Schanler and colleagues[5,6] compared health outcomes for extremely premature infants who received differing doses of human milk throughout the NICU stay. In the first study,[6] health outcomes were compared for 108 infants who received 50 mL/kg/d or more of fortified human milk (n = 62) and those who received exclusive formula feedings (n = 46). Infants who received human milk feedings had fewer days of total parenteral nutrition (TPN); fewer episodes of enteral feed intolerance; a lower incidence of NEC, CLD, and ROP; and a dose-response relationship between the amount of human milk and the number of episodes of late onset sepsis. Even though the human milk-fed infants gained weight more slowly, they were discharged nearly 500 g lighter and 2 weeks earlier than comparison formula-fed infants. The investigators speculated that the earlier discharge was a function of the lower incidence and severity of morbidities in the human milk-fed infants.

In a subsequent study, Schanler and colleagues[5] studied 243 extremely premature infants whose mothers initiated lactation with the intent of providing human milk throughout the infants' NICU stay. If the maternal milk supply was inadequate, the infants were assigned randomly to receive either donor human milk or formula as a supplement to the mother's own milk. Of the 243 infants, 29% received only their own mothers' milk throughout the NICU stay, and the other 71% were distributed equally between the 2 randomized groups. Only minor differences were noticed between the 2 groups randomized to either supplementation with donor human milk or formula, with the donor milk supplemented group demonstrating a slightly lower incidence of CLD and slower weight gain. In contrast, the infants who received only their own mothers' milk during the NICU stay had a lower incidence of all prematurity specific morbidities, and were discharged a week sooner than the infants who required supplementation with either donor human milk or formula.

In a retrospective study of 277 ELBW infants, Patel and colleagues[47] noted a similar trend toward earlier discharge in ELBW infants who received exclusive human milk feedings versus those who received exclusive formula feedings during the NICU stay. Although the human milk fed infants were 1 week less mature (25.2 vs 26.3 weeks) at birth, and demonstrated the same growth velocity from regaining birth weight until NICU discharge (14.5 vs 14.6 g/kg/d), their length of stay in the NICU was 11.7 days shorter (90.2 days vs 101.9 days), and their postmenstrual age at NICU discharge was 2.8 weeks less (38.0 vs 40.8) than the formula-fed infants. In this 5-year, retrospective cohort, Patel and colleagues also described a dose-response relationship between the dose of human milk (mL/kg/d) received during the first 14 days post birth and number of morbidities during the NICU stay.

In a secondary analysis of the National Institute of Child Health and Human Development funded glutamine trial of 1034 ELBW infants cared for in 19 NICUs in the United States,[81] Vohr and colleagues[26] found no differences in hospital-based morbidities or length of NICU stay among formula-fed and human milk–fed infants. However, the investigators reported a dose-response relationship between the amount of human milk received during the NICU stay and developmental outcomes at 18 months[26] and 30 months of age[25] in this cohort. At the 18-month evaluation[26] there was no difference between formula-fed and human milk–fed groups in overall growth. However, the investigators reported that each 10 mL/kg/d of human milk received over the NICU stay was associated with a dose-response increase in scores on standardized neurocognitive and developmental tests, and with a reduced risk of rehospitalization during the first year of life. The most striking differences were observed between the exclusively formula-fed group and the highest quintile of human milk dose received (110 mL/kg/d), with a 5-point IQ advantage for the high human milk group. The investigators concluded that this difference, when considered from a population perspective, translated into significant health care, educational, and societal cost savings over the life span for ELBW infants.

Vohr and colleagues[25] followed this same cohort of infants, and reported outcomes at 30 months of age, corrected for prematurity, for 773 of the original 1034 infants. The relationship between dose of human milk received during the NICU stay and neurocognitive and developmental outcome persisted through this second developmental time point, with each 10 mL/kg/d of human milk ingestion in the NICU adding to infants' scores on standardized tests in a dose-response manner. The risk of rehospitalization remained lower as a function of human milk dose, especially for respiratory illnesses. Thus, it appears that human milk feedings during the NICU stay provide the foundation for better health outcomes during early childhood.

In summary, in 3 of the 4 cohorts of extremely premature or ELBW infants for whom dose of human milk during the NICU stay was measured, investigators reported a lower incidence and severity of morbidities, a shorter length of stay in the NICU, and hospital discharge at lower weights or postmenstrual age in infants who received exclusive or high doses of human milk.[5,6,25,26,47] These data are especially compelling because in the 3 studies, the human milk–fed infants grew either similarly[47] or more slowly[5,6] than comparable infants who received either low doses or no human milk.

In the single cohort for whom health outcomes were measured after the NICU stay, infants in all feeding groups grew similarly during the first 18 and 30 months of life, corrected for prematurity.[25,26] However, a dose-response relationship was described between the amount of human milk feedings received during the NICU stay and scores on tests of neurocognitive and developmental outcome and the risk of rehospitalization at both post-discharge time points. In all 4 cohorts, the most striking differences in outcome were between infants who had received high (or exclusive) doses of human milk and exclusive formula. The findings also suggest that proportionately higher doses of human milk (but not necessarily exclusive or extremely high doses) received over the longer exposure period of the entire course of the NICU stay impact the aforementioned outcomes. Thus, human milk feedings over the NICU stay do not have to be exclusive to confer benefit, but the greatest benefit appears to be linked to high doses or exclusive feedings of human milk.

The specific human milk mechanisms that impact these NICU and post-discharge outcomes are probably both protective and nutritive in nature. Several developmental outcome studies suggest that a lower incidence and severity of morbidities during the NICU stay translate into a shorter NICU stay, lower discharge weight and postmenstrual age, better neurocognitive and developmental outcome, and a lower risk of rehospitalization in premature infants.[10,11,14–16,18–21,49,82,83] By providing primary protection from these morbidities during the early NICU stay, human milk may indirectly impact the associated long-term outcomes.[30]

In addition, many protective components in human milk may be equally, or even more important beyond the first 14 to 28 days post birth, and probably affect these long-term outcomes. Examples of these components include antioxidant activity to counter the untoward effects of oxygen[41]; the "customization" of antibodies via the enteromammary pathway, providing protection from specific pathogens in the NICU environment[84]; oligosaccharides that inhibit the adhesion of pathogens to mucosal membranes in the mouth, throat, and gastrointestinal tract[85] the potential impact of oligosaccharides on neural development[32,86]; and other less studied factors that impact tissue growth and metabolism, such as vascular endothelial growth factor, transforming growth factors, and leptin.[35–37,87,88]

The Impact of Human Milk Feedings After the NICU Stay

Although it can be assumed that premature infants who continue to receive human milk after the NICU stay experience the same short- and long-term benefits as term infants,[89] no well-controlled studies linking these outcomes with either dose or exposure period of human milk have been reported for premature infants after NICU discharge. In contrast, most research in this area has focused on comparing short-term growth velocity and other anthropometric measures for cohorts of premature infants who are discharged in 1 of 3 feeding categories: receiving exclusive human milk, either from the breast, bottle, or a combination of the 2; receiving human milk feedings that are either supplemented with powdered formula or partially replaced with premature formulas; or receiving exclusive formula feedings. The findings from most of these studies suggest that premature infants grow more rapidly with exclusive formula feedings or when human milk feedings are either supplemented or partially replaced with formula. Although no studies have examined the impact of these practices on long-term health outcomes, they are common NICU discharge instructions for human milk–fed premature infants.[90–93]

However, a limitation in all of these post-discharge growth studies is the fact that human milk intake has seldom been measured precisely during breastfeeding, using accurate test-weighing procedures in the home.[91,94–97] even though a series of well-controlled studies indicate that premature infants are vulnerable to underconsumption of milk during exclusive breastfeeding until they achieve term, corrected age.[96,98–101] Similarly, no study has included actual compositional measures of the human milk consumed by the infant, despite the extensive evidence indicating that the caloric content of human milk varies markedly throughout the day and within the same mother.[102–106] Instead, the caloric content of human milk is assumed to be 20 calories per ounce for all feedings, a figure that is inconsistent with the research in this area.[101] Thus, at the present time it is unknown whether exclusively human milk–fed infants grow more slowly because they consume an inadequate volume of milk or because the milk that they consume is inadequate in calories or a specific nutrient such as protein. These are important distinctions, and are diagnosable and manageable for both research and practice, using human milk research technologies that enable an infant to continue receiving high doses of human milk.[42,99,101]

In summary, nothing is known about the long-term implications of feeding either exclusive human milk or human milk supplemented with commercial formula products. Although short-term growth is important, replacement of human milk with formula reduces the overall lifetime dose of human milk for premature infants. Studies with term, healthy infants suggest that many of the long-term health benefits associated with breastfeeding, such as higher scores on intelligence tests and protection from infections, eczema, and adult-onset morbidities, are conferred in a dose-response manner.[89] Thus, replacement of human milk feedings with formula may accelerate short-term growth but has unknown implications for later-onset morbidities.

BEST NICU PRACTICES TO INCREASE DOSE AND EXPOSURE PERIOD OF HUMAN MILK FEEDINGS

This section addresses the best practices for optimizing the dose and exposure period of human milk feeding for premature infants in the NICU. These practices are conceptualized into four aspects of care: encouraging the mother to provide her milk for her infant; providing cost-effective, expert lactation and human milk feeding support for families and staff in the NICU; prioritizing the initiation, establishment, and maintenance of maternal milk volume; and using lactation technologies to manage human milk feeding problems.

Encouraging the Mother to Provide her Milk for her Infant

Exclusive human milk feeding is uniformly recommended as the first food and as the only food during the first months of life by all of the major health organizations with an interest in infant health, including the World Health Organization (WHO),[107] the United States Breastfeeding Committee (USBC),[108] and the American Academy of Pediatrics (AAP).[109] The WHO specifically addresses the importance of colostrum as the first feeding for infants in the immediate post-birth period,[107] and the AAP specifically addresses the importance of human milk feeding for premature infants.[109]

Although the benefits of human milk feeding for premature infants are well documented, many obstetricians, pediatricians, and nurses remain reluctant to encourage mothers to provide their milk and often simply accept the mother's decision to formula feed without further discussion. These professionals often mistakenly assume that they do not have any influence over a mother's feeding decision, or that they will increase the stress for a mother whose infant is in a critical care setting. Finally, some care providers think that it is unethical to encourage mothers to provide milk, and express concern that they are pressuring or coercing mothers at this sensitive time.

Recent research has dispelled many of these concerns and has demonstrated that provider encouragement of human milk feeding for premature infants is effective regardless of the social and ethnic background of families, and that families depend on health care providers to share this information with them.[110–115] A recent review of the ethical issues related to promoting breastfeeding concluded that fully informing mothers of the health benefits of human milk was an ethical responsibility for health care professionals.[111] In addition, concerns that promotion of human milk feeding may make women feel guilty, coerced, or forced into changing their decision were abated in a recent study of 21 mothers of VLBW infants who changed their feeding decision from formula to human milk.[110] The study participants indicated that they changed their decision almost immediately after learning from a health care provider that their milk was a critical component in the overall management of their infants' NICU plan of care.[110] Indeed, one mother was so disturbed that she had not been told of the importance of her milk by professionals in the hospital where she gave birth that she questioned the qualifications of the doctors and nurses who had cared for her and her baby in the referral hospital before her infant's transport to the hospital where this research was conducted.

Although the efficacy and ethics of promoting breastfeeding are documented, the language used to promote the provision of human milk is important when speaking with women and their families. For example, many women do not wish to feed at the breast for several reasons, some of which are extremely sensitive, such as a history of sexual abuse. However, these women may be very amenable to using a breast pump to express their milk so it can be fed by bottle. Similarly, it is more appropriate to focus on providing milk for a limited period of time to "get the baby off to the best start" than to engage in discussions about long-term milk expression or feeding at breast. All decisions about feeding at breast or long-term milk expression can be postponed until the infant's condition is stable and the mother's stress about the premature birth has begun to lessen. These decisions can then be made calmly and thoughtfully with the support of professionals, family members, and friends.

Although this initial discussion with the mother and family should be conducted in a nondirective and noncoercive manner, the benefits of human milk feeding, particularly of the colostrum and early post-birth feedings, should be clearly and scientifically communicated.[30,34,42] Occasionally the terms "noncoercive and nondirective" are misinterpreted to mean that feeding options are presented as if they were two equally safe and efficacious choices. Although the care provider must be supportive and caring in this discussion with families, the scientific evidence about human milk feedings should be shared just like any other NICU therapeutic option that involves family decision making. Examples of talking points that accurately translate scientific terminology about human milk into understandable parent information were summarized in a recent review article.[34] The health care provider who wants to provide encouragement and accurate information about human milk feedings, but who is not a lactation expert, will find this article useful in guiding these discussions with families of NICU infants.

In the Rush Mothers' Milk Club lactation program, the perinatologists, neonatologists, nurses, and dietitians refer to human milk as a "medicine" that only the mother can provide. This explanation is accompanied by appropriate parent focused information packets and handouts that translate the scientific principles about human milk and lactation into understandable words and concepts (Welcome to the Rush Mothers' Milk Club).[116] An additional resource is a recently completed parent focused video about the importance of human milk feedings when an infant is born prematurely. This video, which features real families and infants from the Rush Mothers' Milk Club program, is culturally sensitive, available in Spanish, and can be used in a multitude of health care settings.[116]

Providing Cost-Effective, Expert Lactation and Human Milk Feeding Support for Families and Staff in the NICU

Whereas many maternal-infant health care providers recognize the importance of human milk for premature and NICU infants, individual institutions struggle with respect to implementing evidence-based models of lactation care for this population. Few neonatologists, NICU nurses, and dietitians are experts in the delivery of this care, and frequently turn to lactation consultants whose primary training and expertise is in the management of breastfeeding for term infants and their mothers. As a result, families are often "caught in the middle" with conflicting advice about the importance of human milk and the NICU-specific lactation problems they encounter, such as selecting and using an appropriate breast pump, collecting and storing their milk, and observing clinicians treat their infants' slow weight gain with formula, even when they have an abundance of available milk. The conflicting advice that families receive about providing human milk in the NICU is well documented, is a source of discouragement to mothers, and is a primary reason for lower doses and exposure periods of human milk feedings for recipient infants.[117,118]

The best practice approach to solving inconsistencies in the management of human milk feedings in the NICU is no different from any other care issue: policies and procedures must be based on available scientific evidence rather than individual opinions and attitudes of staff members. This approach includes evidence-based education of personnel, the completion of human milk and lactation competencies, and the development of standardized policies and procedures to guide practice. Similarly, the notion that some staff members are "pro" or "con" human milk should be addressed by NICU administrators in a manner that is consistent with all other NICU therapies. Most NICUs would not tolerate professional staff members providing information to families based on whether they are "pro" or "con" ventilator management or medication regimens, and human milk feedings should be no different. Simply said, the evidence supports the use of human milk in the NICU, and personal attitudes or experiences of individual staff members to the contrary ("I didn't breastfeed my babies and they turned out just fine...") should not be a part of evidence-based practice in the NICU.

Numerous studies have shown that health care professionals have very limited knowledge and skills related to assisting mothers with breastfeeding and providing milk for either healthy or NICU infants.[119–122] However, several recent studies have demonstrated that educational interventions can improve provider knowledge, skills, and attitudes.[123,124] The USBC has developed competencies for breastfeeding and lactation that are applicable to all care providers involved in the care of women and infants.[125] These competencies include skills such as "know how and when to use technology and equipment to support breastfeeding" and "the ability to preserve breastfeeding under adverse conditions."[125] Likewise, the AAP Policy Statement on Breastfeeding details the expectations of pediatricians in promoting, supporting, and protecting breastfeeding.[109] Competencies specific to professionals who provide support to breast pump–dependent mothers and NICU infants have also been developed.[116] Recent research demonstrates that a NICU-specific lactation education program was effective in changing NICU nurses' knowledge and attitudes,[123] and that overall staff breastfeeding education in the NICU resulted in increased human milk feeding rates.[124]

The provision of clinical and educational support for NICU families and professionals is a specialty area that requires education and expertise in complicated NICU situations as well as in the science of lactation and human milk. As such, NICU lactation programs should be under the direction of an advanced practice nurse, dietitian, or neonatologist. This professional needs expertise in the initiation, establishment, and maintenance of maternal milk volume in pump–dependent mothers who have numerous medical complications, and who may be taking multiple medications. Whereas lists of medications that are or are not compatible with breastfeeding are useful in decision making about term, healthy infants who will be breastfeeding exclusively,[126] these decisions must be approached from an individualized risk-benefit perspective for the NICU infant (**Fig. 2**). Similarly, the use of the highest possible dose and longest exposure period of human milk necessitates that this practitioner integrate technologies, such as the creamatocrit and test weights, on a daily basis to prevent, diagnose, and manage common NICU problems with human milk feedings.[42,101] The standardization of this model of practice requires interaction and education of NICU neonatologists, dietitians, nurses, subspecialists, and families.

The optimal lactation team in the NICU can minimize its costs and increase its efficacy by incorporating the use of breastfeeding peer counselors (BPCs). Although the role of the NICU-based BPC is new, research has demonstrated that BPCs in the NICU and in other settings improve human milk and lactation outcomes.[127,128]

Rush Mothers' Milk Club

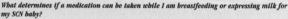

Medications in Mothers' Milk for Babies in Special Care Nursery

Many mothers whose babies are admitted to the Special Care Nursery (SCN) at Rush University Medical Center have pregnancy and birth complications that require they take prescription medications after their babies are born. All families are concerned about whether these medications can be safely taken during breastfeeding or milk expression for their babies. This information sheet is to help you understand how the doctors and nurses in the Rush SCN make decisions about medications in mothers' milk. In addition, your baby's doctor or nurse will talk with you about your specific medications, and discuss them in relation to your baby's individual feeding plan.

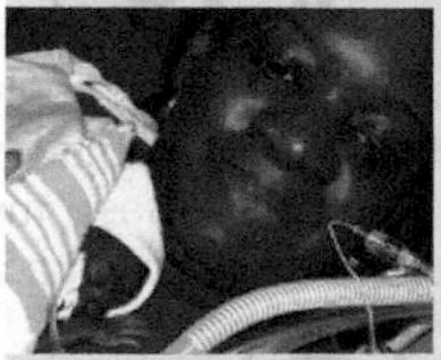

What determines if a medication can be taken while I am breastfeeding or expressing milk for my SCN baby?

Most medications can be safely taken while mothers are breastfeeding or expressing milk for their babies. This is because the medication has to go through several steps before it reaches a baby's blood stream. First, the medication has to be in the mother's blood stream long enough and in high enough amounts that it reaches the milk-making tissue in the breast. Second, the medication has to pass through tiny barriers between the milk-making tissue and the ducts of the breast where milk is removed by the baby or the breast pump. Some medications pass through these barriers more easily than others, and some can't get through at all. Finally, some medications can make it into the milk, but are not easily absorbed into the baby's blood stream from the baby's stomach and intestines.

Are there lists about which medications can be taken during lactation and which ones cannot?

The doctors and nurses in the Rush SCN check mothers' medications with several sources, including recommendations by The American Academy of Pediatrics, and by researchers who specialize in studying medications in mothers' milk. For many medications, these resources compare the amount of medication in the mother's blood stream, her milk, and the baby's blood stream. These resources also alert us to any possible side effects to watch for. Your baby's care provider can share these publications and websites with you if you would like more information.

What other things will influence the doctors' and nurses' decisions about whether a medication can be taken while I provide milk for my baby?

Mothers' milk helps protect babies — especially those born prematurely — from infection and other complications, so the SCN care providers try to balance the risk of **NOT** feeding mothers' milk with possible effects from medications mothers need to take. This is especially true of colostrum, or the milk that is produced during the first days after giving birth. Colostrum is rich in protective substances, but babies receive very small amounts of it when feedings are started. In this way, babies receive maximum protection from the colostrum, and minimum amounts of any medications that may have been released into the milk. For some medications, the SCN care provider may recommend that mothers avoid milk expression during the time of day that the medication is highest in the blood stream. In rare instances, we may recommend that your baby receive partial feedings of mothers' milk and the remainder as formula in order to balance protection from your milk with minimum exposure to medications.

Why do I receive different information from other doctors and nurses about medications that can be taken during lactation?

Medications in mothers' milk is a subspecialty of lactation practice that is relatively new, and many health care providers who work outside of this area may not be aware of the new guidelines and resources listed above. Instead, they often rely on product inserts that accompany a medication, and these inserts almost always advise against combining the medication with lactation. Your baby's SCN care provider is best able to advise you about combining medications and lactation, because we understand both your baby's condition and the transfer of medications into mothers' milk. If you like, we would be happy to personally contact the doctor who prescribed your medications to discuss our recommendations and clarify your baby's feeding plan.

Regardless of conflicting advice, we recommend that you begin expressing and storing your colostrum until we can determine the suitability of the specific medication you are taking. Be sure to write the name and dosage of the medication on the *My Mom Pumps for Me!* milk label on the storage container. We will check the medication and discuss it with you prior to feeding the milk to your baby.

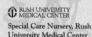

RUSH UNIVERSITY MEDICAL CENTER

Special Care Nursery, Rush University Medical Center

Special Care Nursery
Rush University Medical Center

This parent information sheet was funded by a grant from the Illinois Children's Healthcare Foundation, Hinsdale, IL

Fig. 2. Parent information handout explaining decision-making about medications in mothers' milk for infants in the NICU. (*Available in* English and Spanish, *Courtesy of* Rush Mother's Milk Club, Rush University Medical Center, Chicago, IL.)

The Rush Mothers' Milk Club has incorporated volunteer BPCs since 1997, and has employed BPCs as a part of the NICU lactation team since 2005, when this position was first funded with a foundation grant.[129] These women (and one male counselor) complete a 5-day BPC training program to function as volunteers. Employed BPCs complete an additional 3-month orientation program[116] so that they can acquire the necessary knowledge and skills to practice safely and effectively in the NICU environment. Two of the Rush Mothers' Milk Club BPCs have also met the demanding clinical requirements for non–health care professionals without a college degree to become certified as International Board Certified Lactation Consultants (IBCLCs).

NICU-based BPCs can augment the work of the lactation specialists by performing many of the basic clinical services required in the NICU. For example, they can assume responsibility for teaching all mothers how to use the breast pump, how to clean the collection kit, and how to safely collect, label, store, and transport their milk. However, equally important is that the BPC is a peer of the mother, and can help solve many of the cultural and ethnic lactation and human milk feeding problems that arise. This aspect is particularly important for African American mothers who are significantly more likely to experience preterm birth[130] but less likely to breastfeed or provide their milk.[131,132] A recent study demonstrated that African American mothers experience issues with anxiety and trust when working with nurses and physicians.[133]

A recent study conducted with women in the Rush Mothers' Milk Club demonstrated that the mothers preferred the BPCs to a health care professional when they sought help to address their personal barriers to providing milk for their infants.[134] In addition, the data from this study revealed that the BPC's personal experience with a NICU infant and providing her milk had a profound impact on the new mother and influenced her decision to provide milk for her infant. The mothers who participated in this study also reported that the BPCs provided informational, instrumental, appraisal, and emotional support. The study also demonstrated that BPCs gave the mothers hope that their lives would "eventually return to normal," and made them feel empowered with their decision to initiate and continue providing milk for their infants.

In addition to designated lactation personnel, mothers need basic physical resources in the NICU to provide milk for their infants. These resources include access to a hospital-grade dual electric breast pump and pump kit for adequate milk removal[42,135]; volume-based, rather than ration-based, allocation of containers for storing their expressed milk[42]; refrigerator and freezer space for on-site milk storage of all milk to be fed to the infant during the NICU stay[42]; and access to additional lactation equipment (eg, nipple shields or infant scales to perform test weights) as needed to ensure that infants receive the highest dose of human milk.[42,99] A recent study demonstrated that the cost per 100 mL of maternal human milk is less expensive than donor human milk and specialty formula for NICU infants.[135] These and other health outcome data suggest that the NICU would realize cost savings by promoting maternal human milk feeding over formula or donor human milk feedings.[135] Another large clinical trial is underway to quantify the cost impact to the NICU for providing containers, volume-based refrigerator and freezer space, and additional support equipment.[31]

Prioritizing the Initiation, Establishment, and Maintenance of Maternal Milk Volume

Prioritizing maternal milk volume is the single most important lactation-related responsibility for maternity and neonatal caregivers. An abundant milk volume ensures that the infant has access to exclusive human milk feedings and facilitates the transition to feeding at breast during and after the NICU stay, whereas maternal milk volume problems compromise these goals.[42] Initiating, establishing, and maintaining an adequate milk volume is, however, a demanding task for mothers of premature infants. These mothers are breast pump–dependent, meaning that they must rely on the breast pump to replace the sucking stimulation and milk removal functions of a healthy breastfeeding infant.[136] As such, their needs are very different from those of a mother who is an occasional breast pump user, and can depend on her infant to provide the necessary autocrine stimulus required for milk production.[42]

Several studies have demonstrated that breast pump–dependent women experience problems with delayed lactogenesis and inadequate milk volume,[137–143] with one large study demonstrating that only 29% of mothers with extremely premature infants were able to provide exclusive human milk throughout the NICU stay.[5] However, a recent randomized control trial[136] comparing different breast pump suction patterns suggested that "running out of milk" is at least partially iatrogenic for mothers of VLBW infants, and that implementation of evidence-based best practices may reduce the number of women who do not produce an adequate volume of milk.[42]

The process of developing an adequate milk volume begins during pregnancy, when the breast undergoes several anatomic and physiologic changes in preparation for breastfeeding.[144] Lactogenesis I occurs during the second trimester of pregnancy and is the phase of lactation wherein the mammary glands are sufficiently developed and differentiated to secrete a small amount of colostrum.[52,145] However, the milk secretion is suppressed throughout the remainder of pregnancy by high circulating levels of progesterone.[146] After the delivery of the placenta in the early post-birth period, circulating progesterone levels decline rapidly and, in response, lactogenesis II, the onset of copious milk secretion, occurs and the mother senses the milk "coming in."[52,146–148] Two recent studies[136,149] suggest that specific stimulatory interventions during the transition from lactogenesis I to lactogenesis II may have a programming effect on subsequent maternal milk volume. Whether these interventions exert some effect on the secretory mechanisms in the breast tissue or the neuroendocrine responses is unknown.

Following the onset of lactogenesis II, milk synthesis and secretion are regulated by a combination of autocrine and endocrine processes that depend on regular and effective milk removal via the feedback inhibitor of lactation (FIL) mechanism.[150] For women who exclusively breastfeed a healthy infant, the transition from endocrine to autocrine mechanisms of control occurs seamlessly, because the infant removes available milk and the milk is replaced. Regular and effective milk removal by the infant serves to increase the mean maternal milk volume to approximately 600 to 625 mL/d by the end of the first week post birth.[146] The transition from lactogenesis II to a milk output that is sufficient for exclusive breastfeeding of the infant has been termed "coming to volume" by the authors' research team.[151] This short, but critical transition is the time that most breast pump–dependent mothers experience milk volume problems that require rapid identification and resolution.[42]

In contrast to a term infant who regulates milk synthesis and secretion during this critical transition, breast pump–dependent mothers must undertake frequent and complete breast emptying with a breast pump. Numerous factors that are unique to these women, such as an ineffective breast pump, improperly fitting breast shields, infrequent pump use, or ending a pumping session before all of the available milk is removed, can compromise this transition. Similarly, the intense stress, fatigue, and pain in these early days can down-regulate prolactin via the dopaminergic prolactin inhibiting factor.[52,146] Best practices to prevent, diagnose, and manage milk volume problems in breast pump-dependent women have been summarized in a recent review.[42] However, mothers need measurable milk volume targets and daily monitoring during the critical "coming to volume" transition. In the Rush Mothers' Milk Club program, a BPC contacts each new mother on a daily basis during this period, either in the NICU or by telephone, and reviews with her each item in the brief checklist shown in **Fig. 3**.

Another potential problem experienced by breast pump–dependent mothers during this critical transition is that the administration of hormonal contraceptives in the early

Name: ______________________________ **Infant's DOB:** ______________

Assessment completed by: ______________, **BPC(c) Today's Date**________

☐ in NLFC ☐ in NICU ☐ by telephone ☐ Other

Item 1. Evaluate Maternal Milk Volume

Pumped volume recorded for last 24 hours: ______________ mLs

Number of pumpings last 24 hours: ______________

Total number of minutes pumped last 24 hours ______________

Longest interval between pumpings last 24 hours: ______________

Daily volume is steadily:

☐ Increasing ☐ Staying the same ☐ Decreasing

Item 2. Evaluate Breast Changes

Breasts feel full between pumping	☐ Yes	☐ No
Milk drips or leaks between pumpings	☐ Yes	☐ No
All areas of both breasts empty thoroughly with pumping If no, detail specific areas and plan to see mother	☐ Yes	☐ No
All areas of both breasts are free of local areas of pain and redness If no, detail specific areas and plan to see mother	☐ Yes	☐ No

Item 3. Evaluate Nipple Changes

Both nipples are free of pain or discomfort If no, detail area(s) of nipple(s) affected	☐ Yes	☐ No
Both nipples are free of redness and local pain at juncture of nipple and areola If no, detail which nipple is affected and complete assessment for correctly-fitted breast shields	☐ Yes	☐ No
Both nipples are free of lacerations and bleeding If no, detail which nipple is affected and plan to see mother	☐ Yes	☐ No

Item 4: Evaluate Medications that Impact Milk Volume

All medications and doses are the same as previous day If no, detail changes and discuss with lactation specialist Ask specifically about OTC cold remedies and hormonal birth control	☐ Yes	☐ No

Item 5: Additional Notes and Follow Up Plans:

Fig. 3. "Coming to Volume" checklist to be completed daily for breast pump–dependent mothers of NICU infants until daily milk volume is 350 mL or more for 5 consecutive days.

post-birth period may affect the initiation of lactation and the "coming to volume" transition. Whereas estrogen-containing contraceptives should be avoided in the early post-birth period, the use of progestin contraceptives during this vulnerable period is controversial.[152–156] However, the endocrine mechanism for lactogenesis II is the rapid decline in progesterone in the first days post birth, and conditions that result in elevated progesterone levels, such as retained placental fragments and theca lutein cysts, are known to compromise the initiation of lactation due to the continued progesterone secretion.[157] After lactation has been fully established and the regulation of milk volume occurs via autocrine mechanisms, progestin-containing contraceptives are less likely to have a negative effect.[126]

Although the postponement of a subsequent pregnancy is an important aspect of post-birth care for mothers of premature infants,[158] the selection of a contraceptive must consider the potential impact of the contraceptive on the initiation, establishment, and maintenance of maternal milk volume. At present, the administration of progestin contraceptives such as depot medroxyprogesterone acetate in the immediate post-birth period is inconsistent with the guidelines of the United States Food and Drug Administration,[159] and with recommendations of the WHO[160] and the American Congress of Obstetricians and Gynecologists.[161] Because the obligation of maternal-child health care providers is to protect breastfeeding, progestins should be avoided in the early post-birth period for breast pump–dependent mothers of premature infants until research to support their use in this vulnerable population is available. However, these mothers should receive thorough contraceptive counseling, and nonhormonal methods of contraception should be made available to them.

USING LACTATION TECHNOLOGIES TO MANAGE HUMAN MILK FEEDING PROBLEMS

The prevention, identification, and management of common human milk feeding problems in the NICU is a priority for NICU care providers and lactation specialists so that the infant can receive the highest possible dose of human milk, especially during critical exposure periods. Fortunately, many of the technologies that facilitate these processes have been thoroughly studied by human milk and lactation scientists, and have been adapted for use in the clinical setting. These methods include breast pump technology that is designed to meet the unique needs of breast pump–dependent women[42,136,162]; the creamatocrit technique to accurately and quickly measure the lipid and caloric content in expressed human milk[101,103,163–166]; the use of nipple shields to facilitate milk transfer during breastfeeding[167,168]; and test weights to accurately and precisely measure milk intake during breastfeeding.[94–99] Use of these technologies is easy to learn and should be the standard of care in evidence-based NICU best practices for managing lactation and human milk feeding in the NICU.

Although there is a plethora of scientific literature detailing the scientific foundations and appropriate use of these technologies, they have not been universally integrated into routine NICU care. One reason for this is that many NICU personnel believe that it is just "too much work" to manage human milk feedings and lactation processes so scientifically. For example, many staff members want a simple visual scoring system to estimate milk intake during breastfeeding, or would prefer a single the use of a "default value" (eg, 20 cal/ounce) for the caloric content of expressed human milk. The problem with these less objective mechanisms is that extensive research has demonstrated they are not accurate indicators of either milk intake during breastfeeding[95–97] or caloric density in individual containers of mothers' milk fed in the NICU.[42,101,103,164]

The other primary reason that these effective technologies have not been integrated into NICU best practices is that many lactation proponents believe they are not necessary, and that the focus on "numbers" undermines mothers' confidence. However, research with both test weights[95,96,98] and creamatocrits[163] has shown that NICU mothers can easily learn both techniques, and are reassured by knowing how much milk their infants consume and the caloric content of their milk. Another concern of lactation proponents is that these lactation technologies have been adapted from the research arena to the clinical setting by for-profit industries, so the industry's profit motive versus the "need" for the products is questioned.[169] However, nearly all other NICU products have evolved from industry and have been studied in industry-funded trials because federal dollars are more appropriately directed toward achieving the broader national health objectives for breastfeeding.[170] Rather than focusing on the politics of infant feeding, lactation products should be selected based on the evidence that they are effective in ensuring that infants receive the highest dose of human milk, especially during critical exposure periods.

Use of Breast Pump Technology Designed for and Tested with Breast Pump–Dependent Mothers

Despite the fact that mothers of premature and NICU infants must remain breast pump–dependent for weeks or months, few studies have focused on the effectiveness, efficiency, comfort, and convenience of the hospital-grade electric breast pump that mothers use. In fact, many lactation proponents believe that it is unethical to recommend a specific type of breast pump, despite support from the literature showing that certain breast pumps and breast pump features appear to be superior or more acceptable to pump-dependent mothers than are other pumps.[136,143,149,171,172] In contrast, most of the research in this area has been focused on care practices that influence maternal milk volume such as skin-to-skin holding or pumping regimens (eg, single vs double pumping). However, a breast pump is fundamental to a mother's ability to produce milk, and it is critical that NICU mothers receive the most effective, efficient, comfortable, and convenient breast pump available. Thus, NICU caregivers should provide breast pump recommendations based on the scientific evidence available for the pump, which should include scientific, systematic evaluation of the pump characteristics by breast pump–dependent mothers. Mothers will need to use the pump until their infants consume all milk directly from the breast, which for most infants is when they achieve term, corrected age or slightly later.[98]

Use of the Creamatocrit Technology to Measure Lipid and Calories in Expressed Human Milk

The creamatocrit technique, which involves centrifuging a small specimen of human milk in a capillary tube and then calculating the percentage of total milk volume equal to cream, has been the standard in the research arena since its first description for use with human milk in 1978.[103,165] The creamatocrit provides a quick, inexpensive, easy-to-perform, and accurate method of measuring the lipid and caloric content in expressed human milk[101,103,163–166] Recently the laboratory equipment used in the research arena was adapted into a 2-pound, portable, user-friendly device (Creamatocrit Plus, Medela Inc, McHenry, IL) that is ideal for use in the clinical setting.[101,103] Since it is well established that the lipid and caloric content vary tremendously in individually collected milk samples[103,105,164,166,173–175] and that NICU storage and feeding procedures further reduce baseline lipid and caloric content,[101,176,177] this device should be an essential part of routine NICU care.

A complete review of best NICU practices for preventing, diagnosing, and managing slow weight gain in premature infants that are predominantly or exclusively human milk fed has been published.[101] This review article includes several NICU case studies that detail the use of the creamatocrit technique as part of an overall plan for managing slow weight gain in the NICU setting, without the use of routine supplementation or "rescue" with formula.

Use of Nipple Shields During the Transition to Feeding at Breast for Premature Infants

Few premature infants are able to consume 100% of their feedings from the breast at the time of NICU discharge. A recent study of VLBW infants revealed that while 30.5% of VLBW infants received exclusively human milk at the time of discharge, fewer than 10% were feeding exclusively at the breast.[100] Among the physiologic immaturities on the part of the premature infant is that suction pressures, essential for creating and sustaining the nipple shape during breastfeeding, are not mature until approximately term, corrected age.[99,178] Although positioning techniques that include the mother's hand supporting the infant's head and scapulae can help compensate for the relative weight of the head and the immature suction pressures, many premature infants demonstrate greater milk transfer when feeding with an ultrathin nipple shield.[118,167,179]

The modern nipple shield concentrates the infant's suction pressure in the tunnel of the shield, stimulates the milk flow, and allows the infant to remove milk even with immature suction pressures. Although many lactation proponents think that nipple shields are unnecessary and overused, shorten duration of breastfeeding, and compromise milk transfer to the premature infant, research clearly demonstrates that the nipple shield is advantageous in establishing and maintaining breastfeeding for many premature infants. The indications and correct usage of the nipple shield in preterm and late preterm infants have been summarized in a recent review article.[99]

Use of Test-Weighing Technology to Measure Milk Intake During Breastfeeding

Test-weighing methods, whereby the infant is weighed pre- and post-breastfeeding under identical conditions, have been the standard research technique for measuring milk intake during breastfeeding since the advent of electronic digital scales in the 1980s.[180] In the past decade a lightweight, portable infant scale for measuring test weights has been developed from the more cumbersome research scales of the 1980s.[95] The adapted scale (BabyWeigh, Medela Inc, McHenry, IL, USA), which features the ability to program in the "pre-feed" weight, and to calculate milk intake (1 mL = 1 g) automatically after the infant is weighed post-feed, is ideal for use in the clinical setting or in the infant's home.[98,99,118,179]

Numerous controlled, blinded clinical trials have demonstrated that test weighing is accurate[94,95,180] and acceptable to mothers,[95,96,98] and that breastfeeding effectiveness "tools" or scoring systems do not accurately estimate intake during breastfeeding.[95,96] A review article that summarizes the indications and use of test weights to manage the transition to exclusive feeding at the breast for preterm and late preterm infants has been published.[99] This review features photographs and detailed clinical examples for integrating test weights into an overall post-discharge management plan that includes nipple shield use and breast pump use for this population.

SUMMARY

The evidence about human milk feedings for premature infants in the NICU indicates that there are critical exposure periods post-birth when exclusive or high doses of human milk provide the greatest protection from costly and handicapping morbidities in premature infants. These data should form the basis for research, practice, and quality outcome indicators in the NICU. Best practices to increase the dose and exposure period of human milk feedings in the NICU include: encouraging the mother to provide milk for her infant, providing cost-effective, expert lactation and human milk feeding support for families and staff; prioritizing the initiation, establishment, and maintenance of maternal milk volume; and using lactation technologies to manage human milk feeding problems.

REFERENCES

1. Lucas A, Cole TJ. Breast milk and neonatal necrotising enterocolitis. Lancet 1990;336(8730):1519–23.
2. El-Mohandes A, Picard M, Simmens S. Human milk utilization in the ICN decreases the incidence of bacterial sepsis [abstract]. Pediatr Res 1995;37:306A.
3. Hylander MA, Strobino DM, Dhanireddy R. Human milk feedings and infection among very low birth weight infants. Pediatrics 1998;102(3):E38.
4. Hylander MA, Strobino DM, Pezzullo JC, et al. Association of human milk feedings with a reduction in retinopathy of prematurity among very low birthweight infants. J Perinatol 2001;21(6):356–62.
5. Schanler RJ, Lau C, Hurst NM, et al. Randomized trial of donor human milk versus preterm formula as substitutes for mothers' own milk in the feeding of extremely premature infants. Pediatrics 2005;116(2):400–6.
6. Schanler RJ, Shulman RJ, Lau C. Feeding strategies for premature infants: Beneficial outcomes of feeding fortified human milk versus preterm formula. Pediatrics 1999;103(6 Pt 1):1150–7.
7. Furman L, Taylor G, Minich N, et al. The effect of maternal milk on neonatal morbidity of very low-birth-weight infants. Arch Pediatr Adolesc Med 2003;157(1):66–71.
8. Furman L, Wilson-Costello D, Friedman H, et al. The effect of neonatal maternal milk feeding on the neurodevelopmental outcome of very low birth weight infants. J Dev Behav Pediatr 2004;25(4):247–53.
9. Davidson B, Meinzen-Derr JK, Wagner CL, et al. Fucosylated oligosaccharides in human milk in relation to gestational age and stage of lactation. Adv Exp Med Biol 2004;554:427–30.
10. Hintz SR, Kendrick DE, Stoll BJ, et al. Neurodevelopmental and growth outcomes of extremely low birth weight infants after necrotizing enterocolitis. Pediatrics 2005;115(3):696–703.
11. Stoll BJ, Hansen NI, Adams-Chapman I, et al. Neurodevelopmental and growth impairment among extremely low-birth-weight infants with neonatal infection. JAMA 2004;292(19):2357–65.
12. Hack M. Young adult outcomes of very-low-birth-weight children. Semin Fetal Neonatal Med 2006;11(2):127–37.
13. Hack M, Taylor HG, Drotar D, et al. Chronic conditions, functional limitations, and special health care needs of school-aged children born with extremely low-birth-weight in the 1990s. JAMA 2005;294(3):318–25.
14. Marlow N, Wolke D, Bracewell MA, et al. Neurologic and developmental disability at six years of age after extremely preterm birth. N Engl J Med 2005;352(1):9–19.
15. Payne NR, Carpenter JH, Badger GJ, et al. Marginal increase in cost and excess length of stay associated with nosocomial bloodstream infections in surviving very low birth weight infants. Pediatrics 2004;114(2):348–55.
16. Perlman JM. Neurobehavioral deficits in premature graduates of intensive care—potential medical and neonatal environmental risk factors. Pediatrics 2001;108(6):1339–48.
17. Salhab WA, Perlman JM, Silver L, et al. Necrotizing enterocolitis and neurodevelopmental outcome in extremely low birth weight infants <1000 g. J Perinatol 2004;24(9):534–40.
18. Petrou S, Sach T, Davidson L. The long-term costs of preterm birth and low birth weight: results of a systematic review. Child Care Health Dev 2001;27(2): 97–115.

19. Ehrenkranz RA, Dusick AM, Vohr BR, et al. Growth in the neonatal intensive care unit influences neurodevelopmental and growth outcomes of extremely low birth weight infants. Pediatrics 2006;117(4):1253–61.
20. Ehrenkranz RA, Younes N, Lemons JA, et al. Longitudinal growth of hospitalized very low birth weight infants. Pediatrics 1999;104(2):280–9.
21. Drotar D, Hack M, Taylor G, et al. The impact of extremely low birth weight on the families of school-aged children. Pediatrics 2006;117(6):2006–13.
22. Uraizee F, Gross S. Improved feeding tolerance and reduced incidence of sepsis in sick very low birthweight (VLBW) infants fed maternal milk. Pediatr Res 1989;25:298A [abstract].
23. Simmer K, Metcalf R, Daniels L. The use of breastmilk in a neonatal unit and its relationship to protein and energy intake and growth. J Paediatr Child Health 1997;33(1):55–60.
24. Meinzen-Derr J, Poindexter B, Wrage L, et al. Role of human milk in extremely low birth weight infants' risk of necrotizing enterocolitis or death. J Perinatol 2009;29(1):57–62.
25. Vohr BR, Poindexter BB, Dusick AM, et al. Persistent beneficial effects of breast milk ingested in the neonatal intensive care unit on outcomes of extremely low birth weight infants at 30 months of age. Pediatrics 2007; 120(4):e953–9.
26. Vohr BR, Poindexter BB, Dusick AM, et al. Beneficial effects of breast milk in the neonatal intensive care unit on the developmental outcome of extremely low birth weight infants at 18 months of age. Pediatrics 2006;118(1):e115–23.
27. Sisk PM, Lovelady CA, Dillard RG, et al. Early human milk feeding is associated with a lower risk of necrotizing enterocolitis in very low birth weight infants. J Perinatol 2007;27:428–33 [Epub 2007, Apr 19].
28. Sisk PM, Lovelady CA, Gruber KJ, et al. HM consumption and full enteral feeding among infants who weigh </= 1250 grams. Pediatrics 2008;121(6): e1528–33.
29. Taylor SN, Basile LA, Ebeling M, et al. Intestinal permeability in preterm infants by feeding type: mother's milk versus formula. Breastfeed Med 2009;4(1):11–5.
30. Patel AL, Meier PP, Engstrom JL. The evidence for use of human milk in very low-birthweight preterm infants. Neoreviews 2007;8(11):e459. Accessed April 15, 2009.
31. Meier PP. Health benefits and cost of human milk for very low birthweight infants. 2007;1 R01–NR010009–01.
32. Miller J, McVeagh P. Human milk oligosaccharides: 130 reasons to breast-feed. Br J Nutr 1999;82(55):333–5.
33. Cregan MD, Fan Y, Appelbee A, et al. Identification of nestin-positive putative mammary stem cells in human breastmilk. Cell Tissue Res 2007;329(1):129–36.
34. Rodriguez NA, Miracle DJ, Meier PP. Sharing the science on human milk feedings with mothers of very-low-birth-weight infants. J Obstet Gynecol Neonatal Nurs 2005;34(1):109–19.
35. Diaz-Gomez NM, Domenech E, Barroso F. Breast-feeding and growth factors in preterm newborn infants. J Pediatr Gastroenterol Nutr 1997;24(3):322–7.
36. Dvorak B, Fituch CC, Williams CS, et al. Increased epidermal growth factor levels in human milk of mothers with extremely premature infants. Pediatr Res 2003;54(1):15–9.
37. Dvorak B, Fituch CC, Williams CS, et al. Concentrations of epidermal growth factor and transforming growth factor-alpha in preterm milk. Adv Exp Med Biol 2004;554:407–9.

38. Goldman AS, Chheda S, Keeney SE, et al. Immunologic protection of the premature newborn by human milk. Semin Perinatol 1994;18(6):495–501.
39. Montagne P, Cuilliere ML, Mole C, et al. Immunological and nutritional composition of human milk in relation to prematurity and mother's parity during the first 2 weeks of lactation. J Pediatr Gastroenterol Nutr 1999;29(1):75–80.
40. Ronayne de Ferrer PA, Baroni A, Sambucetti ME, et al. Lactoferrin levels in term and preterm milk. J Am Coll Nutr 2000;19(3):370–3.
41. Shoji H, Shimizu T, Shinohara K, et al. Suppressive effects of breast milk on oxidative DNA damage in very low birthweight infants. Arch Dis Child Fetal Neonatal Ed 2004;89(2):F136–8.
42. Meier PP, Engstrom JL. Evidence-based practices to promote exclusive feeding of human milk in very low-birthweight infants. Neoreviews 2007;8(11):e467 [Accessed April 15, 2009].
43. Claud EC, Walker WA. Bacterial colonization, probiotics, and necrotizing enterocolitis. J Clin Gastroenterol 2008;42(Suppl 2):S46–52.
44. Labbok M, Krasovec K. Toward consistency in breastfeeding definitions. Stud Fam Plann 1990;21(4):226–30.
45. Meier PP, Brown LP. Limitations of the Labbok and Krassovec breastfeeding classification for preterm infants [letter]. J Nurse Midwifery 1997;42: 1259–60.
46. Meinzen-Derr J, Poindexter BB, Donovan EF, et al. Human milk and late-onset sepsis in infants 401-1000 grams: a secondary analysis. International Society for research in human milk and lactation. Proceedings of the Cambridge, UK, 12th International Conference, 2004:44.
47. Patel AL, Engstrom JL, Goldman J, et al. Dose response benefits of human milk in extremely low birth weight premature infants [abstract]. Pediatrlc Academic Societies; 2008.
48. Petrou S, Mehta Z, Hockley C, et al. The impact of preterm birth on hospital inpatient admissions and costs during the first 5 years of life. Pediatrics 2003;112(6 Pt 1):1290–7.
49. Bisquera JA, Cooper TR, Berseth CL. Impact of necrotizing enterocolitis on length of stay and hospital charges in very low birth weight infants. Pediatrics 2002;109(3):423–8.
50. Weimer J. The economic benefits of breastfeeding: a review and analysis. USDA 2001;13:1–14.
51. Neville MC. Anatomy and physiology of lactation. Pediatr Clin North Am 2001; 48(1):13–34.
52. Neville MC, Morton J, Umemura S. Lactogenesis. The transition from pregnancy to lactation. Pediatr Clin North Am 2001;48(1):35–52.
53. Sangild PT, Siggers RH, Schmidt M, et al. Diet- and colonization-dependent intestinal dysfunction predisposes to necrotizing enterocolitis in preterm pigs. Gastroenterology 2006;130(6):1776–92.
54. Sangild PT, Schmidt M, Elnif J, et al. Prenatal development of gastrointestinal function in the pig and the effects of fetal esophageal obstruction. Pediatr Res 2002;52(3):416–24.
55. Sangild PT, Mei J, Fowden AL, et al. The prenatal porcine intestine has low transforming growth factor-beta ligand and receptor density and shows reduced trophic response to enteral diets. Am J Physiol Regul Integr Comp Physiol 2009;296(4):R1053–62.
56. Sangild PT. Gut responses to enteral nutrition in preterm infants and animals. Exp Biol Med (Maywood) 2006;231(11):1695–711.

57. Underwood MA, Gilbert WM, Sherman MP. Amniotic fluid: not just fetal urine anymore. J Perinatol 2005;25(5):341–8.
58. Jensen AR, Elnif J, Burrin DG, et al. Development of intestinal immunoglobulin absorption and enzyme activities in neonatal pigs is diet dependent. J Nutr 2001;131(12):3259–65.
59. Mei J, Zhang Y, Wang T, et al. Oral ingestion of colostrum alters intestinal transforming growth factor-beta receptor intensity in newborn pigs. Livest Sci 2006; 105:214–22.
60. Thymann T, Burrin DG, Tappenden KA, et al. Formula-feeding reduces lactose digestive capacity in neonatal pigs. Br J Nutr 2006;95(6):1075–81.
61. Newburg DS, Walker WA. Protection of the neonate by the innate immune system of developing gut and of human milk. Pediatr Res 2007;61(1):2–8.
62. Vidal K, Donnet-Hughes A. CD14: a soluble pattern recognition receptor in milk. In: Bosze Z, editor. Bioactive components of milk. New York: Springer; 2008. p. 195–216.
63. Labeta MO, Vidal K, Nores JE, et al. Innate recognition of bacteria in human milk is mediated by a milk-derived highly expressed pattern recognition receptor, soluble CD14. J Exp Med 2000;191(10):1807–12.
64. Vidal K, Donnet-Hughes A. CD14: a soluble pattern recognition receptor in milk. Adv Exp Med Biol 2008;606:195–216.
65. Rodriguez NA, Meier PP, Groer MW, et al. Oropharyngeal administration of colostrum to extremely low birth weight infants: theoretical perspectives. J Perinatol 2009;29(1):1–7. Accessed November 24, 2009.
66. Rodriguez NA, Meier PP, Groer MW, et al. A pilot study of the oropharyngeal administration of own mother's colostrum to extremely low birth weight infants. Adv Neonatal Care, in press.
67. Patel AL, Engstrom JL, Meier PP, et al. Effect of human milk feedings on growth velocity and major morbidity in extremely low birth weight infants in the neonatal intensive care unit [abstract]. Chicago: Rush University Forum for Research and Clinical Investigation; 2008
68. Chaud EC, Walker WA. Hypothesis: inappropriate colonization of the premature intestine can cause necrotizing enterocolitis. FASEB J 2001;15: 1398–403.
69. Cotten CM, Taylor S, Stoll B, et al. Prolonged duration of initial empirical antibiotic treatment is associated with increased rates of necrotizing enterocolitis and death for extremely low birth weight infants. Pediatrics 2009;123(1): 58–66.
70. Magne F, Suau A, Pochart P, et al. Fecal microbial community in preterm infants. J Pediatr Gastroenterol Nutr 2005;41(4):386–92.
71. Martin R, Langa S, Reviriego C, et al. Human milk is a source of lactic acid bacteria for the infant gut. J Pediatr 2003;143(6):754–8.
72. Perez PF, Dore J, Leclerc M, et al. Bacterial imprinting of the neonatal immune system: lessons from maternal cells? Pediatrics 2007;119(3):e724–32.
73. Mackie RI, Sghir A, Gaskins HR. Developmental microbial ecology of the neonatal gastrointestinal tract. Am J Clin Nutr 1999;69(5):1035S–45S.
74. Penders J, Thijs C, Vink C, et al. Factors influencing the composition of the intestinal microbiota in early infancy. Pediatrics 2006;118(2):511–21.
75. Harmsen HJ, Wildeboer-Veloo AC, Raangs GC, et al. Analysis of intestinal flora development in breast-fed and formula-fed infants by using molecular identification and detection methods. J Pediatr Gastroenterol Nutr 2000; 30(1):61–7.

76. Rautava S, Walker WA. Commensal bacteria and epithelial cross talk in the developing intestine. Curr Gastroenterol Rep 2007;9(5):385–92.
77. Minekawa R, Takeda T, Sakata M, et al. Human breast milk suppresses the transcriptional regulation of IL-1beta-induced NF-kappaB signaling in human intestinal cells. Am J Physiol, Cell Physiol 2004;287(5):11.
78. Caicedo RA, Schanler RJ, Li N, et al. The developing intestinal ecosystem: implications for the neonate. Pediatr Res 2005;58(4):625–8.
79. Claud EC, Savidge T, Walker WA. Modulation of human intestinal epithelial cell IL-8 secretion by human milk factors. Pediatr Res 2003;53(3):419–25.
80. Schultz C, Temming P, Bucsky P, et al. Immature anti-inflammatory response in neonates. Clin Exp Immunol 2004;135(1):130–6.
81. Poindexter BB, Ehrenkranz RA, Stoll BJ, et al. Parenteral glutamine supplementation does not reduce the risk of mortality or late-onset sepsis in extremely low birth weight infants. Pediatrics 2004;113(5):1209–15.
82. Hack M, Flannery DJ, Schluchter M, et al. Outcomes in young adulthood for very-low-birth-weight infants. N Engl J Med 2002;346(3):149–57.
83. Fanaroff AA, Korones SB, Wright LL, et al. Incidence, presenting features, risk factors and significance of late onset septicemia in very low birth weight infants. the national institute of child health and human development neonatal research network. Pediatr Infect Dis J 1998;17(7):593–8.
84. Brandtzaeg P. The secretory immunoglobulin system: regulation and biological significance: focusing on human mammary glands. In: Davis MK, Isaacs CE, Hanson LA, Wright AL, editors. Integrating population outcomes, biological mechanisms and research methods in the study of human milk and lactation. New York: Plenum Press; 2002. p. 1–16.
85. Andersson B, Porras O, Hanson LA, et al. Inhibition of attachment of *Streptococcus pneumoniae* and *Haemophilus influenzae* by human milk and receptor oligosaccharides. J Infect Dis 1986;153(2):232–7.
86. Nakhla T, Fu D, Zopf D, et al. Neutral oligosaccharide content of preterm human milk. Br J Nutr 1999;82(5):361–7.
87. Siafakas CG, Anatolitou F, Fusunyan RD, et al. Vascular endothelial growth factor (VEGF) is present in human breast milk and its receptor is present on intestinal epithelial cells. Pediatr Res 1999;45(5 Pt 1):652–7.
88. Resto M, O'Connor D, Leef K, et al. Leptin levels in preterm human breast milk and infant formula. Pediatrics 2001;108(1):E15.
89. Ip S, Chung M, Raman G, et al. Breastfeeding and maternal and infant health outcomes in developed countries. Evid Rep Technol Assess 2007;(153):1–186.
90. Schanler RJ. Post-discharge nutrition for the preterm infant. Acta Paediatr Suppl 2005;94(449):68–73.
91. O'Connor DL, Jacobs J, Hall R, et al. Growth and development of premature infants fed predominantly human milk, predominantly premature infant formula, or a combination of human milk and premature formula. J Pediatr Gastroenterol Nutr 2003;37(4):437–46.
92. O'Connor DL, Khan S, Weishuhn K, et al. Growth and nutrient intakes of human milk-fed preterm infants provided with extra energy and nutrients after hospital discharge. Pediatrics 2008;121(4):766–76.
93. Griffin IJ. Postdischarge nutrition for high risk neonates. Clin Perinatol 2002; 29(2):327–44.
94. Meier PP, Lysakowski TY, Engstrom JL, et al. The accuracy of test weighing for preterm infants. J Pediatr Gastroenterol Nutr 1990;10(1):62–5.

95. Meier PP, Engstrom JL, Crichton CL, et al. A new scale for in-home test-weighing for mothers of preterm and high risk infants. J Hum Lact 1994;10(3):163–8.
96. Meier PP, Engstrom JL, Fleming BA, et al. Estimating milk intake of hospitalized preterm infants who breastfeed. J Hum Lact 1996;12(1):21–6.
97. Meier PP, Engstrom JL. Test weighing for term and premature infants is an accurate procedure. Arch Dis Child Fetal Neonatal Ed 2007;92(2):F155–6.
98. Hurst NM, Meier PP, Engstrom JL, et al. Mothers performing in-home measurement of milk intake during breastfeeding of their preterm infants: maternal reactions and feeding outcomes. J Hum Lact 2004;20(2):178–87.
99. Meier PP, Furman LM, Degenhardt M. Increased lactation risk for late preterm infants and mothers: evidence and management strategies to protect breastfeeding. J Midwifery Womens Health 2007;52(6):579–87.
100. Davanzo R, Ronfani L, Brovedani P, et al. Breastfeeding in Neonatal Intensive Care unit Study Group. Breast feeding very-low-birthweight infants at discharge: a multicentre study using WHO definitions. Paediatr Perinat Epidemiol 2009;23(6):591–6.
101. Meier PP, Engstrom JL. Preventing, diagnosing and managing slow weight gain in the human milk-fed very low birthweight infant. Sulla Nutrizione Con Latte Materno 2008;33–47.
102. Ensgtrom JL, Meier PP, Motykowski JE, et al. Effect of human milk storage method and capillary tube type on creamatorcrit (CRCT) values in the neonatal intensive care unit (NICU). Breastfeed Med 2008;3:79.
103. Meier PP, Engstrom JL, Zuleger JL, et al. Accuracy of a user-friendly centrifuge for measuring creamatocrits on mothers' milk in the clinical setting. Breastfeed Med 2006;1(2):79–87.
104. Kent JC, Mitoulas LR, Cregan MD, et al. Volume and frequency of breastfeedings and fat content of breast milk throughout the day. Pediatrics 2006;117(3):e387–95.
105. Spencer SA, Hull D. Fat content of expressed breast milk: a case for quality control. Br Med J 1981;282(6258):99–100.
106. Tyson J, Burchfield J, Sentance F, et al. Adaptation of feeding to a low fat yield in breast milk. Pediatrics 1992;89(2):215–20.
107. World Health Organization. Breastfeeding. Available at: http://www.who.int/topics/breastfeeding/en/. Accessed November 28, 2009.
108. United States Breastfeeding Committee. USBC: a brief history. Available at: http://www.usbreastfeeding.org/AboutUs/History/tabid/62/Default.aspx. Accessed November 28, 2009.
109. American Academy of Pediatrics, Committee on Nutrition. Breastfeeding and the use of human milk. Pediatrics 2005;115(2):496–506.
110. Miracle DJ, Meier PP, Bennett PA. Mothers' decisions to change from formula to mothers' milk for very-low-birth-weight infants. J Obstet Gynecol Neonatal Nurs 2004;33(6):692–703.
111. Miracle DJ, Fredland V. Provider encouragement of breastfeeding: efficacy and ethics. J Midwifery Womens Health 2007;52(6):545–8.
112. Lu MC, Lange L, Slusser W, et al. Provider encouragement of breast-feeding: evidence from a national survey. Obstet Gynecol 2001;97(2):290–5.
113. Pate B. A systematic review of the effectiveness of breastfeeding intervention delivery methods. J Obstet Gynecol Neonatal Nurs 2009;38(6):642–53.
114. Sisk PM, Lovelady CA, Dillard RG, et al. Lactation counseling for mothers of very low birth weight infants: effect on maternal anxiety and infant intake of human milk. Pediatrics 2006;117(1):e67–75.

115. Friedman S, Flidel-Rimon O, Lavie E, et al. The effect of prenatal consultation with a neonatologist on human milk feeding in preterm infants. Acta Paediatr 2004;93(6):775–8.
116. "In Your Hands" Rush Mothers' Milk Club. Rush Mothers' Milk Club. Available at: http://www.rushmothersmilkclub.com. Accessed November 28, 2009.
117. Meier PP, Engstrom JL, Mingolelli SS, et al. The Rush Mothers' Milk Club: breastfeeding interventions for mothers with very-low-birth-weight infants. J Obstet Gynecol Neonatal Nurs 2004;33(2):164–74.
118. Meier PP. Supporting lactation in mothers with very low birth weight infants. Pediatr Ann 2003;32(5):317–25.
119. Freed GL, Clark SJ, Cefalo RC, et al. Breast-feeding education of obstetrics-gynecology residents and practitioners. Am J Obstet Gynecol 1995;173(5):1607–13.
120. Hellings P, Howe C. Breastfeeding knowledge and practice of pediatric nurse practitioners. J Pediatr Health Care 2004;18(1):8–14.
121. Register N, Eren M, Lowdermilk D, et al. Knowledge and attitudes of pediatric office nursing staff about breastfeeding. J Hum Lact 2000;16(3):210–5.
122. Spear HJ. Baccalaureate nursing students' breastfeeding knowledge: a descriptive survey. Nurse Educ Today 2006;26(4):332–7.
123. Bernaix LW, Schmidt CA, Arrizola M, et al. Success of a lactation education program on NICU nurses' knowledge and attitudes. J Obstet Gynecol Neonatal Nurs 2008;37(4):436–45.
124. Merewood A, Philipp BL, Chawla N, et al. The baby-friendly hospital initiative increases breastfeeding rates in a US neonatal intensive care unit. J Hum Lact 2003;19(2):166–71.
125. United States Breastfeeding Committee. Core competencies in breastfeeding care for all health professionals. Available at: http://www.usbreastfeeding.org/LinkClick.aspx?link=Publications%2fCore-Competencies-2009-USBC.pdf%tabid=70&mid=388. Accessed November 28, 2009.
126. Hale TW. Medications and mother's milk. 13th edition. Amarillo (TX): Hale Publishing; 2008.
127. Rossman B. Breastfeeding peer counselors in the united states: helping to build a culture and tradition of breastfeeding. J Midwifery Womens Health 2007;52(6):631–7.
128. Merewood A, Chamberlain LB, Cook JT, et al. The effect of peer counselors on breastfeeding rates in the neonatal intensive care unit: results of a randomized controlled trial. Arch Pediatr Adolesc Med 2006;160(7):681–5.
129. Meier PP. Breastfeeding peer counselors in the NICU: increasing access to care for very low birthweight infants. Hindsdale (IL): Illinois Children's Healthcare Foundation; 2005.
130. Martin JA, Hamilton BE, Sutton PD, et al. Births: final data for 2006. Natl Vital Stat Rep 2009;57(7):1–102.
131. Li R, Fridinger F, Grummer-Strawn L. Racial/ethnic disparities in public opinion about breastfeeding: the 1999–2000 healthstyles surveys in the United States. Adv Exp Med Biol 2004;554:287–91.
132. Li R, Darling N, Maurice E, et al. Breastfeeding rates in the united states by characteristics of the child, mother, or family: the 2002 national immunization survey. Pediatrics 2005;115(1):e31–7.
133. Cricco-Lizza R. Black non-Hispanic mothers' perceptions about the promotion of infant-feeding methods by nurses and physicians. J Obstet Gynecol Neonatal Nurs 2006;35(2):173–80.

134. Rossman B. Breastfeeding peer counselors in the neonatal intensive care unit: maternal perspectives. Chicago: University of Illinois at Chicago; 2009. [Doctoral dissertation].
135. Jegier BJ, Meier PP, Engstrom JL, et al. The initial maternal cost of providing 100 mL of human milk for very low birth weight infants in the neonatal intensive care unit. Breastfeeding Medicine, in press.
136. Meier PP, Engstrom JL, Hurst NM, et al. A comparison of the efficiency, efficacy, comfort, and convenience of two hospital-grade electric breast pumps for mothers of very low birthweight infants. Breastfeed Med 2008;3(3): 141–50.
137. Cregan MD, De Mello TR, Kershaw D, et al. Initiation of lactation in women after preterm delivery. Acta Obstet Gynecol Scand 2002;81(9):870–7.
138. Cregan MD, de Mello TR, Hartmann PE. Pre-term delivery and breast expression: consequences for initiating lactation. Adv Exp Med Biol 2000; 478:427–8.
139. Hill PD, Aldag JC, Zinaman M, et al. Predictors of preterm infant feeding methods and perceived insufficient milk supply at week 12 postpartum. J Hum Lact 2007;23(1):32–8.
140. Hill PD, Aldag JC, Chatterton RT, et al. Comparison of milk output between mothers of preterm and term infants: the first 6 weeks after birth. J Hum Lact 2005;21(1):22–30.
141. Hill PD, Aldag JC, Chatterton RT, et al. Primary and secondary mediators' influence on milk output in lactating mothers of preterm and term infants. J Hum Lact 2005;21(2):138–50.
142. Hill PD, Aldag JC, Chatterton RT. Effects of pumping style on milk production in mothers of non-nursing preterm infants. J Hum Lact 1999;15(3):209–16.
143. Slusher T, Hampton R, Bode-Thomas F, et al. Promoting the exclusive feeding of own mother's milk through the use of hindmilk and increased maternal milk volume for hospitalized, low birth weight infants (< 1800 grams) in Nigeria: a feasibility study. J Hum Lact 2003;19(2):191–8.
144. Lawrence RA, Lawrence RM, editors. Breastfeeding: a guide for the medical profession. 6th edition. Philadelphia: Mosby; 2005. p. 72–3.
145. Kent JC. How breastfeeding works. J Midwifery Womens Health 2007;52(6): 564–70.
146. Neville MC, Morton J. Physiology and endocrine changes underlying human lactogenesis II. J Nutr 2001;131(11):3005S–8S.
147. Chapman D, Perez-Escamilla R. Maternal perception of the onset of lactation: a valid indicator of lactogenesis stage II? Adv Exp Med Biol 2000;478:423–4.
148. Perez-Escamilla R, Chapman D. Can women remember when their milk came in? Adv Exp Med Biol 2001;501:567–72.
149. Morton J, Hall JY, Wong RJ, et al. Combining hand techniques with electric pumping increases milk production in mothers of preterm infants. J Perinatol 2009;29(11):757–64.
150. Knight CH, Peaker M, Wilde CJ. Local control of mammary development and function. Rev Reprod 1998;3(2):104–12.
151. Engstrom JL. The establishment of an adequate maternal milk volume, in press.
152. Rodriguez MI, Kaunitz AM. An evidence-based approach to postpartum use of depot medroxyprogesterone acetate in breastfeeding women. Contraception 2009;80(1):4–6.
153. King J. Contraception and lactation. J Midwifery Womens Health 2007;52(6): 614–20.

154. Halderman LD, Nelson AL. Impact of early postpartum administration of progestin-only hormonal contraceptives compared with nonhormonal contraceptives on short-term breast-feeding patterns. Am J Obstet Gynecol 2002; 186(6):1250–8.
155. Baheiraei A, Ardsetani N, Ghazizadeh S. Effects of progestogen-only contraceptives on breast-feeding and infant growth. Int J Gynecol Obstet 2001; 74(2):203–5.
156. Truitt ST, Fraser AB, Grimes DA, et al. Hormonal contraception during lactation: systematic review of randomized controlled trials. Contraception 2003;68(4): 233–8.
157. Hurst NM. Recognizing and treating delayed or failed lactogenesis II. J Midwifery Womens Health 2007;52(6):588–94.
158. Grisaru-Granovsky S, Gordon ES, Haklai Z, et al. Effect of interpregnancy interval on adverse perinatal outcomes—a national study. Contraception 2009; 80(6):512–8.
159. United State Food and Drug Administration. Physician information for depo provera. Available at: http://www.accessdata.fda.gov/drugsatfda_docs/label/2004/20246s025lbl.pdf. Accessed November 28, 2009.
160. World Health Organization. Medical eligibility criteria for contraceptive use, 4th edition. 2009. Available at: http://whqlibdoc.who.int/publications/2009/9789241563888_eng.pdf. Accessed February 9, 2010.
161. American College of Obstetricians and Gynecologists. Breastfeeding: maternal and infant aspects. ACOG Clin Rev 2007;12(Suppl):1S–16S. Available at: http://www.acog.org/departments/underserved/clinicalReviewv12i1s.pdf. Accessed November 28, 2009.
162. Engstrom JL, Meier PP, Jegier BJ, et al. Comparison of milk output from the right and left breasts during simultaneous pumping in mothers of very low birthweight infants. Breastfeeding Medicine 2007, in press.
163. Griffin TL, Meier PP, Bradford LP, et al. Mothers' performing creamatocrit measures in the NICU: accuracy, reactions, and cost. J Obstet Gynecol Neonatal Nurs 2000;29(3):249–57.
164. Meier PP, Engstrom JL, Murtaugh MA, et al. Mothers' milk feedings in the neonatal intensive care unit: accuracy of the creamatocrit technique. J Perinatol 2002;22(8):646–9.
165. Lucas A, Gibbs JA, Lyster RL, et al. Creamatocrit: simple clinical technique for estimating fat concentration and energy value of human milk. Br Med J 1978; 1(6119):1018–20.
166. Wang CD, Chu PS, Mellen BG, et al. Creamatocrit and the nutrient composition of human milk. J Perinatol 1999;19(5):343–6.
167. Meier PP, Brown LP, Hurst NM, et al. Nipple shields for preterm infants: effect on milk transfer and duration of breastfeeding. J Hum Lact 2000; 16(2):106–14.
168. Chertok IR, Schneider J, Blackburn S. A pilot study of maternal and term infant outcomes associated with ultrathin nipple shield use. J Obstet Gynecol Neonatal Nurs 2006;35(2):265–72.
169. Meier P. Concerns regarding industry-funded trials. J Hum Lact 2005;21(2): 121–3.
170. Brown LP, Bair AH, Meier PP. Does federal funding for breastfeeding research target our national health objectives? Pediatrics 2003;111(4 Pt 1):e360–4.
171. Slusher T, Slusher IL, Biomdo M, et al. Electric breast pump use increases maternal milk volume in African nurseries. J Trop Pediatr 2007;53(2):125–30.

172. Meier PP, Engstrom JL, Janes JE, et al. Comfort and effectiveness of new pumping patterns for the initiation and maintenance of lactation in breast pump-dependent mothers of premature infants, manuscript submitted for publication.
173. Hytten FE. Clinical and chemical studies in human lactation. Br Med J 1954; 1(4855):175–82.
174. Daly SE, Di Rosso A, Owens RA, et al. Degree of breast emptying explains changes in the fat content, but not fatty acid composition, of human milk. Exp Physiol 1993;78(6):741–55.
175. Weber A, Loui A, Jochum F, et al. Breast milk from mothers of very low birthweight infants: variability in fat and protein content. Acta Paediatr 2001;90(7):772–5.
176. Brennan-Behm M, Carlson GE, Meier P, et al. Caloric loss from expressed mother's milk during continuous gavage infusion. Neonatal Netw. J Neonatal Nurs 1994;13(2):27–32.
177. Greer FR, McCormick A, Loker J. Changes in fat concentration of human milk during delivery by intermittent bolus and continuous mechanical pump infusion. J Pediatr 1984;105(5):745–9.
178. Lau C, Alagugurusamy R, Schanler RJ, et al. Characterization of the developmental stages of sucking in preterm infants during bottle feeding. Acta Paediatr 2000;89(7):846–52.
179. Meier PP. Breastfeeding in the special care nursery. prematures and infants with medical problems. Pediatr Clin North Am 2001;48(2):425–42.
180. Woolridge MW, Butte N, Dewey KG, et al. Methods for the measurement of milk volume intake of the breastfed infant. In: Jensen RG, Neville MC, editors. Human lactation: milk components and methodologies. New York: Plenum Press; 1985. p. 5–20.

Decreasing Central Line Associated Bloodstream Infection in Neonatal Intensive Care

Richard J. Powers, MD[a,*], David W. Wirtschafter, MD[b]

KEYWORDS

- Central line associated bloodstream infection
- Nosocomial infection • Bloodstream infection
- Quality improvement

Health care associated infection (HAI) and central line associated bloodstream infection (CLABSI) are major foci of efforts in the realm of safety and error reduction because they represent such an obvious example of a breakdown in the systems of hospital care. Despite the attention that is placed on this topic and the resources expended in research and technology to reduce these infections, the problem persists.

This discussion attempts to shed light on why the problem of CLABSI has not been eliminated as have certain infectious diseases or simple public safety problems. The article discusses the specific evidence-based strategies that have been shown to be effective in reducing CLABSI, the barriers to their adoption in the complex hospital environment, and how they can be successfully overcome.

The authors' goal is to convince readers that the journey toward decreasing CLABSI to zero begins and ends with the reader's appreciation that it is more about *how* we do the right care processes rather than choosing the right processes. The mantra of quality improvement—ensuring that the right process is being used at the right time—is all too often given short shrift as users search for the newest products, policies and best practices. This truism is perhaps best exemplified by model newborn intensive care units (NICUs) throughout the country that have maintained low levels of infection even as patients, products, policies, and practices have so

[a] Good Samaritan Hospital, Newborn Intensive Care Unit, Pediatrix Neonatology Medical Group of San Jose, 3880 South Bascom Avenue, Suite 208, San Jose, CA 95124, USA
[b] David Wirtschafter, MD, Inc, 5523 Voletta Place, Valley View, CA 91607, USA
* Corresponding author.
E-mail address: richard_powers@pediatrix.com

Clin Perinatol 37 (2010) 247–272
doi:10.1016/j.clp.2010.01.014 perinatology.theclinics.com

dramatically changed over 3 decades[1,2] (S. Butler, personal communication, October 2009). Their achievement demonstrates that it is *how* we sustain best practices within the NICU that is critical to continually decreasing CLABSI toward a zero infection rate.[3]

WHY DOES CONTEXT MATTER?

Context refers to the complicated milieu that makes up the unique culture of each NICU. These units are complex workplaces in which hundreds of providers interact either directly or indirectly with large numbers of patients and their families, often for many days or even months. It is not surprising that this merging of various individuals' knowledge, experiences, attitudes, and languages produces many unique and even unstable combinations of these personal factors. The evolution of these combinations is nonlinear and unit-specific. Introducing new processes inevitably stresses these relationships and challenges their evaluation. Studies of organizational learning highlight specific leadership characteristics that are associated with receptivity to change, such as encouraging openness to excellence, learning mechanisms that encourage information flow and aid systems-thinking, and commitment of resources.[4] Each of these factors is uniquely different from center to center. Successful introduction of new processes is thus dependent on understanding the unique human dynamics of each organization. Berwick[5] describes this process as using the construct of "context" as set forth by Pawon and Tilley.[6]

Why Does This Matter to the NICU Patient?

Mortality

Attributable mortality is the proportion of deaths in hospitalized patients who acquire a bloodstream infection that is due to the infection and not the underlying disease. The attributable mortality for bloodstream infection, calculated from case control studies, typically ranges from 15% to 35% for adult patients.[7] Several studies have reported attributable mortality due to HAI in neonates. The rates in these studies vary from 24% in the pre-surfactant era to 11% in the post-surfactant era.[8–10]

Morbidity

The toll of CLABSI in neonates extends beyond the short-term mortality statistics. Newborn sepsis has been shown to be associated with adverse outcomes in multiple systems, the most important of which is the central nervous system (CNS). In short-term and longitudinal follow up studies, the National Institute of Child Health and Human Development (NICHD) Neonatal Research Network and others have shown an association between sepsis, poor growth, and adverse neurodevelopmental outcome at 2 years.[10–12] Abnormalities of the white matter in magnetic resonance imaging studies are reported to be the predominant CNS lesion associated with sepsis.[12,13] This association is supported by emerging evidence that links white matter injury to pre-oligodendroglial cell damage from reactive oxygen species and inflammatory cytokines.[14]

Other systems are also affected by sepsis, most likely through similar mechanisms mediated by inflammatory cytokines. Neonatal sepsis has been associated with longer duration of mechanical ventilation, higher incidence of chronic lung disease, and hepatic fibrosis.[10,15,16] Finally, the cumulative toll of the multisystem injury resulting from sepsis along with the actual short-term morbidity of the sepsis event itself contribute substantially to the duration of hospitalization of affected infants.[10,17,18]

What are the Technical Issues?

Hand colonization

Hand colonization of hospital personnel with pathogenic organisms is associated with transmission of these organisms and HAI.[2,19–21] The role of hand colonization in the transmission of pathogenic organisms has been the subject of numerous cohort and prospective studies, beginning in the nineteenth century with observations by Labarraque and Semmelweis.[22–24] Efforts at reducing hand colonization have led to decreased HAI in hospital-wide studies[25–28] and in the NICU.[29–32] More important are studies that have demonstrated the direct transmission of pathogens from health care workers to catheter material.[24,33,34] This pathway is the key to understanding and appreciating the crucial role of hand colonization in the acquisition of CLABSIs. When hands with high bacterial colony counts come into contact with connections, access ports, or catheter hubs, the organisms become resident in those areas. The potential transformation of individual bacterial colonies to a living planktonic layer or biofilm increases with each exposure.[35,36] Contact with surfaces inside the isolette in the general area of the patient but not part of the central line setup is still problematic, as the accumulation of high pathogenic bacterial counts on these surfaces indirectly contributes to central line contamination when they are touched after hand antisepsis and the central line is subsequently manipulated.[37,38]

Central line colonization

CLABSI prevention is dependent on our ever-changing understanding of the mechanisms of line colonization and subsequent infection. Adult CLABSI studies point to either extraluminal or intraluminal line contamination.[39–42] Accordingly, access techniques and equipment have evolved to obviate open disconnection of lines or, wherever necessary, to ensure decontamination of the hub entry point prior to its entry and continuing sterility during its manipulation. Garland and colleagues[43] performed molecular subtyping of organisms harvested from the skin surrounding neonatal peripherally inserted central catheter (PICC) insertion sites, their hubs, the catheter tips, and blood cultures, finding, as did the earlier observation by Salzman and colleagues,[44] that hub colonization was often present and the organism was concordant with simultaneously drawn blood cultures (80% and 71%, respectively). Garland and colleagues concluded that at least 67% of the CLABSIs were intraluminally acquired. These studies form the scientific basis for using techniques and equipment that address each of these vulnerabilities, for example, insertion site decontamination, closed vascular access systems, needleless connectors, and scrupulous hub decontamination prior to entry.

How is CLABSI Defined?

Different definitions of bloodstream infections (BSI) or CLABSI have evolved as the subject has been increasingly studied. Regarding the actual definition of a *bloodstream infection*, the gold standard is a positive blood culture. The term *nosocomial infection* often includes hospital acquired pneumonia and urinary tract infections, and the term *sepsis* usually describes a clinical presentation not requiring a positive blood culture. A *central line associated bloodstream infection* is a bloodstream infection that occurs with a central line in place or within 48 hours of a central line being removed when no other source of infection is identified.[45]

The other essential factor to be addressed in defining BSI is how to distinguish between a true infection and a contaminated specimen when a blood culture is positive with the growth of a common contaminant, eg, Coagulase-negative *Staphylococcus* (CONS). Various strategies are suggested to make this distinction, either based on multiple cultures or the time to detection as a proxy for the quantity of organisms in the original sample. Studies in neonates suggest that as many as 33% to 50% of positive blood cultures with CONS are contaminants.[2,46]

MICROBIOLOGY

The distribution of organisms associated with neonatal BSIs has been reported by the NICHD (15 United States neonatal ICUs) and by the Israel Neonatal Network, representing 28 Israeli neonatal ICUs[10,47] (**Table 1**). Both large networks report a similar pattern of pathogens, with gram-positive organisms predominating. In both series the most common single organism associated with BSI was CONS (47% and 55% for Israel and the NICHD, respectively). This finding underscores the importance of incorporating specific criteria in the definition of laboratory confirmed bloodstream infection to account for the prevalence of this skin contaminant as a frequent source of infection. Both networks use the same composite definition of sepsis with CONS, requiring a positive blood culture and the presence of specific clinical symptoms.

Beyond the impact of CONS, gram-negative organisms, coagulase-positive *Staphylococcus*, and *Candida* species are the remaining pathogens commonly associated with neonatal bloodstream infection. Gram-negative organisms play an important role due to their obvious source coming from the maternal genitourinary tract with colonization at or shortly after birth. The gram-positive organisms, especially coagulase-positive and coagulase-negative staphylococci, are most often acquired from skin colonization, on the skin of both the patient and the health care workers' hands.[19,20] The gram-negative organisms and *Candida* species are also introduced into the patient's bloodstream via the patient's or health care worker's skin as the primary source of colonization.

Successful Programs Address a Mix of Technical and Contextual Factors

Care "bundles" describe multiple interventions that are disseminated nearly simultaneously to address one or more interrelated clinical or administrative problems. The concept was popularized by the Institute for Healthcare Improvement (IHI)[48] and has served as an important means to further innovation, especially with regard to preventing HAI.[49] Their potential efficacy derives from 3 streams of evolving understandings about the challenges in preventing and controlling HAI: (1) the appreciation that consensus statements of "provisional best practices," also termed guidelines, are an effective way to translate complex knowledge into effective practices; (2) the epidemiologic perspective that there are many contributing factors to HAI; and (3) the demonstrated utility of "bundled" interventions in the NICU to promote multiple, simultaneous, and effective changes in practices.[2,50–56]

Guidelines have been a means to define medical and nursing practice consensus for decades.[57] Reviews of their evolution, in particular with regard to their scientific quality, efficacy, and effectiveness, have been commented on by Sinuff and colleagues[58] in general, by Boluyt and colleagues[59] with regard to pediatrics, and by Merritt and colleagues[60,61] with regard to neonatal examples. Guideline noncompliance studies have noted factors that impede implementation such as ambiguous evidence, perception of irrelevance to individual patient or contextual situations, and so forth.[62,63] Nonetheless, on balance, systematic evaluations suggest that they are effective, especially when addressing multidimensional problem-solving tasks such as preventing CLABSI.

Heavy skin colonization, line placement with limited use of sterile barriers, site of line placement, line replacement over a guide wire, contamination of the catheter hub, line

Table 1
Distribution of Pathogens Associated with Bloodstream Infections in Very Low Birthweight Infants

	Israel Neonatal Network		NICHD Network	
Organism	**N**	**(%)**	**N**	**(%)**
Gram-positive organisms	**1043**	**55.4**	**922**	**70.2**
Coagulase-negative Staph	899	47.3	629	47.9
Coagulase-positive Staph	74	3.9	103	7.8
Enterococcus/group D Strep	54	2.9	43	3.3
Group B Streptococcus	6	0.3	30	2.3
Other	20	1.1	117	8.9
Gram-negative organisms	**593**	**31.2**	**231**	**17.6**
Klebsiella	277	14.7	52	4
Pseudomonas	80	4.2	35	2.7
Enterobacter	72	3.8	33	2.5
Escherichia coli	53	2.8	64	4.9
Acinetobacter	44	2.3	-	-
Other	67	3.6	47	3.5
Mixed organisms	**34**	**1.8**	-	-
Gram-negative and Gram-negative	18	0.9	-	-
Gram-negative and Gram-positive	10	0.5	-	-
Bacteria and fungi	6	0.3	-	-
Candida	**210**	**11.1**	-	-
Candida albicans	49	2.6	76	5.8
Candida parapsilosis	36	1.9	54	4.1
Unspecified Candida/Fungal sp.	125	6.6	30	2.3
Total	**1880**	**100**	**1313**	**100**

Stoll 2002 and Makhoul 2002.

placement greater than 7 days, inexperienced marginally skilled operators, and host susceptibility are among the many significant factors identified with the risk of a CLABSI in general.[64] Neonatal reviews have identified additional factors: poor skin integrity and prolonged line necessity.[53,65] Interventions that focus on only one challenge, even critically important ones such as hand hygiene, may not be associated with sustained gains; hence the need to implement changes simultaneously.[48]

Table 2 compares major dimensions of reported "bundle" implementations in NICUs during the last decade. Their assessment is problematic for several reasons. The NICUs do not all share the same metrics: some report *all* BSI regardless of deduced cause and then have varied the denominator by total admissions or by total patient days. Also, the CLABSI definition has been refined and then made more stringent[66] over the last decade, making it impossible to compare rates from before 2008 to those reported subsequently. The latest changes have caused rates to decrease, based solely on definitional changes, by at least one-third.[67] Because the reports span eras of rapidly falling baseline rates, processes associated with initial gains are no longer considered innovative changes that merit reporting, as NICUs implement additional changes in the quest to achieve "zero" infection levels.[68]

Table 2
Bundle implementation in NICUs

References	Kil03[2,167]	Gol02[50]	And05[51]	Aly05[52]	Sch06[53]	Wir09[54]	Lee09[55]	Cur09[168]
Processes specifically addressed								
Diagnostic processes	■	░	░	░	░	■	░	░
Hand hygiene optimization	■		■		■	■	■	■
Chlorhexidene use			■			■	■	■
Skin breaks management							■	
Vascular access								
Maximal barrier precautions					■	■	■	■
PICC team inserts lines	■	■	■		■	■	■	■
PICC team manages lines		■				■	?	■
Dressing change management		■		■		■	■	■
Line necessity review	■		■		■	■		■
Closed vascular systems	■			■		■		
Line entry management	■			■	■	■	■	■
Unit Culture: audit & feedback						■		■
Unit Culture: multi-disciplinary	■				■	■		■

Other related process								
Earlier enteral feeds	■				■	■		
Ventilator circuit management							■	
Antibiotic use							■	
Visit restrictions							■	
Outcomes								
Design	p/p	p/p	p/p	p/p	p/p	p/p	rct	p/p
% Reduction	34.0%	62%	57%	87%	55%	25%	32%	93%
Level at end of process	16.5%	5.8*	9%	2.0[a]	3.8[b]	3.2[a]	17.4[c]	0.2[d]

The black squares indicate that NICUs emphasized additional efforts to ensure compliance with existing standard CDC definition. The gray squares indicate use of existing standard definition without mention of additional efforts to ensure compliance.

Abbreviations: p/p, pre-/post-study design; rct, randomized controlled trial.

[a] BSI/1000 line days pre 08 CDC definition.

[b] BSI/1000 patient days pre 08 CDC definition.

[c] all BSI per 100 patients pre 08 CDC definition.

[d] CLABSI per 1000 line days 08 CDC definition.

Finally, the thematic presentation of an intervention begs the question of "context" and "the devil in the details" surrounding each described intervention. Aboelela and colleagues[69] completed a systematic review of bundle implementations and noted the scarcity of data about component compliance or, when reported, the wide variance of compliance rates making evaluation of any particular intervention's efficacy problematic. Even simple extrapolation from a list of interventions described by the collaborative's leadership may only indicate an idealization of what may have been implemented. For instance, in the Canadian NICU dissemination trial, there were 34 recommended processes to be implemented by the 5 study NICUs, making a total of 170 possible practices to be implemented.[55] Of these, 36% were already in place before the study, 38% were implemented during the study, and 25% of them were ignored. Notwithstanding these caveats, as well as recognizing that many items included in "bundles" have not, or cannot, be evaluated using conventional randomized controlled trial methodology, the authors propose that the following processes contribute to prevention and control of CLABSI in NICUs based on the compilation shown in **Table 2**, the additional evidence noted in this discussion, and their personal experiences with 3 prevention networks.

Improve Your Unit's "Safe Culture" Measures

The landmark reports from the Institute of Medicine, *To Err is Human* and *Crossing the Quality Chasm*, brought together the foundations of and galvanized the future agenda for efforts to improve patient safety. Although safety efforts affect all patient processes, the discussion here is limited to summarizing the relevance of these efforts to decreasing CLABSIs as demonstrated by the successful efforts of Pronovost and colleagues[70] in the Michigan Keystone ICU Project. Their efforts started with reflecting on how we would know that patients are safer. Pronovost and colleagues proposed a balance of "immature" measures: 2 rate-based measures (CLABSI rate and percentage compliance with a ventilator-associated pneumonia prevention bundle) and 2 qualitative measures (how often the authors learn from defects and whether a unit has a safe culture). These investigators used the measure of safety culture tool validated by their colleague Sexton.[71] As noted in its communication, the 5-point Likert scaled question: "In this ICU, it is difficult to speak up if I perceive a problem with patient care" has the strongest correlation with the complete questionnaire's scoring of teamwork climate. More dramatically, the CLABSI decreases noted in the 108 participating ICUs were highly correlated with improvements in the "Teamwork Climate" scale of the simultaneously administered safety attitude questionnaire associated with a targeted program to improve the units' safety climate.[72–74] Thus, the authors recommend that units make this issue an integral part of their initial effort. Possibly their hospital will have implemented a house-wide effort that can satisfy this need. Alternatively, the authors have found that NICUs can implement program metrics as simple as periodically distributing the single question shown above on the staff's sense of safely voicing concerns, akin to the famous Toyota "Stop the Line" mantra, and use it to monitor their efforts to improve the culture of safety in their units.[75]

Implementation of Evidence-Based Practices

Hand hygiene

Perform hand hygiene before contact with central lines Hand antisepsis must be performed before and after contact with the patient and any equipment that comes in contact with the patient, or touching contaminated objects in the environment. If gloves have been used, hand antisepsis should be performed on their removal.

Hand antisepsis refers to the use of either a waterless alcohol product or an antiseptic detergent containing chlorhexidine gluconate (CHG) or triclosan.

Alcohol-based waterless agents have been shown to be at least as effective as or in some studies more effective than CHG and triclosan, against gram-positive and gram-negative bacteria and most viruses.[24,76–79] Soaps containing CHG or triclosan are necessary when hands are visibly soiled to remove the organic material, and they have a theoretical advantage in that both agents have a residual effect after rinsing. Alcohol is nevertheless a very effective antiseptic agent, despite the lack of residual effect. Alcohol has been shown in numerous clinical studies to be more effective than antiseptic washes due to its ease of use, ready availability, and reduced skin irritation.[78,80–83] It is the recommended agent of choice in the hospital setting, including the NICU. Effective alcohol products contain either isopropyl alcohol (IPA) or ethyl alcohol (EA) at 60% to 95%. These products also have emollients that substantially improve their tolerance by health care workers.

Ensure compliance with hand hygiene expectations Despite the strong recommendations and educational campaigns urging health care workers to perform appropriate hand hygiene before and after patient contact, studies have repeatedly documented that compliance is well below expectations. Health care workers are aware of the science of pathogen transmission, but are often overwhelmed in their minute-to-minute tasks of routine patient care and responding to bedside emergencies related to patient instability. It has been shown that there are up to 20 opportunities for hand hygiene per hour[84] and that hand hygiene compliance approximates 40%.[19] Barriers to hand hygiene compliance are related to lack of ready access to hand hygiene products, skin irritation of health care workers' hands, understaffing, overcrowding, and lack of any direct consequence for noncompliance.[84,85]

Hand hygiene interventions are most effective in reducing CLABSIs if they focus on the processes related to central line manipulation, ie, insertion, maintenance, and access to these lines. This approach has been demonstrated in examples of successful central line bundle implementation, where the hand hygiene survey processes are specifically aimed at these interventions.[54,70] Targeting the central line manipulations provides a more concentrated effort in the area where consequences of nonadherence to hand hygiene regimens are the greatest.

Insertion of central lines

Use maximal barrier precautions for insertion of central catheters Maximal barrier precautions require the use of sterile cap, mask, gown, gloves, and drape. The rationale for this practice is the reduction of contamination during insertion of an indwelling catheter. The benefits of this approach have been demonstrated in prospective randomized trials with adult critical care patients. In a randomized controlled trial, Mermel studied maximal barrier precautions during the insertion of pulmonary artery catheters and showed a significant effect of this practice on the reduction of CLABSI.[86]

Perform skin antisepsis at the catheter entry site Use of a CHG solution is recommended in this situation. The residual effect of CHG-containing preparations gives them preference for prolonged antimicrobial action to inhibit extraluminal migration of organisms colonizing the skin surface once the catheter is placed. In numerous studies with adult patients, CHG-containing solutions have been shown to be superior to povidone-iodine in reducing the incidence of bloodstream infection.[87] Garland and colleagues[88] also showed a similar advantage of CHG over povidone-iodine in neonates. Concerns over sensitivity reactions with CHG have been raised,[51] but these should be weighed against the relative benefits of this agent over those without residual effect and the fact that all skin antiseptics have relative adverse effects, for example, systemic absorption with iodine causing thyroid suppression and local skin reactions along with systemic absorption of alcohol in neonates.[89] CHG is the recommended skin antisepsis agent in the Association of Women's Health, Obstetric and Neonatal Nurses/National Association of Neonatal Nurses skin guideline and is specified in the Central Line Bundle adapted from the IHI used in the Michigan Keystone ICU Project.[70,90] Local skin reactions can be mitigated by rinsing with sterile water after a 30-second application, as the residual effect will still remain.[77] Due to ongoing concerns over local reactions, many centers limit the use of CHG preparations in the most premature infants, at least in the immediate perinatal period, choosing povidone instead.

Use a dedicated team Use a dedicated team of individuals who have received special training for insertion, maintenance, and monitoring of central lines. Numerous studies have demonstrated the advantages of this approach. By assuring that proper technique is used by those with the most expertise in the technical aspects as well as clinical decision-making regarding management of line complications, lines are placed with fewer attempts and CLABSI rates have been decreased.[91–94]

Select the appropriate site Catheter insertion site is emphasized by the Centers for Disease Control and Prevention (CDC) in the 2002 Guideline and is a prominent component of the IHI Central Line Bundle.[19] Factors influencing these recommendations are the association of phlebitis with CLABSIs along with the known association of phlebitis with lines placed in the lower extremities compared with the upper extremities. The density of skin flora is another factor behind this recommendation, with the subclavian site preferable over the internal jugular or femoral sites, due to the lower density of skin colonization. These factors are less relevant in neonates as lower extremity catheters have actually been shown to have fewer infectious complications than those in upper extremities. Intuitively, the density of colonization at the insertion site should be a factor in umbilical lines, but Butler-O'Hara and colleagues[95] have shown that umbilical lines left in for 28 days have the same infection rate compared with the practice of removal at 7 days followed by placement of a PICC line for 21 days.

Maintenance of central lines

Minimize access ports Line setups should be designed to minimize the number of ports/connections. Each port of entry and connector must be viewed as an independent opportunity for line contamination. The intuitive notion that minimizing entry points will reduce opportunities for violating technique is strengthened by a prospective randomized clinical trial in which a significantly higher rate of CLABSI events was associated with the use of triple-lumen catheters than with single-lumen catheters.[96] Needleless ports are recommended because they do not require opening to provide access, and they can be cleaned thoroughly before entry.[19] Closed medication systems decrease opportunities for contamination, especially when connecting ports are placed far from areas contaminated by diapers.[52]

Change line setups and access ports in a timely fashion Intravenous administration sets should be changed at recommended intervals: parenteral solutions containing dextrose or amino acids every 72 hours; lipid-containing solutions and sets used for administration of blood products every 24 hours.[97–101] Needleless access ports should be changed at least as often as administration sets. Some manufacturers may recommend a longer interval for changing, but in vivo clinical studies point to contamination of these ports as a source of CLABSI[102–104] and demonstrate the presence of bacterial biofilm on the connectors by 72 hours in a majority of patients studied.[105]

Manage the insertion site Dressings covering the catheter insertion site are important in securing the line, which prevents migration, dislodgement, or breakage, and aids in preventing the entry of microorganisms at the insertion site. Sterile gauze or sterile transparent dressings have been studied and neither material has been shown to be superior in preventing CLABSIs.[106,107] Transparent occlusive dressings are used more commonly as they allow one the ability to inspect the insertion site for local complications and potential line dislodgement, but they are more difficult to manage if blood is oozing from the insertion site. The CDC recommends changing the dressing if it becomes damp, loosened, or visibly soiled.[19] It is also recommended to be changed every 48 hours if it is a gauze or tape dressing, if there is a gauze beneath an occlusive dressing, or if a transparent dressing is no longer adherent to the skin.[108–110] Surgical cap, mask, and sterile gloves should be worn by the personnel making the dressing change. In addition to these CDC minimum recommendations, a sterile gown is suggested by others, primarily based on expert opinion.[108] The same method of skin antisepsis recommended for initial insertion, that is, CHG solution, is recommended for the dressing change, due to the residual effect.

Sterilize access ports before entry The original studies showed efficacy with disinfection of needless access devices with IPA, but recent guidelines suggest that CHG/IPA combinations may be better.[98,102,103,111] Menyhay and Maki[112] evaluated 3 needleless valve connectors by exposing each to a known load of contaminating bacteria. Of the 30 connectors accessed after conventional disinfection (3–5 second swabbing using a sterile swab of 70% IPA), 67% were found to have significant growth of colony-forming units in the broth recovered from subsequent flushing. Donlan and colleagues[105] showed a 63% incidence of biofilm contamination composed primarily of CONS in a series of needleless connectors collected from patients on a bone marrow transplant unit. Kaler[113] compared disinfection of 3 different needleless devices using 15-second hub scrubs with either 3% CHG/70% IPA or 70% IPA, and found them to be equally effective. These data motivate current recommendations to scrub connectors for 15 seconds before and after entry. CHG or IPA are both recommended as noted here, but CHG is increasingly being described as the preferred disinfecting agent, perhaps because of its demonstrated persistence. The UK National Health Service Hospitals Guideline advises that an alcoholic chlorhexidine gluconate solution (preferably 2% CHG in 70% IPA) should be used and allowed to dry when decontaminating the injection port or catheter hub before and after it has been used to access the system.[114] Soothill and colleagues[115] describe a pediatric transplant service's 75% decrease in CLABSI after switching connection disinfectants to 2% CHG/70% IPA from 70% IPA in accord with this recommendation. Recently, manufacturers have introduced new self-swabbing disinfecting caps, although further evaluations of how these various products can be effectively implemented are needed.[116]

Bacteria, following entry into a device, can develop biofilm within the device that extends throughout the catheter. Scanning electron microscopy of needleless connectors shows the typical features of both bacterial cells and apparent extracellular polymeric substances within the device[36,105,117] (**Figs. 1–3**). Bacteria gain adherence to the smooth catheter surfaces through a process termed conditioning, whereby organic molecules such as proteins are absorbed by the polymer and then alter its mechanical characteristics. Murga and colleagues[118] demonstrated how blood, when drawn back

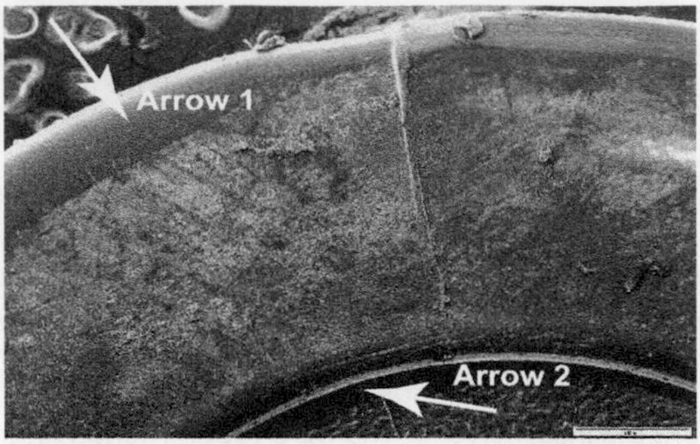

Fig. 1. Scanning electron microscopy images show the rim (*arrow 1*) and a small part of the access port (*arrow 2*) of a connector that has been used on an intensive care patient. (*From* Ryder M. Improve CRBSI prevention: target intraluminal risks. Executive Healthcare Management 2009; Issue 8; with permission. Available at: http://www.executivehm.com/article/Improve-CRBSI-Prevention-Target-Intraluminal-Risks/.)

and forth through a catheter, can serve as an adequate source of conditioning materials to promote biofilm formation by gram-negative bacteria. Donlan and colleagues[105,119] have reviewed alternative means to eradicate biofilm: antibiotic lock protocols are presently available and effective for sensitive bacteria, but less so for fungi; other means, such as ultrasound, bacteriophages, quorum-sensing inhibitors, or enzymes are currently being developed and evaluated.

Lastly, needleless connector design has gone through several phases and it is still not clear if, and how, the design features affect the likelihood of these connectors becoming contaminated.[117,120] Investigation of outbreaks associated with needleless connectors suggest that particular design characteristics may be associated with more frequent contamination when used in actual clinical environments as distinguished from evaluations under laboratory conditions.[121,122] The previously mentioned Society for Healthcare Epidemiology of America/Infectious Diseases Society of America strategies statement cautions users of positive-pressure needleless connectors to weigh their risks and benefits,[111] which has in turn generated controversy.[39,123] The unsettled state of these technologies obliges clinicians to

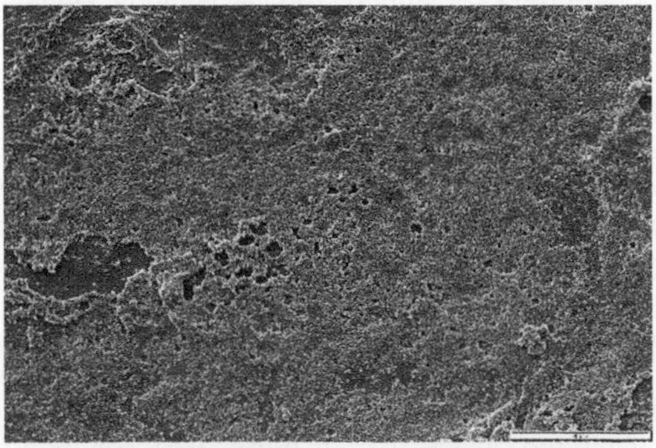

Fig. 2. Higher magnifications reveal that large areas of the rim are covered with a dense biofilm. (*From* Ryder M, Schaudinn C, Gorur A, et al. Microscopic evaluation of microbial colonization on needleless connectors. Publication Number 5-36, APIC Annual Education Conference, Denver, CO 2008; with permission.)

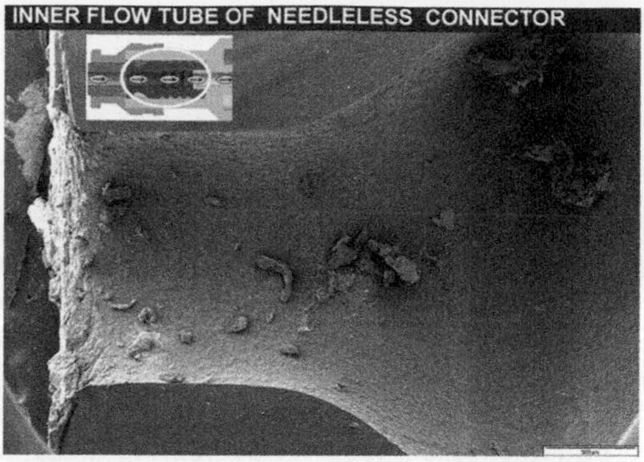

Fig. 3. Biofilm visible inside needleless connector. (*From* Ryder M. Improve CRBSI prevention: target intraluminal risks. Executive Healthcare Management 2009; Issue 8; with permission. Available at: http://www.executivehm.com/article/Improve-CRBSI-Prevention-Target-Intraluminal-Risks/.)

maintain a constant vigilance for emerging technologies and their evaluations under both laboratory and clinical conditions.

Monitor the necessity of central lines The longer a central line is in place, the greater is the risk of infection. This observation has been confirmed in several studies in newborns.[10,124–126] In the largest of these studies, Stoll and colleagues[10] showed that use beyond 22 days was a critical threshold for all types of central lines, after which the risk of infection increased substantially. Chathas and colleagues[124] showed the same increased risk at 21 days. The primary purpose and ongoing need for the central catheter should be assessed on a daily basis to facilitate its removal in a timely manner.

Ensure compliance with line management expectations Compliance-enhancing measures include continuing efforts to ensure adequate initial training to perform the procedures, provision of adequate supplies for their execution, and ongoing programs to encourage and monitor their implementation. Kilbride and colleagues[2] reported that institutional NICU cohesion around these practices was observed to be very high, and epitomized implementation of the concept of "unit culture" as a necessary ingredient for successful practice of a care process, especially when that process requires frequent daily repetitions, often for weeks to months, by many different personnel.

Evaluate and Incorporate Quality Improvement Methods into your Unit's Operation

Sustained quality improvement is highly dependent on successful administration of both the adoption and application of technical processes within the NICUs. Medical and nursing professionals may underestimate the necessity of addressing this factor because of the difficulty in addressing it or, worse, denigrate it because of the lack of randomized controlled trials to validate it. A recent critical review of Six Sigma, Lean, and Studer Group transformational strategies in health care found no studies using randomized controlled trial evaluation designs and only a few studies using pre-/post-interventional evaluative designs.[127] Despite the weakness of the published reports, the market acceptance and adoption of these transformational strategies suggests a large body of experiential evidence driving their acceptance as fulfilling this administrative need.

Griffiths and colleagues[128] evaluated studies of organizational factors affecting successful infection control programs and reached similar conclusions: lack of high-quality studies but prerequisites to achieving infection control must include processes that address senior and ward leadership, staff morale, and stability. Specific implemented techniques include the use of the "Toyota Production System" ideas in the successful CLABSI prevention work described at the Allegheny General Hospital[129] and at the University of Washington Children's Hospital.[130] Studer Group ideas were used in the HAI prevention work described by Murphy.[131] Nelson and colleagues,[132,133] who have developed the concept of the "clinical microsystem" as the building block for understanding the management and transformation of clinical practice and have provided excellent tools for addressing these tasks. Edwards, as Director of Dartmouth-Hitchcock NICU, has collaborated with them in adapting and demonstrating the utility of these concepts to the NICU environment and HAI prevention.[134,135]

Manage your project leadership using the "Plan-Do-Study-Act" methodology

Alternatively, variations of the "Plan-Do-Study-Act" (PDSA) methodology have been promoted as effective means for managing practice adoption. PDSA is the methodology advocated principally by the influential IHI (see IHI Improvement Methods at http://www.ihi.org/ihi/topics/improvement/improvementmethods/). Caldwell, in *Mentoring Strategic Change in Health Care*,[136] provides very practical advice on how to manage change using the Plan-Do-Check-Act model. For instance, the California Perinatal Quality Care Collaborative (CPQCC) Toolkit[137] incorporates and models these recommended steps in its guide for NICU CLABSI prevention project management. Other neonatal CLABSI prevention projects have used the PDSA model to guide their efforts.[2,55,138] The authors recommend PDSA methods, especially in the context of NICUs whose quality improvement methodology is not tied to other methods adopted hospital-wide in their medical centers.

Build internal and external levels of collaboration as a means to participate in learning communities

Collaboration is at the heart of team learning. Bohmer and Edmondson[139] have highlighted differences between individual and team learning: whereas the former describes the individual's learning as a one-way knowledge transfer, learning as "keeping up," and repetition as the path to best practice, team learning occurs at multiple levels involving all those who participate in the process, is an ongoing process that develops and refines knowledge-in-use, and is one in which reflection rather than repetition is the critical process.

At the tactical level, team learning should be an integral part of each NICU's daily processes. Effectively applied learning processes, such as the aforementioned PDSA cycles or clinical microsystem development, exemplify some of the ways that this can be realized, and they should become the norm for unit learning. The authors recommend that each NICU seek to involve increasing numbers of their staff in these team-learning processes and, in consideration of this structural quality improvement goal, that units include a metric to reflect their progress toward this goal.

At the operational level, CLABSI prevention requires successful collaboration with many individuals and departments based outside of the NICU hierarchy. Each of these entities needs to be tactfully and respectfully approached to ensure appropriate understanding as to how each functionary can best work to serve the patient's interests. Practical points, such as how lines can be arranged prior to off-NICU procedures so as to anticipate the anesthesiologist's, surgeon's, or radiologist's needs, can avoid unintended breaks in line care during these procedures. Likewise, all visiting consultants, house staff, and technicians need to understand how they can comply with the unit's policies for protecting lines and maintaining the patient's environment. The magnitude and the challenges of these learning processes cannot be overestimated, nor their overemphasized.

At the strategic level, collaboration among like-minded colleagues from other institutions, both near and far, is increasingly being seen as a more effective way of spreading useful ideas between centers. Successful collaboratives cultivate mutual trust, support nonlinear development of problem-solving strategies, and focus on process and outcome measurement to drive change.[140] There are now many productive neonatal collaboratives, whether based on voluntary relationships, for example, VON, or structural affinities, CPQCC and Pediatrix Medical Group, which exemplify the utility and feasibility for each NICU to participate in one or more collaborative relationships.

Ensure audit and feedback

Audit and feedback are time-honored methods to define objectives and measure their achievement,[141] which build on the notion that standardization is the foundation of excellence.[142] Audits can address care processes, outcomes, or both. Process audits can be viewed as retrospective mirrors of prospectively deployed checklists. For instance, auditing hand hygiene practice has been a mainstay of HAI prevention.[143] Audit results drove the adoption of alcohol-based hand rubs to improve hand hygiene compliance in busy ICUs.[144] However, further consideration has led to understanding how poorly global hand hygiene audits reflect actual performance. "Secret shoppers" have been used to obtain unobtrusive observations,[145] but their utility is mitigated by difficulties in assuring the observer's continuing anonymity and staff expense proxy measures, such as the volume of consumed disinfectants have been used with some effect.[146] Of greater concern is recent evidence that compliance falls off during multi-step complex tasks, suggesting that observation schedules should be weighted more toward complex events.[37]

These experiences form the basis for the authors' recommendation that NICU managers take a broader view to identifying the process steps critical to achieving lowered CLABSI rates.[129,130] At a minimum, periodic audits of line set-up and line entry should be incorporated into the NICU routine in a manner similar to the accepted norms for hand hygiene compliance, as was recently demonstrated in a California collaborative.[54,67,136] This collaborative demonstrated how to periodically audit for a range of essential HAI prevention processes and noted prompt compliance improvement.

Feedback needs to be both objective and subjective but, more importantly, on time and frequent. Objective displays of progress as manifested by various process and outcome metrics serve to enable everyone in the NICU to "know the score." Leaders can model their concern by including simple inquiries during their rounds about "what's the score," for example, how many days has it been since our last CLABSI? Annotated "run charts," that is, statistical process control charts that include pointers describing the dates of key initiatives, serve to reinforce the staff's understanding that positive change does occur. There can never be enough recognition of achievements, whether individual or by the group, especially when delivered by higher management levels. And celebrations, accompanied by "healthy" foods, are always welcomed by NICU staff members!

Implement a real-time positive blood culture review process

Reflecting on adverse events is a key characteristic of high reliability organizations (HRO).[147–150] CLABSI events deservedly rate this type of attention, starting with the first receipt in the NICU of a positive blood culture report.[129] The authors have used an investigative technique that seeks to gather circumstantial evidence surrounding each event, based on published and personal experiences of implicated associations with CLABSIs.[137] Anecdotal reports indicate that users found these focused reviews well worth their time. Perhaps the most important user observation has been that investigations beginning at the first report of a positive culture enable far richer verbal recollection of antecedent events than when inquiries are limited solely to chart reviews. These observations then need to be followed by critical thinking as to what system changes could have prevented the sequence of events leading to the infection. Their value is enhanced when the experiences and learning are shared anonymously with peers in a collaborative, as each description can often generate new hypotheses or productive solutions.

Monitor Emerging Practices

The aforementioned interventions are discussed in the context of the central line bundle, reflecting the common strategies that have proven to be effective when introduced simultaneously. As such, these practices are focused and short term, chosen in many cases for their more rapid effect. There still are potentially useful interventions that should be considered in designing a unit-specific strategy to reduce CLABSI, even though they may not yield gains in the relatively short term of bundle interventions.

Intravenous immunoglobulin

Nineteen randomized controlled trials of prophylactic intravenous immunoglobulin (IVIG) including approximately 5000 infants were reviewed in a meta-analysis by Ohlsson and Lacy,[151] showing a significant decrease in incidence of infection with an overall reduction of 3%. However, because of the potential morbidity of this treatment and its high cost relative to a small treatment effect, IVIG is not generally recommended.

Vancomycin prophylaxis

Strategies incorporating prophylactic systemic vancomycin have shown efficacy in reducing overall sepsis and CONS sepsis rates.[152] Garland and colleagues[153] reported a randomized trial demonstrating the efficacy of a vancomycin-heparin lock solution in reducing the incidence of CLABSI. Due to concern over selection of vancomycin-resistant organisms, these strategies are not widely recommended, although in certain situations where staphylococcal sepsis is prevalent they may be justified.

Human milk feedings

Three small randomized controlled trials and several observational studies have been reported in which human milk feedings were compared with formula for protection against neonatal sepsis.[154] Human milk was shown to have a protective effect, but the overall quality of the studies is poor. Human milk feeding has numerous other nutritional benefits along with any shown in these studies, and is recommended even in the absence of quality data proving its benefit in reducing sepsis. Early introduction of human milk may also promote earlier establishment of full enteral nutrition, thus contributing to shorter duration of central line use.[155,156]

Reduced intravenous lipid duration

Lipids have been shown in 2 observational studies to be associated with increased CONS bacteremia.[157,158] The association is thought to be due to an immunosuppressive effect of intravenous lipids as well as the propensity to support microbial growth.[159] The nutritional value of the extra energy provided by lipids should be balanced by their potential risk for CLABSI.

Technical innovation

Important technological developments are constantly underway. These include antibiotic impregnated catheters,[160–164] antibiotic dressings for central lines with either CHG or silver,[165–167] new designs of needleless connectors with features to minimize the opportunity for biofilm development, antibiotic releasing caps, and specialized scrubbers for needleless connectors.[114,119,120] These developments are often first reported in trade journals before publication in the medical literature, illustrating the importance of monitoring development in these areas as well as traditional sources. However, caution should be exercised with adoption of new technologies, as there may be harmful side effects more prevalent in vulnerable premature infants or incompatibilities of materials leading to their dysfunction.

SUMMARY

CLABSI results in increased mortality and adverse outcomes related to multiple systems with lifelong consequences. CLABSIs have come to be recognized as preventable adverse events that result from lapses in technique at multiple levels of care. This recognition is essential to instill the appropriate sense of personal accountability for individual health care workers necessary to motivate change. Strategies to reduce CLABSI have been described in the literature over the past decades. Successful changes have incorporated these strategies into bundles of practice that are more effective when introduced simultaneously. New clinical and technological studies demonstrate that the science of CLABSI reduction is dynamic, with ongoing modifications in technique and innovations in hardware elements. Equally important in efforts at CLABSI reduction is a thoughtful and systematic approach tailored to the unique elements that comprise an individual NICU, addressing the social as well as the scientific elements of change.

REFERENCES

1. Unger A, Goetzman BW, Chan C, et al. Nutritional practices and outcome of extremely premature infants. Am J Dis Child 1986;140:1027–33.
2. Kilbride HW, Powers R, Wirtschafter DD, et al. Evaluation and development of potentially better practices to prevent neonatal nosocomial bacteremia. Pediatrics 2003;111:e504–18.
3. Kilbride HW, Wirtschafter DD, Powers RJ, et al. Implementation of evidence-based potentially better practices to decrease nosocomial infections. Pediatrics 2003;111(4 Pt 2):e519–33.
4. Carroll JS, Edmondson AC. Leading organisational learning in health care. Qual Saf Health Care 2002;11:51–6.
5. Berwick DM. The science of improvement. JAMA 2008;299:1182–4.
6. Pawson R, Tilley N. Realistic evaluation. London, England: Sage Publications, Ltd; 1997.
7. Wenzel RP. Perspective: attributable mortality: the promise of better antimicrobial therapy. J Infect Dis 1998;178:917–9.
8. Townsend TR, Wenzel RP. Nosocomial bloodstream infections in a newborn intensive care unit: a case-matched control study of morbidity, mortality and risk. Am J Epidemiol 1981;114:73–80.

9. Pessoa-Silva CL, Miyasaki CH, de Almeida MF, et al. Neonatal late-onset bloodstream infection: attributable mortality, excess of length of stay and risk factors. Eur J Epidemiol 2001;17:715–20.
10. Stoll BJ, Hansen N, Fanaroff AA, et al. Late-onset sepsis in very low birth weight neonates: the experience of the NICHD Neonatal Research Network. Pediatrics 2002;110:285–91.
11. Stoll BJ, Hansen NI, Adams-Chapman I, et al. Neurodevelopmental and growth impairment among extremely low-birth-weight infants with neonatal infection. JAMA 2004;292:2357–65.
12. Shah DK, Doyle LW, Anderson PJ, et al. Adverse neurodevelopment in preterm infants with postnatal sepsis or necrotizing enterocolitis is mediated by white matter abnormalities on magnetic resonance imaging at term. J Pediatr 2008; 153:170–5, 5 e1.
13. Glass HC, Bonifacio SL, Chau V, et al. Recurrent postnatal infections are associated with progressive white matter injury in premature infants. Pediatrics 2008; 122:299–305.
14. Back SA. Perinatal white matter injury: the changing spectrum of pathology and emerging insights into pathogenetic mechanisms. Ment Retard Dev Disabil Res Rev 2006;12:129–40.
15. Lahra MM, Beeby PJ, Jeffery HE. Intrauterine inflammation, neonatal sepsis, and chronic lung disease: a 13-year hospital cohort study. Pediatrics 2009;123:1314–9.
16. Hermans D, Talbotec C, Lacaille F, et al. Early central catheter infections may contribute to hepatic fibrosis in children receiving long-term parenteral nutrition. J Pediatr Gastroenterol Nutr 2007;44:459–63.
17. Payne NR, Carpenter JH, Badger GJ, et al. Marginal increase in cost and excess length of stay associated with nosocomial bloodstream infections in surviving very low birth weight infants. Pediatrics 2004;114:348–55.
18. Mahieu LM, Buitenweg N, Beutels P, et al. Additional hospital stay and charges due to hospital-acquired infections in a neonatal intensive care unit. J Hosp Infect 2001;47:223–9.
19. O'Grady NP, Alexander M, Dellinger EP, et al. Guidelines for the prevention of intravascular catheter-related infections. Centers for Disease Control and Prevention. MMWR Recomm Rep 2002;51:1–29.
20. Milisavljevic V, Wu F, Cimmotti J, et al. Genetic relatedness of *Staphylococcus epidermidis* from infected infants and staff in the neonatal intensive care unit. Am J Infect Control 2005;33:341–7.
21. Larson EL. APIC guideline for handwashing and hand antisepsis in health care settings. Am J Infect Control 1995;23:251–69.
22. Labarraque AG. Instructions and observations regarding the use of chlorides of soda and lime. New Haven (CT): Baldwin and Treadway; 1829.
23. Elek SD. Semmelweis commemoration. Semmelweis and the oath of Hippocrates. Proc R Soc Med 1966;59:346–52.
24. Ehrenkranz NJ, Alfonso BC. Failure of bland soap handwash to prevent hand transfer of patient bacteria to urethral catheters. Infect Control Hosp Epidemiol 1991;12:654–62.
25. Casewell MW, Dalton MT, Webster M, et al. Gentamicin-resistant *Klebsiella aerogenes* in a urological ward. Lancet 1977;2:444–6.
26. Maki DG. The use of antiseptics for handwashing by medical personnel. J Chemother 1989;1(Suppl 1):3–11.
27. Simmons M. Complexity theory in the management of communicable diseases. J Hosp Infect 2003;54:87–92.

28. Doebbeling BN, Stanley GL, Sheetz CT, et al. Comparative efficacy of alternative hand-washing agents in reducing nosocomial infections in intensive care units. N Engl J Med 1992;327:88–93.
29. Webster J, Faoagali JL, Cartwright D. Elimination of methicillin-resistant *Staphylococcus aureus* from a neonatal intensive care unit after hand washing with triclosan. J Paediatr Child Health 1994;30:59–64.
30. Zafar AB, Butler RC, Reese DJ, et al. Use of 0.3% triclosan (Bacti-Stat) to eradicate an outbreak of methicillin-resistant *Staphylococcus aureus* in a neonatal nursery. Am J Infect Control 1995;23:200–8.
31. Larson EL, Early E, Cloonan P, et al. An organizational climate intervention associated with increased handwashing and decreased nosocomial infections. Behav Med 2000;26:14–22.
32. Sharek PJ, Benitz WE, Abel NJ, et al. Effect of an evidence-based hand washing policy on hand washing rates and false-positive coagulase negative staphylococcus blood and cerebrospinal fluid culture rates in a level III NICU. J Perinatol 2002;22(2):137–43.
33. Marples RR, Towers AG. A laboratory model for the investigation of contact transfer of micro-organisms. J Hyg (Lond) 1979;82:237–48.
34. Mackintosh CA, Hoffman PN. An extended model for transfer of micro-organisms via the hands: differences between organisms and the effect of alcohol disinfection. J Hyg (Lond) 1984;92:345–55.
35. Costerton JW, Stewart PS, Greenberg EP. Bacterial biofilms: a common cause of persistent infections. Science 1999;284:1318–22.
36. Ryder M. Improve CRBSI prevention: target intraluminal risks. 2009;(8). Available at: http://www.executivehm.com/article/Improve-CRBSI-Prevention-Target-Intraluminal-Risks/. Accessed January 8, 2010.
37. Eveillard M, Joly-Guillou ML. 'Measurement and interpretation of hand hygiene compliance rates: importance of monitoring entire care episodes': reply to Professor Gould. J Hosp Infect 2009;72(3):211–7.
38. Bhalla A, Pultz NJ, Gries DM, et al. Acquisition of nosocomial pathogens on hands after contact with environmental surfaces near hospitalized patients. Infect Control Hosp Epidemiol 2004;25:164–7.
39. Mermel LA, Allon M, Bouza E, et al. Clinical practice guidelines for the diagnosis and management of intravascular catheter-related infection: 2009 Update by the Infectious Diseases Society of America. Clin Infect Dis 2009;49:1–45.
40. Salzman MB, Isenberg HD, Rubin LG. Use of disinfectants to reduce microbial contamination of hubs of vascular catheters. J Clin Microbiol 1993;31:475–9.
41. Mahieu LM, De Dooy JJ, Lenaerts AE, et al. Catheter manipulations and the risk of catheter-associated bloodstream infection in neonatal intensive care unit patients. J Hosp Infect 2001;48:20–6.
42. Mahieu LM, De Muynck AO, Ieven MM, et al. Risk factors for central vascular catheter-associated bloodstream infections among patients in a neonatal intensive care unit. J Hosp Infect 2001;48:108–16.
43. Garland JS, Alex CP, Sevallius JM, et al. Cohort study of the pathogenesis and molecular epidemiology of catheter-related bloodstream infection in neonates with peripherally inserted central venous catheters. Infect Control Hosp Epidemiol 2008;29:243–9.
44. Salzman MB, Isenberg HD, Shapiro JF, et al. A prospective study of the catheter hub as the portal of entry for microorganisms causing catheter-related sepsis in neonates. J Infect Dis 1993;167:487–90.

45. Edwards JR, Peterson KD, Andrus ML, et al. National Healthcare Safety Network (NHSN) Report, data summary for 2006 through 2007, issued November 2008. Am J Infect Control 2008;36:609–26.
46. St Geme JW 3rd, Harris MC. Coagulase-negative staphylococcal infection in the neonate. Clin Perinatol 1991;18:281–302.
47. Makhoul IR, Sujov P, Smolkin T, et al. Epidemiological, clinical, and microbiological characteristics of late-onset sepsis among very low birth weight infants in Israel: a national survey. Pediatrics 2002;109:34–9.
48. Nolan T, Berwick DM. All-or-none measurement raises the bar on performance. JAMA 2006;295:1168–70.
49. Levy MM, Pronovost PJ, Dellinger RP, et al. Sepsis change bundles: converting guidelines into meaningful change in behavior and clinical outcome. Crit Care Med 2004;32:S595–7.
50. Golombek SG, Rohan AJ, Parvez B, et al. "Proactive" management of percutaneously inserted central catheters results in decreased incidence of infection in the ELBW population. J Perinatol 2002;22:209–13.
51. Andersen C, Hart J, Vemgal P, et al. Prospective evaluation of a multi-factorial prevention strategy on the impact of nosocomial infection in very-low-birth-weight infants. J Hosp Infect 2005;61:162–7.
52. Aly H, Herson V, Duncan A, et al. Is bloodstream infection preventable among premature infants? A tale of two cities. Pediatrics 2005;115:1513–8.
53. Schelonka RL, Scruggs S, Nichols K, et al. Sustained reductions in neonatal nosocomial infection rates following a comprehensive infection control intervention. J Perinatol 2006;26:176–9.
54. Wirtschafter DD, Pettit J, Kurtin P, et al. A statewide quality improvement collaborative to reduce neonatal central line-associated blood stream infections. J Perinatol 2010;30:170–81.
55. Lee SK, Aziz K, Singhal N, et al. Improving the quality of care for infants: a cluster randomized controlled trial. CMAJ 2009;181:469–76.
56. Lachman P, Yuen S. Using care bundles to prevent infection in neonatal and paediatric ICUs. Curr Opin Infect Dis 2009;22:224–8.
57. NIH consensus Development Conference on critical care medicine. Crit Care Med 1983;11:466–9.
58. Sinuff T, Patel RV, Adhikari NK, et al. Quality of professional society guidelines and consensus conference statements in critical care. Crit Care Med 2008;36:1049–58.
59. Boluyt N, Lincke CR, Offringa M. Quality of evidence-based pediatric guidelines. Pediatrics 2005;115:1378–91.
60. Merritt TA, Palmer D, Bergman DA, et al. Clinical practice guidelines in pediatric and newborn medicine: implications for their use in practice. Pediatrics 1997; 99:100–14.
61. Merritt TA, Gold M, Holland J. A critical evaluation of clinical practice guidelines in neonatal medicine: does their use improve quality and lower costs? J Eval Clin Pract 1999;5:169–77.
62. Cabana MD, Rand CS, Powe NR, et al. Why don't physicians follow clinical practice guidelines? A framework for improvement. JAMA 1999;282:1458–65.
63. Gurses AP, Seidl KL, Vaidya V, et al. Systems ambiguity and guideline compliance: a qualitative study of how intensive care units follow evidence-based guidelines to reduce healthcare-associated infections. Qual Saf Health Care 2008;17:351–9.
64. Safdar N. Bloodstream infection: an ounce of prevention is a ton of work. Infect Control Hosp Epidemiol 2005;26:511–4.

65. Borghesi A, Stronati M. Strategies for the prevention of hospital-acquired infections in the neonatal intensive care unit. J Hosp Infect 2008;68:293–300.
66. NHSN patient safety component protocol. January 2008. Available at: http://www.dhcs.ca.gov/provgovpart/initiatives/nqi/Documents/NHSNManPSPCurr.pdf. Accessed January 8, 2010.
67. Schulman J, Wirtschafter DD, Kurtin P. Neonatal intensive care unit collaboration to decrease hospital-acquired bloodstream infections: from comparative performance reports to improvement networks. Pediatr Clin North Am 2009;56: 865–92.
68. Warye KL, Murphy DM. Targeting zero health care-associated infections. Am J Infect Control 2008;36:683–4.
69. Aboelela SW, Stone PW, Larson EL. Effectiveness of bundled behavioural interventions to control healthcare-associated infections: a systematic review of the literature. J Hosp Infect 2007;66:101–8.
70. Pronovost P, Needham D, Berenholtz S, et al. An intervention to decrease catheter-related bloodstream infections in the ICU. N Engl J Med 2006;355: 2725–32.
71. Sexton JB, Helmreich RL, Neilands TB, et al. The Safety Attitudes Questionnaire: psychometric properties, benchmarking data, and emerging research. BMC Health Serv Res 2006;6:44.
72. Pronovost PJ, Berenholtz SM, Goeschel C, et al. Improving patient safety in intensive care units in Michigan. J Crit Care 2008;23:207–21.
73. Pronovost P, Sexton B. Assessing safety culture: guidelines and recommendations. Qual Saf Health Care 2005;14:231–3.
74. Pronovost PJ, Weast B, Bishop K, et al. Senior executive adopt-a-work unit: a model for safety improvement. Jt Comm J Qual Saf 2004;30:59–68.
75. Thompson DN, Wolf GA, Spear SJ. Driving improvement in patient care: lessons from Toyota. J Nurs Adm 2003;33:585–95.
76. Ojajarvi J. Effectiveness of hand washing and disinfection methods in removing transient bacteria after patient nursing. J Hyg (Lond) 1980;85:193–203.
77. Ayliffe GA, Babb JR, Davies JG, et al. Hand disinfection: a comparison of various agents in laboratory and ward studies. J Hosp Infect 1988;11:226–43.
78. Larson EL, Laughon BE. Comparison of four antiseptic products containing chlorhexidine gluconate. Antimicrobial Agents Chemother 1987;31:1572–4.
79. Kjolen H, Andersen BM. Handwashing and disinfection of heavily contaminated hands—effective or ineffective? J Hosp Infect 1992;21:61–71.
80. Larson EL, Eke PI, Laughon BE. Efficacy of alcohol-based hand rinses under frequent-use conditions. Antimicrobial Agents Chemother 1986;30:542–4.
81. Winnefeld M, Richard MA, Drancourt M, et al. Skin tolerance and effectiveness of two hand decontamination procedures in everyday hospital use. Br J Dermatol 2000;143:546–50.
82. Boyce JM, Kelliher S, Vallande N. Skin irritation and dryness associated with two hand-hygiene regimens: soap-and-water hand washing versus hand antisepsis with an alcoholic hand gel. Infect Control Hosp Epidemiol 2000;21:442–8.
83. Larson EL, Aiello AE, Bastyr J, et al. Assessment of two hand hygiene regimens for intensive care unit personnel. Crit Care Med 2001;29:944–51.
84. Pittet D, Hugonnet S, Harbarth S, et al. Effectiveness of a hospital-wide programme to improve compliance with hand hygiene. Infection Control Programme. Lancet 2000;356:1307–12.
85. Goldmann D. System failure versus personal accountability—the case for clean hands. N Engl J Med 2006;355:121–3.

86. Mermel LA, McCormick RD, Springman SR, et al. The pathogenesis and epidemiology of catheter-related infection with pulmonary artery Swan-Ganz catheters: a prospective study utilizing molecular subtyping. Am J Med 1991;91:197S–205S.
87. Chaiyakunapruk N, Veenstra DL, Lipsky BA, et al. Chlorhexidine compared with povidone-iodine solution for vascular catheter-site care: a meta-analysis. Ann Intern Med 2002;136:792–801.
88. Garland JS, Buck RK, Maloney P, et al. Comparison of 10% povidone-iodine and 0.5% chlorhexidine gluconate for the prevention of peripheral intravenous catheter colonization in neonates: a prospective trial. Pediatr Infect Dis J 1995;14:510–6.
89. Upadhyayula S, Kambalapalli M, Harrison CJ. Safety of anti-infective agents for skin preparation in premature infants. Arch Dis Child 2007;92:646–7.
90. Lund CH, Kuller J, Lane AT, et al. Neonatal skin care: evaluation of the AWHONN/NANN research-based practice project on knowledge and skin care practices. Association of Women's Health, Obstetric and Neonatal Nurses/National Association of Neonatal Nurses. J Obstet Gynecol Neonatal Nurs 2001;30:30–40.
91. BeVier PA, Rice CE. Initiating a pediatric peripherally inserted central catheter and midline catheter program. J Intraven Nurs 1994;17:201–5.
92. Kyle KS, Myers JS. Peripherally inserted central catheters. Development of a hospital-based program. J Intraven Nurs 1990;13:287–90.
93. Soifer NE, Borzak S, Edlin BR, et al. Prevention of peripheral venous catheter complications with an intravenous therapy team: a randomized controlled trial. Arch Intern Med 1998;158:473–7.
94. Linck DA, Donze A, Hamvas A. Neonatal peripherally inserted central catheter team. Evolution and outcomes of a bedside-nurse-designed program. Adv Neonatal Care 2007;7:22–9.
95. Butler-O'Hara M, Buzzard CJ, Reubens L, et al. A randomized trial comparing long-term and short-term use of umbilical venous catheters in premature infants with birth weights of less than 1251 grams. Pediatrics 2006;118:e25–35.
96. McCarthy MC, Shives JK, Robison RJ, et al. Prospective evaluation of single and triple lumen catheters in total parenteral nutrition. JPEN J Parenter Enteral Nutr 1987;11:259–62.
97. Sitges-Serra A, Linares J, Perez JL, et al. A randomized trial on the effect of tubing changes on hub contamination and catheter sepsis during parenteral nutrition. JPEN J Parenter Enteral Nutr 1985;9:322–5.
98. Arduino MJ, Bland LA, Danzig LE, et al. Microbiologic evaluation of needleless and needle-access devices. Am J Infect Control 1997;25:377–80.
99. Josephson A, Gombert ME, Sierra MF, et al. The relationship between intravenous fluid contamination and the frequency of tubing replacement. Infect Control 1985;6:367–70.
100. Maki DG, Botticelli JT, LeRoy ML, et al. Prospective study of replacing administration sets for intravenous therapy at 48- vs 72-hour intervals. 72 hours is safe and cost-effective. JAMA 1987;258:1777–81.
101. Snydman DR, Donnelly-Reidy M, Perry LK, et al. Intravenous tubing containing burettes can be safely changed at 72 hour intervals. Infect Control 1987;8:113–6.
102. Brown JD, Moss HA, Elliott TS. The potential for catheter microbial contamination from a needleless connector. J Hosp Infect 1997;36:181–9.
103. Luebke MA, Arduino MJ, Duda DL, et al. Comparison of the microbial barrier properties of a needleless and a conventional needle-based intravenous access system. Am J Infect Control 1998;26:437–41.

104. Cookson ST, Ihrig M, O'Mara EM, et al. Increased bloodstream infection rates in surgical patients associated with variation from recommended use and care following implementation of a needleless device. Infect Control Hosp Epidemiol 1998;19:23–7.
105. Donlan RM, Murga R, Bell M, et al. Protocol for detection of biofilms on needleless connectors attached to central venous catheters. J Clin Microbiol 2001;39: 750–3.
106. Maki DG, Ringer M. Evaluation of dressing regimens for prevention of infection with peripheral intravenous catheters. Gauze, a transparent polyurethane dressing, and an iodophor-transparent dressing. JAMA 1987;258:2396–403.
107. Hoffmann KK, Weber DJ, Samsa GP, et al. Transparent polyurethane film as an intravenous catheter dressing. A meta-analysis of the infection risks. JAMA 1992;267:2072–6.
108. Sharpe EL. Tiny patients, tiny dressings: a guide to the neonatal PICC dressing change. Adv Neonatal Care 2008;8:150–62 [quiz: 63–4].
109. Pettit J, Wyckoff M, editors. NANN (National Association of Neonatal Nurses) peripherally inserted central catheters guideline for practice. 2nd edition. Glenview (IL): National Association of Neonatal Nurses; 2007.
110. Infusion Nurses Society. Infusion nursing standards of practice. J Infus Nurs 2006;29:1–92.
111. Marschall J, Mermel LA, Classen D, et al. Strategies to prevent central line-associated bloodstream infections in acute care hospitals. Infect Control Hosp Epidemiol 2008;29(Suppl 1):S22–30.
112. Menyhay SZ, Maki DG. Disinfection of needleless catheter connectors and access ports with alcohol may not prevent microbial entry: the promise of a novel antiseptic-barrier cap. Infect Control Hosp Epidemiol 2006;27:23–7.
113. Kaler W. Successful disinfection of needleless access ports: a matter of time and friction. JAVA 2007;12:142.
114. Pratt RJ, Pellowe CM, Wilson JA, et al. Epic2: National evidence-based guidelines for preventing healthcare-associated infections in NHS hospitals in England. J Hosp Infect 2007;65(Suppl 1):S1–64.
115. Soothill JS, Bravery K, Ho A, et al. A fall in bloodstream infections followed a change to 2% chlorhexidine in 70% isopropanol for catheter connection antisepsis: a pediatric single center before/after study on a hemopoietic stem cell transplant ward. Am J Infect Control 2009;37:626–30.
116. Moureau N. Winning the War on CLABSIs: the role of education and new technology. Infection Control Today 2009;Oct:32–6. Available at: http://www.infectioncontroltoday.com/articles/clabsi-education-and-technology.html. Accessed January 8, 2010.
117. Ryder M, Schaudinn C, Gorur A, et al. Microscopic evaluation of microbial colonization on needleless connectors.2008
118. Murga R, Miller JM, Donlan RM. Biofilm formation by gram-negative bacteria on central venous catheter connectors: effect of conditioning films in a laboratory model. J Clin Microbiol 2001;39:2294–7.
119. Donlan RM. Biofilms on central venous catheters: is eradication possible? Curr Top Microbiol Immunol 2008;322:133–61.
120. Hanchett M. Needleless connectors and bacteremia: is there a relationship 2009;1–8. Available at: http://www.vpico.com/articlemanager/printerfriendly.aspx?article=60652. Accessed January 8, 2010.
121. Salgado CD, Chinnes L, Paczesny TH, et al. Increased rate of catheter-related bloodstream infection associated with use of a needleless mechanical valve

device at a long-term acute care hospital. Infect Control Hosp Epidemiol 2007; 28:684–8.
122. Seymour VM, Dhallu TS, Moss HA, et al. A prospective clinical study to investigate the microbial contamination of a needleless connector. J Hosp Infect 2000;45:165–8.
123. Edgar KJ. Does the evidence support the SHEA-IDSA recommendation on the use of positive-pressure mechanical valves? Infect Control Hosp Epidemiol 2009;30:402–3 [author reply: 3–4].
124. Chathas MK, Paton JB, Fisher DE. Percutaneous central venous catheterization. Three years' experience in a neonatal intensive care unit. Am J Dis Child 1990; 144:1246–50.
125. Durand M, Ramanathan R, Martinelli B, et al. Prospective evaluation of percutaneous central venous silastic catheters in newborn infants with birth weights of 510 to 3,920 grams. Pediatrics 1986;78:245–50.
126. Cairns PA, Wilson DC, McClure BG, et al. Percutaneous central venous catheter use in the very low birth weight neonate. Eur J Pediatr 1995;154:145–7.
127. Vest JR, Gamm LD. A critical review of the research literature on Six Sigma, Lean and StuderGroup's Hardwiring Excellence in the United States: the need to demonstrate and communicate the effectiveness of transformation strategies in healthcare. Implement Sci 2009;4:35.
128. Griffiths P, Renz A, Hughes J, et al. Impact of organisation and management factors on infection control in hospitals: a scoping review. J Hosp Infect 2009; 73:1–14.
129. Shannon RP, Frndak D, Grunden N, et al. Using real-time problem solving to eliminate central line infections. Jt Comm J Qual Saf 2006;32:479–87.
130. Stapleton FB, Hendricks J, Hagan P, et al. Modifying thc Toyota Production System for continuous performance improvement in an academic children's hospital. Pediatr Clin North Am 2009;56:799–813.
131. Murphy B. Evidence-based leadership for reduced risk. Managing Infection Control 2007;(7):64–72.
132. Nelson EC, Batalden PB, Godfrey MM. Quality by design-a clinical microsystems approach. Hoboken (NJ): John Wiley and Sons, Inc.; 2007.
133. Clinical microsystems. Available at: http://dms.dartmouth.edu/cms/. Accessed November 1, 2009.
134. Batalden PB, Nelson EC, Edwards WH, et al. Microsystems in health care: Part 9. Developing small clinical units to attain peak performance. Jt Comm J Qual Saf 2003;29:575–85.
135. Edwards WH. Preventing nosocomial bloodstream infection in very low birth weight infants. Semin Neonatol 2002;7:325–33.
136. Caldwell C. Mentoring strategic change in health care: an action guide. Milwaukee (WI): ASQC Quality Press; 1995.
137. California Perinatal Quality Care Collaborative. Quality Improvement. Available at: http://www.cpqcc.org/quality_improvement. Accessed November 1, 2009.
138. Horbar JD, Plsek PE, Leahy K. NIC/Q 2000: establishing habits for improvement in neonatal intensive care units. Pediatrics 2003;111:e397–410.
139. Bohmer RM, Edmondson AC. Organizational learning in health care. Health Forum J 2001;44:32–5.
140. Ayers LR, Beyea SC, Godfrey MM, et al. Quality improvement learning collaboratives. Qual Manag Health Care 2005;14:234–47.
141. Randolph G, Esporas M, Provost L, et al. Model for improvement—Part two: measurement and feedback for quality improvement efforts. Pediatr Clin North Am 2009;56:779–98.

142. Kurtin P, Stucky E. Standardize to excellence: improving the quality and safety of care with clinical pathways. Pediatr Clin North Am 2009;56:893–904.
143. Haas JP, Larson EL. Measurement of compliance with hand hygiene. J Hosp Infect 2007;66:6–14.
144. Allegranzi B, Pittet D. Role of hand hygiene in healthcare-associated infection prevention. J Hosp Infect 2009;73(4):305–15.
145. van de Mortel T, Murgo M. An examination of covert observation and solution audit as tools to measure the success of hand hygiene interventions. Am J Infect Control 2006;34(3):95–9.
146. McGuckin M, Waterman R, Govednik J. Hand hygiene compliance rates in the United States—a one-year multicenter collaboration using product/volume usage measurement and feedback. Am J Med Qual 2009;24:205–13.
147. Luria JW, Muething SE, Schoettker PJ, et al. Reliability science and patient safety. Pediatr Clin North Am 2006;53:1121–33.
148. Shapiro MJ, Jay GD. High reliability organizational change for hospitals: translating tenets for medical professionals. Qual Saf Health Care 2003;12: 238–9.
149. Berenholtz SM, Hartsell TL, Pronovost PJ. Learning from defects to enhance morbidity and mortality conferences. Am J Med Qual 2009;24:192–5.
150. Pronovost PJ, Berenholtz SM, Goeschel CA, et al. Creating high reliability in health care organizations. Health Serv Res 2006;41:1599–617.
151. Ohlsson A, Lacy JB. Intravenous immunoglobulin for preventing infection in preterm and/or low-birth-weight infants. Cochrane Database Syst Rev 2001;(2):CD000361.
152. Craft A, Finer N. Nosocomial coagulase negative staphylococcal (CoNS) catheter-related sepsis in preterm infants: definition, diagnosis, prophylaxis, and prevention. J Perinatol 2001;21:186–92.
153. Garland JS, Alex CP, Henrickson KJ, et al. A vancomycin-heparin lock solution for prevention of nosocomial bloodstream infection in critically ill neonates with peripherally inserted central venous catheters: a prospective, randomized trial. Pediatrics 2005;116:e198–205.
154. de Silva A, Jones PW, Spencer SA. Does human milk reduce infection rates in preterm infants? A systematic review. Arch Dis Child Fetal Neonatal Ed 2004; 89:F509–13.
155. Ben XM. Nutritional management of newborn infants: practical guidelines. World J Gastroenterol 2008;14:6133–9.
156. Troche B, Harvey-Wilkes K, Engle WD, et al. Early minimal feedings promote growth in critically ill premature infants. Biol Neonate 1995;67:172–81.
157. Freeman J, Goldmann DA, Smith NE, et al. Association of intravenous lipid emulsion and coagulase-negative staphylococcal bacteremia in neonatal intensive care units. N Engl J Med 1990;323:301–8.
158. Avila-Figueroa C, Goldmann DA, Richardson DK, et al. Intravenous lipid emulsions are the major determinant of coagulase-negative *staphylococcal bacteremia* in very low birth weight newborns. Pediatr Infect Dis J 1998;17:10–7.
159. Melly MA, Meng HC, Schaffner W. Microbiol growth in lipid emulsions used in parenteral nutrition. Arch Surg 1975;110:1479–81.
160. Abdelkefi A, Achour W, Ben Othman T, et al. Use of heparin-coated central venous lines to prevent catheter-related bloodstream infection. J Support Oncol 2007;5:273–8.
161. Shah PS, Shah N. Heparin-bonded catheters for prolonging the patency of central venous catheters in children. Cochrane Database Syst Rev 2007;(4):CD005983.

162. Williams D. Catheters, materials and infection. Med Device Technol 2002;13: 8–11.
163. Yasukawa T, Fujita Y, Sari A. Antimicrobial-impregnated central venous catheters. N Engl J Med 1999;340:1762.
164. Ranucci M, Isgro G, Giomarelli PP, et al. Impact of Oligon central venous catheters on catheter colonization and catheter-related bloodstream infection. Crit Care Med 2003;31:52–9.
165. Garland JS, Alex CP, Mueller CD, et al. Local reactions to a chlorhexidine gluconate-impregnated antimicrobial dressing in very low birth weight infants. Pediatr Infect Dis J 1996;15:912–4.
166. Crnich CJ, Maki DG. The promise of novel technology for the prevention of intravascular device-related bloodstream infection. I. Pathogenesis and short-term devices. Clin Infect Dis 2002;34:1232–42.
167. Khattak AZ, Ross, RE, Arnold, C, et al. A randomized controlled trial of the safety of silver alginate (Algidex) patches in very low birth weight (VLBW) infants with central lines. J Perinatol 2009. [Epub ahead of print].
168. Curry S, Honeycutt M, Goins G, et al. Catheter-associated bloodstream infections in the NICU: getting to zero. Neonatal Netw 2009;28(3):151–5.

Quality Improvement in Respiratory Care: Decreasing Bronchopulmonary Dysplasia

Robert H. Pfister, MD[a,b], Jay P. Goldsmith, MD[c,d,*]

KEYWORDS

- Chronic lung disease • Quality improvement
- Respiratory care • Bronchopulmonary dysplasia

NOMENCLATURE AND DEFINITION

Chronic lung disease (CLD) is 1 of the most common long-term complications in very preterm infants. Bronchopulmonary dysplasia (BPD), initially characterized by Northway and colleagues[1] in 1967, is the most common cause of CLD occurring in infancy. BPD was originally defined as the presence of clinical symptoms, the need for supplemental oxygen to treat hypoxemia, and an abnormal chest radiograph at 28 days of age, later revised to 36 weeks postmenstrual age (PMA).[2,3] In 2001, the National Institutes of Health developed a consensus definition of BPD to help compare the incidence of the disease among institutions and evaluate potential preventive strategies and treatments. This definition was based on gestational age at birth, time of assessment, and severity of disease (**Table 1**).[4] More recently, a new physiologic description by Walsh and colleagues[2] has been proposed: the inability to maintain an oxygen saturation of 90% or greater in room air. This definition is particularly useful for centers implementing quality improvement (QI) methods to improve pulmonary outcomes because of its objectivity. However, none of these definitions uses P_{CO_2} levels in defining the severity of the disease, and this value at 36 weeks PMA may be the best predictor of future respiratory morbidity.

[a] Department of Pediatrics, The University of Vermont, Burlington, VT, USA
[b] Fletcher Allen Health Care, Smith 556, 111 Colchester Avenue, Burlington, VT 05401, USA
[c] Department of Pediatrics, Tulane University Medical School, 1430 Tulane Avenue, New Orleans, LA 70112-2699, USA
[d] 1625 Joseph Street, New Orleans, LA 70115, USA
* Corresponding author. 1625 Joseph Street, New Orleans, LA 70115.
E-mail address: goldsmith.jay@gmail.com

Clin Perinatol 37 (2010) 273–293
doi:10.1016/j.clp.2010.01.015
perinatology.theclinics.com
0095-5108/10/$ – see front matter

Table 1
Diagnostic criteria for BPD

Gestational Age	<32 wk	≥32 wk
Time of assessment	36 wk PMA or discharge to home, whichever comes first	>28 d but <56 d postnatal age or discharge to home, whichever comes first
Mild BPD	Oxygen>21% for at least 28 d plus: breathing room air at 36 wk PMA or discharge, whichever comes first	Breathing room air by 56 d postnatal age or discharge, whichever comes first
Moderate BPD	Need for <30% oxygen at 36 wk PMA or discharge, whichever comes first	Need for <30% oxygen at 56 d postnatal age or discharge, whichever comes first
Severe BPD	Need for ≥30% oxygen or positive pressure,(PPV or NCPAP) at 36 wk PMA or discharge, whichever comes first	Need for ≥30% oxygen or positive pressure (PPV or NCPAP) at 56 d postnatal age or discharge, whichever comes first

Abbreviations: NCPAP, nasal continuous positive airway pressure; PMA, postmenstrual age; PPV, positive pressure ventilation.

Data from Jobe AH, Bancalari E. NICHD/NHLBI/ORD workshop summary: bronchopulmonary dysplasia. Am J Respir Crit Care Med 2001;163:1723–9.

BPD was originally described as a complication of respiratory distress syndrome (RDS) and included the influence of 3 key factors: lung immaturity, acute lung injury, and disordered repair of the original lung injury. This classic BPD was noted during an era when mechanical ventilation was just beginning to be used to treat preterm infants with respiratory distress and was characterized by airway injury, smooth muscle hypertrophy, and areas of lung parenchymal fibrosis alternating with areas with emphysematous changes. Improvements in prenatal care, such as the use of antenatal steroids, combined with improvements in respiratory management, such as the use of pulmonary surfactants, have resulted in the successful treatment of increasingly smaller infants with less resulting BPD as it was originally described. However, in lieu of the classic BPD, modern neonatal respiratory care has witnessed the emergence of a new BPD. This new BPD may occur with little acute lung injury, or after resolution of lung injury, and is believed to be affected by other factors such as inflammation (secondary to sepsis or chorioamnionitis) and the presence of a patent ductus arteriosus (PDA).[3,5,6] Compared with classic BPD, preterm infants who have new BPD have decreased fibrosis and emphysema but also have a marked decrease in alveolar septation and microvascular development (**Table 2**).

CLD encompasses both the classic and the new BPD but also recognizes that lung injury can occur not only in preterm infants but in term infants who need aggressive ventilatory support for severe lung disease and develop lung injury as a result. In addition, the term CLD is used to reflect that, although the primary pathology is related to the lungs, CLD is a multisystem disease. Extremely-low-birth-weight (ELBW) infants with CLD suffer not only more pulmonary morbidity but also more neurodevelopmental problems, nutritional deficiencies, and prolonged lengths of hospital stay compared with infants without CLD.[7–9]

CLINICAL PRESENTATION AND PATHOPHYSIOLOGY

On physical examination, infants with CLD have certain characteristic features. Tachypnea with shallow breathing, retractions, and a paradoxic breathing pattern is

Table 2
Classic versus new BPD

Classic BPD	New BPD
Premature and term infants before steroids, surfactants	Very-low-birth-weight and extremely-low-birth-weight infants
Short periods of high ventilatory support: baro- and volutrauma	Modest ventilatory support over months
Hyperventilation with normal or low P_{CO_2}	Permissive hypercapnia but inability to wean off assisted ventilation
Associated with pulmonary air leaks, meconium aspiration syndrome, and pneumonia	Associated with chorioamnionitis, sepsis, PDA; poor nutrition (vitamin deficiencies)
Inflammation, fibrosis prominent; areas of atelectasis alternating with areas of emphysema	Less prominent inflammation, fibrosis; dilated alveolar ducts
Injury/repair sequence	Maldevelopment sequence: ↓ alveolar septation, ↓ alveolar surface area, ↓ microvascular development

Data from Jobe AH, Ikegami M. Mechanisms initiating lung injury in the preterm. Early Hum Dev 1998;53(1):81–94.

common. On auscultation, nonspecific, but atypical, breath sounds that include rhonchi, rales, and wheezes may all be heard. The heterogeneous damage to airways and lungs results in variable time constants and increasing ventilation-perfusion mismatch. Dynamic lung compliance is often diminished secondary to fibrosis and edema.[10] Increased airway resistance of small and larger airways has been reported.[11] Tracheomalacia is often present and may be exacerbated by bronchodilator therapy.[12] As the course of CLD progresses, initial low lung volumes secondary to atelectasis are often at least partially replaced by hyperinflation and gas trapping.

CLD is marked by distortion and dysfunction of the pulmonary circulation in parallel to pulmonary parenchymal injury. Epithelial lesions, fibroblast proliferation, and smooth muscle hyperplasia have been observed. These structural changes result in a pulmonary vascular bed that is markedly reduced compared with normal. Abnormally marked vasoconstriction in response to hypoxia often accompanies these structural abnormalities, further increasing pulmonary vascular resistance.[13] The structural and functional changes contribute to the rapid development of progressive and often severe pulmonary hypertension. This finding, in turn, may lead to poor right ventricular function, diminished cardiac output, and impaired oxygen delivery, and is a predictor of mortality in affected infants.[14] A pathognomonic sign of this end stage of the disease is a thickened protruding tongue, sometimes called "clubbing" of the tongue, which is probably caused by the reduced ability of venous blood to return to the thorax (**Fig. 1**). Other cardiovascular abnormalities associated with CLD include systemic hypertension, left ventricular hypertrophy, and development of systemic-pulmonary collateral vessels.[15]

Factors that Affect Pathogenesis of BPD

CLD has a multifactorial cause. Northway and colleagues[1] originally documented the presence of cytotoxic oxygen free radicals and postulated that oxygen toxicity was a major cause of CLD. Mechanical ventilators, although an important tool for management of critically ill newborns, are universally implicated in the development of

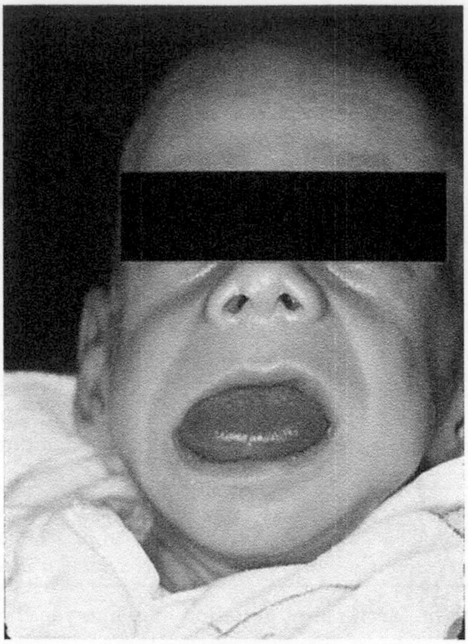

Fig. 1. Clubbing of the tongue seen in end-stage BPD.

CLD.[16,17] Barotrauma and volutrauma from mechanical ventilation combined with oxygen toxicity contribute to inflammatory reactions that contribute to the development of CLD and persist past the immediate neonatal period.[18–21] Inflammation contributing to the development of CLD may also occur after chorioamnionitis, fetal infection, sepsis, and ventilator-associated or nosocomial pneumonia.[22–28] Infection may also exacerbate evolving CLD and result in increased lung injury secondary to release of proteolytic enzymes. The link between fluid overload and the presence of a symptomatic PDA with CLD can potentially be explained by an increased need for mechanical ventilation in these infants.[5] CLD occurs in about one-fifth of ventilated newborns, with risk inversely proportional to birth weight and gestational age. Although most infants developing CLD are premature, about 75% of affected infants have birth weight less than 1000 g and only 5% of those affected have birth weight greater than 1500 g.[29] Genetic factors have been implicated in the severity of acute respiratory disease and the development of CLD.[22,23]

Antenatal factors have also been implicated in the pathogenesis of CLD. Antenatal steroids are believed to be protective from CLD through the amelioration of RDS (although epidemiologic studies do not support this association).[24–26] Inadequate nutrition is believed to lead to decreased alveolar development, impaired surfactant production, and a catabolic state that inhibits growth and repair of the premature lung.

WHY QI TO REDUCE CLD?

Despite the many interventions that have been shown to be efficacious in reducing CLD, the incidence of CLD has remained stable during the past 2 decades.[27,28] The Vermont Oxford Network (VON) 2008 Database Summary reports a 25.5% incidence of BPD at discharge on infants whose birth weight was less than 1500 g. This observation represents a decrease of almost 3% from the previous 3 years in this large cohort of approximately 50,000 infants from 700 centers. Despite this slow but encouraging drop in the incidence of BPD, many of the reported best practice interventions have not been effectively translated into practice in many neonatal intensive care units (NICUs) in the United States. CLD rates in individual institutions vary from a 5% to 65% incidence within the VON. Risk adjustment for confounders such as birth weight, gestational age, race, antenatal steroid administration frequency, and RDS severity reduce the variation between centers but do not eliminate it. Shrunken estimates that adjust for NICU volume and random variation similarly do not account for all of the wide variation noted. This variation also exists when correcting for the risk of chance. Given that neither case mix (disease severity) nor chance explains the variation that exists between centers, treatment practices must be a large contributing reason behind the variation in outcomes.

Recognition of wide variability in the rates of CLD among centers has existed since the 1980s and persisted into the present decade.[30,31] Van Marter and colleagues's[31] comparison of 2 Boston hospitals with Columbia Babies' Hospital shows the stark differences in approaches to use of mechanical ventilation, surfactant, and nasal continuous positive airway pressure (NCPAP) and the resultant wide variation in BPD rates; however, survival in the comparison institutions was not statistically different (**Fig. 2**). This wide variation in outcomes, even among highly respected centers, which cannot be explained by other factors, is the justification for the use of QI methods as an ideal method for CLD reduction. Because there remains a gap between what is known and what is done, QI programs are increasingly being used as a method for incorporating evidence into practice.

Specific Prevention/Treatment Practices and Their Evidence

When neonatal centers decide to use QI methods in an effort to decrease CLD, they have a myriad of practice options from which to choose. Because many factors contribute to the pathogenesis of CLD, QI efforts typically use a bundle of interventions together; each practice used has varying levels of supporting evidence. Although it might seem intuitive that clinicians would embrace practices supported by the highest level of evidence (LOE), this is not uniformly the case.[32] Any practice to be implemented should be carefully researched and the underpinning evidence should be

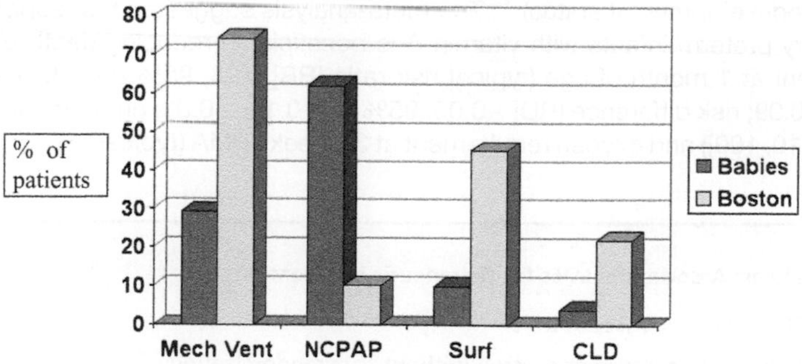

Fig. 2. Variation in practice and outcomes for VLBW infants: Columbia Babies' Hospital (New York) versus 2 Boston hospitals. *Abbreviations:* Mech vent, mechanical ventilation; NCPAP, nasal continuous positive airway pressure; Surf, surfactant use; CLD, chronic lung disease. (*From* Van Marter LJ, Allred EN, Pagano M, et al. Do clinical markers of barotrauma and oxygen toxicity explain interhospital variation in rates of chronic lung disease? The Neonatology Committee for the Developmental Network. Pediatrics 2000;105(6):1194–201; with permission.)

assessed. Because very few practices in neonatology are supported by the highest LOE, these practices are sometimes called potentially better practices (PBPs).

There are several systems for grading the LOE for a practice.[33,34] High LOEs are more likely to yield a true estimate of the effects of an intervention, and lower levels less likely to do so. In such hierarchies, expert opinion, which was historically considered to be the best source of evidence, is relegated to the lowest level. The pinnacle of the hierarchy is now occupied by large, well-designed and conducted, randomized, controlled trials (RCTs), or systematic reviews of multiple RCTs (meta-analysis). However, when attempting to decrease the incidence of a complication such as CLD, which is known to have a multifactorial cause, the effect of 1 or more changes in practice may have no effect on the desired goal even though the practices chosen have a high LOE for a particular outcome. For example, use of prophylactic exogenous surfactant to decrease the severity of RDS and shorten days on mechanical ventilatory support has an LOE of 1 for these outcomes. Intuitively, this effect would seem to also reduce the incidence of BPD, but this intervention alone has not been shown to alter the incidence of this disease.

Many organizations have attempted to categorize LOEs for the systematic evaluation of published scientific manuscripts. The system used by the American Heart Association, modeled on the original Oxford system, is widely used and is seen in **Box 1**.[35]

PREVENTATIVE MEASURES TO LOWER THE INCIDENCE OF CLD: PBPS

This section briefly reviews some of the more common PBPs, which include preventative measures and treatment interventions for CLD. LOEs are noted in parentheses.

Vitamin A (LOE 1)

BPD has multiple causes and influencing factors, including factors inhibiting normal epithelial healing. Vitamin A is an important nutrient during recovery from epithelial lung injury; however, preterm infants have low vitamin A levels at birth.[36] This vitamin A–deficient state may contribute to an increased risk of developing BPD. A Cochrane systematic review examined the effect of vitamin A supplementation in infants with birth weight of 1500 g or less and reported clinical outcomes (death, BPD, long-term neurodevelopmental status).[37] The meta-analysis suggested that supplementation of very preterm infants with vitamin A is beneficial in reducing death or oxygen requirement at 1 month of age (typical risk ratio [RR] 0.93, 95% confidence interval [CI] 0.88, 0.99; risk difference [RD] −0.05, 95% CI −0.10, −0.01; number need to treat [NNT] 20 [10, 100]) and oxygen requirement at 36 weeks PMA (typical RR 0.87, 95% CI

Box 1
American Heart Association: LOEs for therapeutic interventions

LOE 1: RCTs or meta-analyses of RCTs

LOE 2: Studies using concurrent controls without true randomization (eg, pseudorandomization or meta-analysis of such studies)

LOE 3: Studies using retrospective controls

LOE 4: Studies without a control group (eg, case series)

LOE 5: Studies not directly related to the specific patient/population (eg, different patient/population, animal models, mechanical models, and so forth.

0.77, 0.98; RD −0.08, 95% CI −0.14, −0.01; NNT 13 [7, 100]). The results of the meta-analysis are heavily influenced by one multi-institutional study by Tyson and colleagues[38] that is the largest randomized study of vitamin A supplementation reported, having a sample size more than twice that of all other studies combined. This trial included infants with birth weight of 401 to 1000 g. Another trial, by Ambalavanan and colleagues,[39] which compared different intramuscular dosing regimes, suggests that, at least for infants with birth weight between 401 and 1000 g, the optimal dose seems to be 5000 IU 3× weekly for 4 weeks.

Prophylactic or Early Surfactant Treatment (LOE 1–2)

Evidence supports the provision of pulmonary surfactant by prophylactic or early treatment strategies to prevent acute lung injury and to reduce mortality.[40,41] How this translates into improvements in terms of reductions in rates of CLD is less clear. Prophylactic strategies that provide exogenous pulmonary surfactant in the initial 20 minutes of life to infants deemed at risk for developing RDS have shown efficacy at limiting RDS severity, but this gain has not been shown to translate into decreases in rates of CLD (RR = 0.96, 95% CI 0.82, 1.12).[40] Given the clear improvement in initial respiratory status, a reduction in CLD would seem plausible. However, this failure to reduce CLD is, at least in part, a result of the development of CLD among extremely small, ill-surviving infants who might otherwise have died. Although CLD is not reduced, prophylactic surfactant has been shown to be beneficial in increasing survival without CLD (RR = 0.85, 95% CI 0.76, 0.95). Compared with delayed treatment, surfactant administration strategies that deliver surfactant in the first 2 hours of life to patients with established RDS have been efficacious in limiting CLD (RR = 0.70, 95% CI 0.55, 0.88).[41] Because of this finding and the increasing usefulness of CPAP, one viable approach is to attempt to stabilize infants initially on NCPAP and provide early surfactant only if the infants deteriorate.

Antenatal Steroids (LOE 3)

Antenatal steroids have been shown to be remarkably effective at reducing mortality and decreasing RDS; however, these gains have not translated into meaningful decreases in rates of CLD.[24–26] At least 2 mechanisms exist to explain this phenomenon. Antenatal steroids, like pulmonary surfactant administration, may be keeping patients alive who would have otherwise died, but at the cost of developing CLD. A second possible explanation for this lack of effect is that antenatal steroids improve lung function initially, but impair alveolar development.[42] Given that the survival and early fetal lung maturation benefits of maternally administered corticosteroids are well documented, centers should consider perinatal programs aimed at increasing the rates of administration of antenatal steroids to mothers threatening to deliver before 34 weeks' gestation. When administered, betamethasone is preferred, rather than dexamethasone.[43,44]

Optimal Nutrition (LOE 3)

Preterm infants with CLD have nutritional deficits that may contribute to short- and long-term morbidity and mortality. Although no studies exist that examine the effects of increased energy intake, early parental protein, early introduction of lipids, or provision of breast milk for preterm infants with (or developing) CLD, most experts believe that optimal nutritional support is important for premature lung maturation and repair.

Optimal Oxygen Therapy (LOE 2–3)

The optimal target range for blood oxygen tension (Pa_{O_2}) or oxygen saturation (Sp_{O_2}) in premature infants has not been determined, although it is generally accepted that extremes are injurious.[45] Premature lungs have decreased defense mechanisms against oxygen toxicity. In addition, alveolar macrophages and surfactant-producing type II pneumocytes are adversely affected by hyperoxia. Even low levels of inspired oxygen and arterial Pao_2 levels of 50 to 80 mm Hg are higher than levels in the fetus and potentially toxic. For example, Askie and colleagues[45] compared the effects of standard targeted oxygen saturations (91%–94%) with high saturations (95%–98%) amongst infants born after less than 30 weeks' gestation. The high-saturation group had higher rates of BPD and higher rates of home-based oxygen therapy. In the STOP-ROP trial of higher (96%–99%) versus conventional (89%–94%) pulse oximetry targets, the group receiving higher inspired oxygen had higher rates of BPD, diuretic use, and longer hospital stays.[46]

Both studies evaluated infants who were not in the immediate postnatal period. Early in the course of RDS, expert opinion is not unified as to the optimal oxygen saturation range; however, it is probably appropriate to maintain the oxygen saturation at less than 95% and the arterial oxygen tension at less than 90 mm Hg. If BPD is already established, higher targets may be prudent to avoid the development of cor pulmonale.[47] Compliance with intended pulse oximetry targets is typically poor, with most noncompliance greater than the intended range. Success with maintaining the intended pulse oximeter saturation range has been shown to vary markedly among centers, among patients within centers, and for individual patients over time.[48] Regardless of the intended range of targeted oxygen saturations, it is of vital importance to achieve buy-in and a culture motivated toward compliance among staff at the local grassroots level to achieve the desired target ranges with any degree of consistency.[49]

Conventional Mechanical Ventilation Strategies

All types of mechanical ventilation are injurious to the premature lung. Ventilator-induced lung injury (VILI) is associated with alveolar structural damage, pulmonary edema, inflammation, and fibrosis. Causes of this injury include high airway pressure (barotrauma),[50] excessive gas volumes (volutrauma),[51–53] alveolar collapse and re-expansion (atelectotrauma),[54] and increased inflammation (biotrauma).[55] When using conventional ventilation, a strategy for minimizing lung injury is to limit the duration of mechanical ventilation and provide optimal lung volumes using gentle ventilation techniques, as reflected by moderate permissive hypercapnia. In practice, this entails optimal positive expiratory end pressure (PEEP)[51] for lung recruitment and ventilation with low lung tidal volumes (4–6 mL/kg). Hypocapnia is clearly to be avoided as it has been shown to be associated with increased rates of BPD, intraventricular hemorrhage (IVH), and periventricular leukomalacia (PVL).[56–58] A small study by Mariani and colleagues[59] suggested that ventilation strategies amongst very-low-birth-weight (VLBW) infants who had received surfactant and were maintained mildly hypercapnic ($Paco_2$ 45–55 mm Hg) were safe (ie, no increased rates of IVH or PVL) and reduced the duration of mechanical ventilation. A larger, multicenter, randomized trial reported that $Paco_2$ targeted at 52 mm Hg resulted in a reduction in mechanical ventilation at 36 weeks PMA but did not decrease death or BPD.[60]

In the early phase of RDS, it is appropriate to maintain a $Paco_2$ of 45 to 55 mm Hg with a pH greater than 7.20 to 7.25. By postnatal day 3 to 4, metabolic compensation gradually develops, which permits a higher $Paco_2$ for the same pH. Volume-targeted ventilation allows for the peak inflating pressure (PIP) to respond to changes in lung compliance and patient respiratory effort and may deliver desired tidal volumes more consistently at lower pressures.[61] Although targeted tidal volume ventilation may be useful in avoiding injurious over-distention and reduction of hypocapnea, there are no long-term data to support its routine use.[62] Patient-triggered ventilation, when used in the recovery phase of RDS, significantly shortens the weaning from mechanical ventilation.[63]

Some of the strongest evidence for an effective prevention strategy to decrease BPD includes limiting the duration of mechanical ventilation.[6,31,64] Very premature infants who have been intubated and provided surfactant may often be successfully extubated to NCPAP quickly.[65] A Cochrane systematic review reported that NCPAP reduces extubation failure and BPD.[66] Nasal intermittent positive pressure ventilation (NIPPV) has been shown to increase the effectiveness of CPAP in extubated infants, leading to a decrease in reintubation rates and a trend toward decreased BPD.[67] Administration of methylxanthines, such as caffeine citrate, to very preterm infants for treatment of apnea of prematurity, reduces the need for mechanical ventilation and has recently been shown to significantly reduce need for reintubation and the rate of BPD.[68,69]

High-frequency Oscillation (LOE 3)

The results of RCTs and even meta-analyses of studies of high-frequency ventilation as a primary mode of respiratory support have been inconsistent. The 2 largest neonatal studies that both enrolled infants who received antenatal steroids and surfactant, and that used an alveolar recruitment strategy, had different results.[70,71] Meta-analytical techniques have been similarly conflicting: 1 showed a modest reduction in BPD,[72] whereas another showed no benefit.[73]

NCPAP (LOE 2–3)

CPAP applied at birth reduces lung injury and improves lung volumes after birth.[64] Several observational studies suggest that preterm infants treated with early CPAP have a reduced need for intubation, mechanical ventilation, and incidence of BPD without increasing morbidity.[30,74–79] The COIN trial, which compared outcomes of 25- to 28-week gestation infants receiving NCPAP at birth with those receiving intubation, surfactant administration, and ventilation, showed that not all preterm infants in this gestational age range need to be intubated at birth. Infants receiving CPAP without intubation had a decreased incidence of death or oxygen need at 28 days, although they had similar rates of these outcomes by 36 weeks' gestation.[80] However, infants treated initially with CPAP who failed and required intubation, had a higher incidence of pulmonary air leaks. Ammari and colleagues[74] reported that larger preterm infants (751–1250 g) were more successful (76% did not require intubation) when stabilized on CPAP than smaller ones. Fifty percent of the smaller infants in that study (<751 g) ultimately required intubation. Evidence also suggests that infants treated with early CPAP who also have higher oxygen requirements (FiO_2>45%) have reduced complications if transiently intubated and treated with surfactant.[81] Technique and experience applying the NCPAP prongs with a snug fit and using a chin strap to minimize air leak influence success. The VON Delivery Room Management study (DRM) was designed to compare the effects of 3 distinct methods of postdelivery stabilization and subsequent respiratory care on BPD and survival in premature infants at high risk of RDS. The 3 approaches to postdelivery care include (1) intubation, prophylactic surfactant administration shortly after delivery, and subsequent stabilization on ventilator support; (2) early stabilization on CPAP with selective intubation and surfactant administration for clinical indications; and (3) intubation, prophylactic surfactant administration shortly after delivery, and rapid extubation to CPAP. Until the results of this and other trials are completed, a strategy of applying NCPAP selectively to spontaneously breathing VLBW infants with characteristics suggesting sufficient surfactant pools and success on CPAP should be considered. The selection of these patients is crucial, because omitting intubation and surfactant administration may allow the development of atelectasis and a higher risk of pneumothorax if intubation is required. Patient selection for CPAP alone should consider gestational age, weight, completion of antenatal steroids, presence of infection (chorioamnionitis), and signs of asphyxia, all factors that affect the production of endogenous surfactant.

T-Piece Resuscitator (LOE 3)

In the delivery room, clinicians are prone to contributing to volutrauma secondary to vigorous ventilation of infants transitioning poorly. Uncontrolled excessively large or small tidal volumes are injurious to the developing lung. Measuring and controlling tidal volumes in the delivery room, including the use of a T-piece resuscitator, may be desirable but are unproven in terms of prevention of CLD.[17,82,83]

Treatment of Symptomatic PDA (LOE 3)

The presence of a symptomatic PDA in VLBW infants has been shown to be predictive of the need for supplemental oxygen and prolonged ventilation.[84] Treatment of a symptomatic PDA has been shown to prevent the decrease in alveolar septation and microvascular development that characterizes the new BPD but has not been shown to reduce the risk of developing BPD.[85] Surgical closure of a symptomatic PDA increases the risk of BPD and is associated with adverse neurodevelopmental outcomes.[86] However, this finding may be because of the adverse selection of infants who require surgical, as opposed to pharmacologic or medical, treatment alone.

Fluid Restriction (LOE 3)

Excessive intravenous fluid administration, colloid administration, and early sodium supplementation increase the risk of CLD.[87,88] In addition, infants who lose less weight and receive more intravenous fluids immediately after birth have an increased risk for development of CLD.[89,90] However, it is not clear that fluid restriction reduces the incidence of BPD.[91] Given these data, careful restriction of water intake so that physiologic needs are met without allowing significant dehydration seems prudent.

Prevention from Infection (LOE 2–3)

Nosocomial bacteremia increases the risk of developing CLD.[92,93] Nosocomial pneumonia contributes to increased lung injury and BPD secondary to polymorphonuclear leukocyte infiltration and release of protelolytic enzymes.[94] Prevention of sepsis or pneumonia will result in decreased inflammation and decreased time on mechanical ventilation and should be a goal of every center. Programs to reduce ventilator associated pneumonia (VAP) have been advocated and commercial bundles are marketed; however, no data have shown that these programs reduce the incidence of CLD.

Methylxanthines (LOE 1)

Traditional pharmacologic intervention for apnea of prematurity has included methylxanthine medications, such as caffeine citrate. These medications decrease the frequency of apnea events and decrease the need for reintubation and mechanical ventilation.[68] Recently, it has been shown that these short-term gains also translate into long-term benefits. In a well-conducted study of 2006 infants, Schmidt and colleagues[69] reported the effect of caffeine citrate, administered to infants born weighing between 500 and 1250 g, for any of the following purposes: to prevent apnea, to treat apnea, and to facilitate extubation. This study reported decreased time on ventilatory support, decreased oxygen use, decreased corticosteroid administration, and decreased need for transfusions. Most importantly, a significant reduction in the rate of development of BPD (adjusted odds ratio [OR] 0.64, 95% CI 0.52–0.78) was noted in the treatment group.[69]

Postnatal Corticosteroids

Few interventions for CLD have received as much attention and controversy as the administration of corticosteroids to premature infants. Studies have reported that inhaled and systemic steroids improve lung mechanics and gas exchange and reduce inflammation.[95,96] Systemic corticosteroids have been used early ($\leq$7 days) to prevent the development of CLD and late (>7 days) to treat established lung disease. Early and late corticosteroids significantly reduce the incidence of CLD.[97,98] However, there are important concerns regarding adverse events associated with systemic steroids. Although immediate pulmonary benefit is realized, increased alveolar simplification is reported.[99] Other adverse events include systemic hypertension, hypertrophic cardiomyopathy, infection, hyperglycemia, gastrointestinal bleeding, and perforation.[97,98,100] In addition, long-term follow-up studies of infants who received early steroids report an increased risk of abnormal neurologic examination and cerebral palsy.[97] However, major neurosensory disability, and the combined rate of death or major neurosensory disability, were not significantly different between steroid and control groups in infants randomized to receive late steroids.[98] The adverse events associated with steroids are generally based on data from studies that used high doses of dexamethasone for long periods of time and questions remain over the potential safety of other steroids and for smaller doses given for shorter periods of time.[15,101] Because of concerns regarding these adverse events, the American Academy of Pediatrics and the Canadian Pediatric Society recommended against the routine use of systemic steroids to treat or prevent CLD.[102] The clinician must weigh the potential risks of short-term late or rescue use of steroids versus the potential benefits of potentiating extubation in those infants who are still ventilator dependent or on high concentrations of inspired oxygen after several weeks of therapy.

To avoid the adverse effects of systemic steroids, inhaled steroids have been tested and found to have no significant advantage with respect to prevention or treatment of CLD compared with systemic steroids.[103,104] No long-term neurodevelopmental outcome data are available regarding inhaled steroids. One trial reported a decrease in the perceived need for systemic steroids after inhaled steroid administration.[105]

Other Potential Better Practices to Reduce BPD

Several other practices have been proposed to reduce the incidence of BPD in an individual hospital. These include practices which are difficult to test and for which there are few data. Some of these practices include Golden Hour care, during which the resuscitation team for a VLBW infant has a scripted protocol for resuscitation and the team is graded in some standard way after the first hour of life; standard protocols for ventilatory management; standard extubation criteria; avoidance of unplanned extubation; standard nutritional protocols; and others. Each of these has some scientific rationale, but none has been shown to individually reduce the incidence or severity of BPD. However, the involvement of the entire NICU team in QI protocols establishes a unit rapport, identifies problem outcomes, and heightens the awareness of members of the care team to new techniques and methods of care. Here the Hawthorne effect may be advantageous even if the individual PBP is not.

QI: METHODS FOR IMPLEMENTATION AND SUCCESS

The Institute for Health Care Improvement (IHI) first adopted and described many of the QI methods widely used. These landmark methods, called the Breakthrough Series, showed how collaborative improvement models bring health care professionals together to focus on the gap between evidence-based practices and implementation of these practices, and to accelerate the pace of improvement in their organizations.[106] Key to any QI movement is multidisciplinary grassroots involvement and effective leadership. Successful QI efforts require conscious emphasis on 4 key habits as described by Plsek.[107] The first of these is to view the clinical process at hand as a system that involves many factors and many participants. Understanding that any improvement strategy is a complex process or system that involves multiple disciplines and influences is vital to making meaningful change. The second habit, fostering teamwork from a variety of disciplines to improve collaborative learning, has been shown to hasten implementation and success of QI efforts.[108] Meetings, conference calls, Internet meeting rooms, and list serves are all integral to the success of any QI movement. A fun and social atmosphere can be important in energizing the process. The third habit involves the need for adoption and adherence to evidence-based practice. Understanding the importance and the limits of the literature behind any potential change in practice is compelling. The habit for change should be embraced. Significant resistance to change will uniformly exist in almost all cultures. Centers that embrace change will be more successful in terms of initiating change. Because the QI process is a progressive, repetitive process, Plan-Do-Study-Act (PDSA; see the article by Ellsbury and Ursprung elsewhere in this issue) cycles are frequently used.[109] These cycles are frequently embraced by QI teams and emphasize continuous improvement through change, analysis of this change, and feedback.

QI requires consistent accurate data on performance and outcomes. Data from an individual hospital's NICU are essential in identification of individual practices and outcomes that need improvement. Comparisons of outcomes and processes with those of high-performing centers (benchmarking) and with large databases are important to the improvement process. The comparison databases to which centers may have access include those available from the California Perinatal Quality Care Collaborative (CPQCC), the National Association of Children's Hospitals and Related Institutions (NACHRI), the National Institute for Child Health and Development (NICHD), the Pediatrix Medical Group Data Warehouse, and the VON.

The VON NIC/Q Experience

The VON has participated and led several successive QI collaborative efforts framed around the IHI method, called NIC/Q. These collaboratives have often focused on improvement of respiratory care practices to reduce CLD. The initial VON NIC/Q collaborative represented the initial use of QI in neonates.[110] Participating hospitals received instruction in QI, reviewed performance data, identified common improvement goals, and implemented PBPs developed through analysis of the processes of care, literature review, and site visits. The term PBP was chosen to indicate that, although the interventions had supporting evidence and internal validity, they needed to be proven effective via implementation and local customization.

The initial NIC/Q experience identified 9 PBPs adopted by 4 participating centers and showed a 12% decrease in CLD, although significant heterogeneity of outcome was noted. The 2000 NIC/Q Collaborative that focused on reduction in CLD was successful in identifying and implementing 9 PBPs but did not document improvement in the rates of CLD.[106,111,112] The 2002 NIC/Q group, also referred to as the

Breathsavers Group, identified and implemented 13 PBPs. They noted improvements in process outcomes including time on mechanical ventilation, steroid use, time to initial surfactant administration, and increased use of NCPAP. These changes were responsible for a decrease in the rates of CLD in 14 of 18 participating centers and a 27% overall reduction in the incidence of CLD between 2001 and 2003 in a cohort of approximately 1800 infants per year.[113,114] Among the NIC/Q collaboratives aimed at reducing CLD, individual centers had markedly varying results. Some participating NICUs witnessed paradoxic increases in CLD rates; however, these centers were often among the hospitals with the lowest rates of CLD at the outset, reflecting a regression toward the mean phenomenon. The question of why the NIC/Q 2002 collaborative was successful may potentially be explained by several factors. The PBPs identified were different from those selected by the NIC/Q 2000 group and had critically appraised evidence. In addition, the NIC/Q 2002 group members benefited from previous experience in the VON QI process. Many of the participant hospitals had participated in the initial NIC/Q effort and NIC/Q 2000.

Other Groups

Other groups have documented and published their attempts to reduce CLD using similar QI methods. One recent study by Birenbaum and colleagues[115] described the experience of one center that compared cohorts before and after changes in clinical management implemented in their hospital by using QI methods. Although this center did not participate in the VON Breathsavers Group, their focused interventions were similar to those adopted by many centers in the VON Group: lower, tighter pulse oximeter limits; a selective intubation and prophylactic surfactant policy; delivery room stabilization using CPAP via T-piece resuscitator; and initial treatment in the NICU with NCPAP. The group was successful in terms of improvement in process outcomes: more use of the T-piece resuscitator in the delivery room, more use of NCPAP delivered in the delivery room, and less time on the ventilator. These changes may have contributed to a reduction in the incidence of CLD in the center from 46.5% in 2002 to 20.5% in 2005, representing an overall relative risk reduction of 55.8%. Limitations of the study are that it is an unblinded retrospective cohort review from a single center. In addition, because it was a before-and-after study, the possibility exists that other unrecognized changes were taking place concurrently with the study.

A second recent attempt to use QI methods to decrease CLD has been documented by Nowadzky and colleagues.[116] This group focused on implementation of a single intervention, use of nasal bubble CPAP to facilitate a reduction in mechanical ventilation and ultimately a reduction in CLD. This group was successful in implementing the planned intervention: more infants received bubble NCPAP during the study period. This clinical change did translate into a reduction in the use of conventional ventilation but did not yield an improvement in the incidence of CLD. However, an increase in the rates of ROP was observed. This study is similarly limited by its designs as an unblended retrospective cohort review from a single center. It should be noted that the study occurred in a center at high altitude (Denver, CO, USA), where the incidence of BPD defined by the need for oxygen at 36 weeks PMA is much higher than at sea level.

There is inherent difficulty in limiting the exposure to bias that comes with retrospective studies. Many different factors may inject bias into a model. In addition, it is often difficult for a center to concurrently provide 2 varying methods of caring for an infant. Because of these limitations, several prospective cluster-RCTs, which use single NICU centers instead of individual patients as the unit of randomization, have been performed. The earliest attempt of cluster trial techniques to test QI methods in reducing CLD was performed by the VON. They conducted a cluster-RCT that tested whether centers that were exposed to a multifaceted collaborative QI intervention could be successful in earlier surfactant administration and thereby reduce CLD.[117] One-hundred and fourteen member hospitals (which treated 6039 infants of 23–29 weeks' gestation) within the VON participated in the trial. The intervention consisted of audit and feedback regarding surfactant administration practices, evidence-based workshops with didactic sessions and QI exercises, and collaboration with participating centers via conference calls and an e-mail discussion list. Compared with infants from control hospitals, infants in the intervention hospitals received their first dose of surfactant sooner after birth (median time of 21 minutes vs 78 minutes, $P<.0010$).[117] The intervention did not create a statistically significant change in the rate of CLD or mortality, but was successful at changing the behavior of neonatologists toward more evidence-based practice.

The National Institute of Child Health and Human Development Neonatal Research Network published the findings of a cluster-randomized trial of benchmarking and QI techniques for high-risk infants in 2007.[118] This study contained 17 centers within the network and enrolled 4093 infants with birth weight less than 1250 g. Three of the 17 centers were identified as best performers based on their high rates of survival without CLD. These centers were used as benchmarks; their respiratory practices were examined and emulated at 7 centers (the intervention group) using QI methods. Seven other centers did not initiate a respiratory QI program (control centers). Intervention centers were successful in implementing PBPs that were similar to the benchmark centers, including reduced oxygen saturation targets and reduced exposure to mechanical ventilation. Changes in rates of survival free of CLD between the 7 intervention centers and 7 control centers were not observed in the 3-year study period.

A third cluster trial to reduce CLD was published in 2009 that tested QI methods emphasizing the role of evidence in QI.[119] Twelve NICUs in the Canadian Neonatal Network participated in the study; 6 aimed at reduction of nosocomial infection and 6 focused on reduction of CLD. Infants in the group attempting to limit infection were used as the control comparison for the CLD group and vice versa All infants born at less than 32 weeks' gestation were included. The participant hospitals in the study used a method (the Evidence-based Practice for Improving Quality) that focused on critical appraisal of evidence and examination of individual hospital data to identify hospital-specific practice changes and strategies. The study ran for 3 years and enrolled 3070 infants in the arm dedicated to reduction of CLD. No decrease in the rate of CLD was observed in the nosocomial infection (control) group but in the pulmonary group, a 15% decrease from baseline was observed in the study period. The investigators concluded that their QI method is effective in reducing the incidence of CLD in NICUs. The study was halted before the goal sample size and 1 large NICU withdrew from the study while it was ongoing. In addition, the potential for the Hawthorne effect (the effect that being observed has on the behaviors of individuals and the potential for bias) in this study limits its generalizability. Nevertheless, this report represents the first study to incorporate QI methods using a cluster trial technique, with the hospital as the unit of reference, to successfully reduce the incidence of CLD.

WHY HAVE QI INITIATIVES NOT BEEN UNIFORMLY SUCCESSFUL IN REDUCING CLD RATES?

Controversy exists on whether QI techniques can be successful on disease processes with heterogeneous causes and influences such as CLD. QI methods have given mixed results when studied systematically. Estimates of the effectiveness of specific

QI strategies may be limited by difficulty in classifying complex interventions, insufficient numbers of studies, publication bias, and selection bias.[120]

There are multiple contributing factors to the development of CLD. Nonetheless, the wide disparity of center-based BPD incidence (varying in the VON databank by a factor of 10) of a fairly homogenous population of premature infants (birth weight 400–1500 g) seems to highlight the varying implementation of evidence-based practices in individual hospitals. Clinicians may be hampered by the choice of multiple possible interventions and treatment strategies to reduce the incidence of BPD. Controversy exists on whether QI methods that implement multiple interventions will be effective in limiting pathology with multiple causes. Methods for continuous QI have been used to improve and change processes more easily and consistently than outcomes. Complex outcomes, such as CLD, often require changes in multiple practices over an extended hospitalization that involves multiple disciplines and caretakers. It may be that PBPs taken from the benchmarking centers with admired outcomes may not be beneficial to each center with less-than-desired outcomes. This concept may be especially possible in the cases for which only weak supporting evidence exists to support these practices. Of the multitude of interventions, processes, and strategies implemented by any given center, it is unknown which (or what combinations) contribute to improved outcomes. Critical appraisal of evidence is thereby of utmost importance. In addition, the importance of local customization of individual practices cannot be overemphasized. Interventions or strategies useful in one setting may not make clinically significant improvements in a separate setting. Lastly, centers aiming toward QI are susceptible to the Hawthorne effect: the NICUs that chose to participate in QI projects are self-selected, highly interested and motivated, and willing participants. Improvement in performance, especially in terms of intermediate and process measures, is noted when performance receives additional scrutiny. As noted earlier, these intermediate performance measures will not always translate to improved outcomes. Accordingly, caution in generalization of QI findings is encouraged. Finally, QI methods toward improvement in CLD or any other outcome should not be considered as a substitute for formal RCTs but as a tool for implementing evidence and studying the effects of change in complex adaptive systems.[121]

REFERENCES

1. Northway WH Jr, Rosan RC, Porter DY. Pulmonary disease following respirator therapy of hyaline-membrane disease. Bronchopulmonary dysplasia. N Engl J Med 1967;276(7):357–68.
2. Walsh MC, Wilson-Costello D, Zadell A, et al. Safety, reliability, and validity of a physiologic definition of bronchopulmonary dysplasia. J Perinatol 2003; 23(6):451–6.
3. Charafeddine L, D'Angio CT, Phelps DL. Atypical chronic lung disease patterns in neonates. Pediatrics 1999;103(4 Pt 1):759–65.
4. Jobe AH, Bancalari E. NICHD/NHLBI/ORD workshop summary: bronchopulmonary dysplasia. Am J Respir Crit Care Med 2001;163:1723–9.
5. Bancalari E. Changes in the pathogenesis and prevention of chronic lung disease of prematurity. Am J Perinatol 2001;18(1):1–9.
6. Jobe AH, Ikegami M. Mechanisms initiating lung injury in the preterm. Early Hum Dev 1998;53(1):81–94.
7. Hack M, Wilson-Costello D, Friedman H, et al. Neurodevelopment and predictors of outcomes of children with birth weights of less than 1000 g: 1992–1995. Arch Pediatr Adolesc Med 2000;154(7):725–31.

8. Hoekstra RE, Ferrara TB, Couser RJ, et al. Survival and long-term neurodevelopmental outcome of extremely premature infants born at 23–26 weeks' gestational age at a tertiary center. Pediatrics 2004;113(1 Pt 1):e1–6.
9. Tyson JE, Parikh NA, Langer J, et al. Intensive care for extreme prematurity–moving beyond gestational age. N Engl J Med 2008;358(16):1672–81.
10. Bryan MH, Hardie MJ, Reilly BJ, et al. Pulmonary function studies during the first year of life in infants recovering from the respiratory distress syndrome. Pediatrics 1973;52(2):169–78.
11. Wolfson MR, Bhutani VK, Shaffer TH, et al. Mechanics and energetics of breathing helium in infants with bronchopulmonary dysplasia. J Pediatr 1984; 104(5):752–7.
12. Tepper RS, Morgan WJ, Cota K, et al. Expiratory flow limitation in infants with bronchopulmonary dysplasia. J Pediatr 1986;109(6):1040–6.
13. Mourani PM, Ivy DD, Gao D, et al. Pulmonary vascular effects of inhaled nitric oxide and oxygen tension in bronchopulmonary dysplasia. Am J Respir Crit Care Med 2004;170(9):1006–13.
14. Goodman G, Perkin RM, Anas NG, et al. Pulmonary hypertension in infants with bronchopulmonary dysplasia. J Pediatr 1988;112(1):67–72.
15. Kinsella JP, Greenough A, Abman SH. Bronchopulmonary dysplasia. Lancet 2006;367(9520):1421–31.
16. Kraybill EN, Runyan DK, Bose CL, et al. Risk factors for chronic lung disease in infants with birth weights of 751 to 1000 grams. J Pediatr 1989;115(1):115–20.
17. Bjorklund LJ, Ingimarsson J, Curstedt T, et al. Manual ventilation with a few large breaths at birth compromises the therapeutic effect of subsequent surfactant replacement in immature lambs. Pediatr Res 1997;42(3):348–55.
18. Munshi UK, Niu JO, Siddiq MM, et al. Elevation of interleukin-8 and interleukin-6 precedes the influx of neutrophils in tracheal aspirates from preterm infants who develop bronchopulmonary dysplasia. Pediatr Pulmonol 1997;24(5):331–6.
19. Pierce MR, Bancalari E. The role of inflammation in the pathogenesis of bronchopulmonary dysplasia. Pediatr Pulmonol 1995;19(6):371–8.
20. Groneck P, Speer CP. Inflammatory mediators and bronchopulmonary dysplasia. Arch Dis Child Fetal Neonatal Ed 1995;73(1):F1–3.
21. Ozdemir A, Brown MA, Morgan WJ. Markers and mediators of inflammation in neonatal lung disease. Pediatr Pulmonol 1997;23(4):292–306.
22. Nickerson BG, Taussig LM. Family history of asthma in infants with bronchopulmonary dysplasia. Pediatrics 1980;65(6):1140–4.
23. Clark DA, Pincus LG, Oliphant M, et al. HLA-A2 and chronic lung disease in neonates. JAMA 1982;248(15):1868–9.
24. Wright LL, Verter J, Younes N, et al. Antenatal corticosteroid administration and neonatal outcome in very low birth weight infants: the NICHD Neonatal Research Network. Am J Obstet Gynecol 1995;173(1):269–74.
25. Roberts D, Dalziel S. Antenatal corticosteroids for accelerating fetal lung maturation for women at risk of preterm birth. Cochrane Database Syst Rev 2006;(3): CD004454.
26. Horbar JD. Antenatal corticosteroid treatment and neonatal outcomes for infants 501 to 1500 gm in the Vermont-Oxford Trials Network. Am J Obstet Gynecol 1995;173(1):275–81.
27. Young TE, Kruyer LS, Marshall DD, et al. Population-based study of chronic lung disease in very low birth weight infants in North Carolina in 1994 with comparisons with 1984. The North Carolina Neonatologists Association. Pediatrics 1999; 104(2):e17.

28. Marshall DD, Kotelchuck M, Young TE, et al. Risk factors for chronic lung disease in the surfactant era: a North Carolina population-based study of very low birth weight infants. North Carolina Neonatologists Association. Pediatrics 1999;104(6):1345–50.
29. Rojas MA, Gonzalez A, Bancalari E, et al. Changing trends in the epidemiology and pathogenesis of neonatal chronic lung disease. J Pediatr 1995;126(4): 605–10.
30. Avery ME, Tooley WH, Keller JB, et al. Is chronic lung disease in low birth weight infants preventable? A survey of eight centers. Pediatrics 1987;79(1):26–30.
31. Van Marter LJ, Allred EN, Pagano M, et al. Do clinical markers of barotrauma and oxygen toxicity explain interhospital variation in rates of chronic lung disease? The Neonatology Committee for the Developmental Network. Pediatrics 2000;105(6):1194–201.
32. Lenfant C. Shattuck lecture. Clinical research to clinical practice–lost in translation? N Engl J Med 2003;349(9):868–74.
33. Gray JAM. Evidence-based healthcare. Edinburgh. 2nd edition. New York: Churchill Livingston; 2001. p. xxix, 444.
34. Center_for_Evidence_Based_Medicine. Available at: http://www.cebm.net/index.aspx?o=1025. Accessed January 8, 2010.
35. American Heart Association. ILCOR, c2010 evidence evaluation worksheet guidelines. Available at: www.americanheart.org/ILCOR. Accessed January 8, 2010.
36. Shenai JP, Chytil F, Jhaveri A, et al. Plasma vitamin A and retinol-binding protein in premature and term neonates. J Pediatr 1981;99(2):302–5.
37. Darlow BA, Graham PJ. Vitamin A supplementation to prevent mortality and short and long-term morbidity in very low birthweight infants. Cochrane Database Syst Rev 2007;(4):CD000501.
38. Tyson JE, Wright LL, Oh W, et al. Vitamin A supplementation for extremely-low-birth-weight infants. National Institute of Child Health and Human Development Neonatal Research Network. N Engl J Med 1999;340(25):1962–8.
39. Ambalavanan N, Wu TJ, Tyson JE, et al. A comparison of three vitamin A dosing regimens in extremely-low-birth-weight infants. J Pediatr 2003;142(6):656–61.
40. Soll RF, Morley CJ. Prophylactic versus selective use of surfactant in preventing morbidity and mortality in preterm infants. Cochrane Database Syst Rev 2001;(2):CD000510.
41. Yost CC, Soll RF. Early versus delayed selective surfactant treatment for neonatal respiratory distress syndrome. Cochrane Database Syst Rev 2000;(2):CD001456.
42. Jobe AH. Antenatal factors and the development of bronchopulmonary dysplasia. Semin Neonatol 2003;8(1):9–17.
43. Feldman DM, Carbone J, Belden L, et al. Betamethasone vs dexamethasone for the prevention of morbidity in very-low-birthweight neonates. Am J Obstet Gynecol 2007;197(3):284, e1–4.
44. Lee BH, Stoll BJ, McDonald SA, et al. Adverse neonatal outcomes associated with antenatal dexamethasone versus antenatal betamethasone. Pediatrics 2006;117(5):1503–10.
45. Askie LM, Henderson-Smart DJ, Irwig L, et al. Oxygen-saturation targets and outcomes in extremely preterm infants. N Engl J Med 2003;349(10):959–67.
46. Supplemental Therapeutic Oxygen for Prethreshold Retinopathy Of Prematurity (STOP-ROP), a randomized, controlled trial. I: primary outcomes. Pediatrics 2000;105(2):295–310.

47. Ambalavanan N, Carlo WA. Ventilatory strategies in the prevention and management of bronchopulmonary dysplasia. Semin Perinatol 2006;30(4):192–9.
48. Hagadorn JI, Furey AM, Nghiem TH, et al. Achieved versus intended pulse oximeter saturation in infants born less than 28 weeks' gestation: the AVIOx study. Pediatrics 2006;118(4):1574–82.
49. Goldsmith JP, Greenspan J. NICU oxygen management: a team effort. Pediatrics 2007;119(6):1195–6.
50. Palta M, Gabbert D, Weinstein MR, et al. Multivariate assessment of traditional risk factors for chronic lung disease in very low birth weight neonates. The Newborn Lung Project. J Pediatr 1991;119(2):285–92.
51. Clark RH, Gerstmann DR, Jobe AH, et al. Lung injury in neonates: causes, strategies for prevention, and long-term consequences. J Pediatr 2001;139(4):478–86.
52. Garland JS, Buck RK, Allred EN, et al. Hypocarbia before surfactant therapy appears to increase bronchopulmonary dysplasia risk in infants with respiratory distress syndrome. Arch Pediatr Adolesc Med 1995;149(6):617–22.
53. Dreyfuss D, Saumon G. Barotrauma is volutrauma, but which volume is the one responsible? Intensive Care Med 1992;18(3):139–41.
54. Taskar V, John J, Evander E, et al. Surfactant dysfunction makes lungs vulnerable to repetitive collapse and reexpansion. Am J Respir Crit Care Med 1997;155(1):313–20.
55. Attar MA, Donn SM. Mechanisms of ventilator-induced lung injury in premature infants. Semin Neonatol 2002;7(5):353–60.
56. Ehlert CA, Truog WE, Thibeault DW, et al. Hyperoxia and tidal volume: Independent and combined effects on neonatal pulmonary inflammation. Biol Neonate 2006;90(2):89–97.
57. Greisen G, Vannucci RC. Is periventricular leucomalacia a result of hypoxic-ischaemic injury? Hypocapnia and the preterm brain. Biol Neonate 2001;79(3–4):194–200.
58. Fabres J, Carlo WA, Phillips V, et al. Both extremes of arterial carbon dioxide pressure and the magnitude of fluctuations in arterial carbon dioxide pressure are associated with severe intraventricular hemorrhage in preterm infants. Pediatrics 2007;119(2):299–305.
59. Mariani G, Cifuentes J, Carlo WA. Randomized trial of permissive hypercapnia in preterm infants. Pediatrics 1999;104(5 Pt 1):1082–8.
60. Carlo WA, Stark AR, Wright LL, et al. Minimal ventilation to prevent bronchopulmonary dysplasia in extremely-low-birth-weight infants. J Pediatr 2002;141(3):370–4.
61. Keszler M. Volume-targeted ventilation. J Perinatol 2005;25(Suppl 2):S19–22.
62. McCallion N, Davis PG, Morley CJ. Volume-targeted versus pressure-limited ventilation in the neonate. Cochrane Database Syst Rev 2005;(3):CD003666.
63. Greenough A, Milner AD, Dimitriou G. Synchronized mechanical ventilation for respiratory support in newborn infants. Cochrane Database Syst Rev 2001;(1):CD000456.
64. Jobe AH, Kramer BW, Moss TJ, et al. Decreased indicators of lung injury with continuous positive expiratory pressure in preterm lambs. Pediatr Res 2002;52(3):387–92.
65. Verder H, Albertsen P, Ebbesen F, et al. Nasal continuous positive airway pressure and early surfactant therapy for respiratory distress syndrome in newborns of less than 30 weeks' gestation. Pediatrics 1999;103(2):E24.

66. Davis PG, Henderson-Smart DJ. Nasal continuous positive airways pressure immediately after extubation for preventing morbidity in preterm infants. Cochrane Database Syst Rev 2003;(2):CD000143.
67. Davis PG, Lemyre B, de Paoli AG. Nasal intermittent positive pressure ventilation (NIPPV) versus nasal continuous positive airway pressure (NCPAP) for preterm neonates after extubation. Cochrane Database Syst Rev 2001;(3):CD003212.
68. Henderson-Smart DJ, Steer P. Methylxanthine treatment for apnea in preterm infants. Cochrane Database Syst Rev 2001;(3):CD000140.
69. Schmidt B, Roberts RS, Davis P, et al. Caffeine therapy for apnea of prematurity. N Engl J Med 2006;354(20):2112–21.
70. Courtney SE, Durand DJ, Asselin JM, et al. High-frequency oscillatory ventilation versus conventional mechanical ventilation for very-low-birth-weight infants. N Engl J Med 2002;347(9):643–52.
71. Johnson AH, Peacock JL, Greenough A, et al. High-frequency oscillatory ventilation for the prevention of chronic lung disease of prematurity. N Engl J Med 2002;347(9):633–42.
72. Henderson-Smart DJ, Cools F, Bhuta T, et al. Elective high frequency oscillatory ventilation versus conventional ventilation for acute pulmonary dysfunction in preterm infants. Cochrane Database Syst Rev 2007;(3):CD000104.
73. Thome UH, Carlo WA, Pohlandt F. Ventilation strategies and outcome in randomised trials of high frequency ventilation. Arch Dis Child Fetal Neonatal Ed 2005; 90(6):F466–73.
74. Ammari A, Suri M, Milisavljevic V, et al. Variables associated with the early failure of nasal CPAP in very low birth weight infants. J Pediatr 2005;147(3):341–7.
75. De Klerk AM, De Klerk RK. Nasal continuous positive airway pressure and outcomes of preterm infants. J Paediatr Child Health 2001;37(2):161–7.
76. Gittermann MK, Fusch C, Gittermann AR, et al. Early nasal continuous positive airway pressure treatment reduces the need for intubation in very low birth weight infants. Eur J Pediatr 1997;156(5):384–8.
77. Jonsson B, Katz-Salamon M, Faxelius G, et al. Neonatal care of very-low-birthweight infants in special-care units and neonatal intensive-care units in Stockholm. Early nasal continuous positive airway pressure versus mechanical ventilation: gains and losses. Acta Paediatr Suppl 1997;419:4–10.
78. Kamper J, Wulff K, Larsen C, et al. Early treatment with nasal continuous positive airway pressure in very low-birth-weight infants. Acta Paediatr 1993;82(2): 193–7.
79. Thomson MA. Continuous positive airway pressure and surfactant; combined data from animal experiments and clinical trials. Biol Neonate 2002;81(Suppl 1):16–9.
80. Morley CJ, Davis PG, Doyle LW, et al. Nasal CPAP or intubation at birth for very preterm infants. N Engl J Med 2008;358(7):700–8.
81. Stevens TP, Harrington EW, Blennow M, et al. Early surfactant administration with brief ventilation vs. selective surfactant and continued mechanical ventilation for preterm infants with or at risk for respiratory distress syndrome. Cochrane Database Syst Rev 2007;(4):CD003063.
82. Ingimarsson J, Björklund LJ, Curstedt T, et al. Incomplete protection by prophylactic surfactant against the adverse effects of large lung inflations at birth in immature lambs. Intensive Care Med 2004;30(7):1446–53.
83. Bennett S, Finer NN, Rich W, et al. A comparison of three neonatal resuscitation devices. Resuscitation 2005;67(1):113–8.
84. Cotton RB, Stahlman MT, Kovar I, et al. Medical management of small preterm infants with symptomatic patent ductus arteriosus. J Pediatr 1978;92(3):467–73.

85. Clyman RI. Mechanisms regulating the ductus arteriosus. Biol Neonate 2006; 89(4):330–5.
86. Chorne N, Leonard C, Piecuch R, et al. Patent ductus arteriosus and its treatment as risk factors for neonatal and neurodevelopmental morbidity. Pediatrics 2007;119(6):1165–74.
87. Kavvadia V, Greenough A, Dimitriou G, et al. Randomised trial of fluid restriction in ventilated very low birthweight infants. Arch Dis Child Fetal Neonatal Ed 2000; 83(2):F91–6.
88. Hartnoll G, Betremieux P, Modi N. Randomised controlled trial of postnatal sodium supplementation on oxygen dependency and body weight in 25–30 week gestational age infants. Arch Dis Child Fetal Neonatal Ed 2000;82(1):F19–23.
89. Bell EF, Acarregui MJ. Restricted versus liberal water intake for preventing morbidity and mortality in preterm infants. Cochrane Database Syst Rev 2008;(1):CD000503.
90. Oh W, Poindexter BB, Perritt R, et al. Association between fluid intake and weight loss during the first ten days of life and risk of bronchopulmonary dysplasia in extremely low birth weight infants. J Pediatr 2005;147(6):786–90.
91. Kavvadia V, Greenough A, Dimitriou G, et al. Randomized trial of two levels of fluid input in the perinatal period–effect on fluid balance, electrolyte and metabolic disturbances in ventilated VLBW infants. Acta Paediatr 2000;89(2):237–41.
92. Stoll BJ, Hansen N, Fanaroff AA, et al. Late-onset sepsis in very low birth weight neonates: the experience of the NICHD Neonatal Research Network. Pediatrics 2002;110(2 Pt 1):285–91.
93. Liljedahl M, Bodin L, Schollin J. Coagulase-negative staphylococcal sepsis as a predictor of bronchopulmonary dysplasia. Acta Paediatr 2004;93(2): 211–5.
94. Polin RA, Polin RA, Yoder MC. Workbook in practical neonatology. 4th edition. Philadelphia: Saunders/Elsevier; 2007. p. xii, 500.
95. Yoder MC Jr, Chua R, Tepper R. Effect of dexamethasone on pulmonary inflammation and pulmonary function of ventilator-dependent infants with bronchopulmonary dysplasia. Am Rev Respir Dis 1991;143(5 Pt 1):1044–8.
96. Halliday HL. Clinical trials of postnatal corticosteroids: inhaled and systemic. Biol Neonate 1999;76(Suppl 1):29–40.
97. Halliday HL, Ehrenkranz RA, Doyle LW. Early (<8 days) postnatal corticosteroids for preventing chronic lung disease in preterm infants. Cochrane Database Syst Rev 2009;(1):CD001146.
98. Halliday HL, Ehrenkranz RA, Doyle LW. Late (>7 days) postnatal corticosteroids for chronic lung disease in preterm infants. Cochrane Database Syst Rev 2009;(1):CD001145.
99. Jobe AH, Bancalari E. Bronchopulmonary dysplasia. Am J Respir Crit Care Med 2001;163(7):1723–9.
100. Watterberg KL, Gerdes JS, Cole CH, et al. Prophylaxis of early adrenal insufficiency to prevent bronchopulmonary dysplasia: a multicenter trial. Pediatrics 2004;114(6):1649–57.
101. Tin W, Wiswell TE. Adjunctive therapies in chronic lung disease: examining the evidence. Semin Fetal Neonatal Med 2008;13(1):44–52.
102. Postnatal corticosteroids to treat or prevent chronic lung disease in preterm infants. Pediatrics 2002;109(2):330–8.
103. Shah V, Ohlsson A, Halliday HL, et al. Early administration of inhaled corticosteroids for preventing chronic lung disease in ventilated very low birth weight preterm neonates. Cochrane Database Syst Rev 2007;(4):CD001969.

104. Shah SS, Ohlsson A, Halliday H, et al. Inhaled versus systemic corticosteroids for the treatment of chronic lung disease in ventilated very low birth weight preterm infants. Cochrane Database Syst Rev 2007;(4):CD002057.
105. Cole CH, Colton T, Shah BL, et al. Early inhaled glucocorticoid therapy to prevent bronchopulmonary dysplasia. N Engl J Med 1999;340(13):1005–10.
106. Burch K, Rhine W, Baker R, et al. Implementing potentially better practices to reduce lung injury in neonates. Pediatrics 2003;111(4 Pt 2):e432–6.
107. Plsek PE. Quality improvement methods in clinical medicine. Pediatrics 1999; 103(1 Suppl E):203–14.
108. Shine KI. Health care quality and how to achieve it. Acad Med 2002;77(1):91–9.
109. Shewhart WA. Economic control of quality of manufactured product. New York: D. Van Nostrand Company, Inc; 1931. p. xiv, 501.
110. Horbar JD, Rogowski J, Plsek PE, et al. Collaborative quality improvement for neonatal intensive care. NIC/Q Project Investigators of the Vermont Oxford Network. Pediatrics 2001;107(1):14–22.
111. Sharek PJ, Baker R, Litman F, et al. Evaluation and development of potentially better practices to prevent chronic lung disease and reduce lung injury in neonates. Pediatrics 2003;111(4 Pt 2):e426–31.
112. Kaempf JW, Campbell B, Sklar RS, et al. Implementing potentially better practices to improve neonatal outcomes after reducing postnatal dexamethasone use in infants born between 501 and 1250 grams. Pediatrics 2003;111(4 Pt 2):e534–41.
113. Payne NR, LaCorte M, Sun S, et al. Evaluation and development of potentially better practices to reduce bronchopulmonary dysplasia in very low birth weight infants. Pediatrics 2006;118(Suppl 2):S65–72.
114. Payne NR, LaCorte M, Karna P, et al. Reduction of bronchopulmonary dysplasia after participation in the Breathsavers Group of the Vermont Oxford Network Neonatal Intensive Care Quality Improvement Collaborative. Pediatrics 2006; 118(Suppl 2):S73–7.
115. Birenbaum HJ, Dentry A, Cirelli J, et al. Reduction in the incidence of chronic lung disease in very low birth weight infants: results of a quality improvement process in a tertiary level neonatal intensive care unit. Pediatrics 2009;123(1): 44–50.
116. Nowadzky T, Pantoja A, Britton JR. Bubble continuous positive airway pressure, a potentially better practice, reduces the use of mechanical ventilation among very low birth weight infants with respiratory distress syndrome. Pediatrics 2009;123(6):1534–40.
117. Horbar JD, Carpenter JH, Buzas J, et al. Collaborative quality improvement to promote evidence based surfactant for preterm infants: a cluster randomised trial. BMJ 2004;329(7473):1004.
118. Walsh M, Laptook A, Kazzi SN, et al. A cluster-randomized trial of benchmarking and multimodal quality improvement to improve rates of survival free of bronchopulmonary dysplasia for infants with birth weights of less than 1250 grams. Pediatrics 2007;119(5):876–90.
119. Lee SK, Aziz K, Singhal N, et al. Improving the quality of care for infants: a cluster randomized controlled trial. CMAJ 2009;181(8):469–76.
120. Shojania KG, Ranji SR, McDonald KM, et al. Effects of quality improvement strategies for type 2 diabetes on glycemic control: a meta-regression analysis. JAMA 2006;296(4):427–40.
121. Berwick DM. The science of improvement. JAMA 2008;299(10):1182–4.

Index

Note: Page numbers of article titles are in **boldface** type.

Clin Perinatol 37 (2010) 295–305
doi:10.1016/S0095-5108(10)00031-X
perinatology.theclinics.com